NUTRITION in EXERCISE and SPORT

Edited by Ira Wolinsky and James F. Hickson, Jr.

Published Titles

Exercise and Disease,
Ronald R. Watson and Marianne Eisinger

Nutrients as Ergogenic Aids for Sports and Exercise,
Luke Bucci

Nutrition in Exercise and Sport, Second Edition,
Ira Wolinsky and James F. Hickson, Jr.

Nutrition Applied to Injury Rehabilitation and Sports Medicine,
Luke Bucci

Nutrition for the Recreational Athlete,
Catherine G. Ratzin Jackson

NUTRITION in EXERCISE and SPORT

Edited by Ira Wolinsky

Published Titles

Sports Nutrition: Minerals and Electrolytes,
Constance V. Kies and Judy A. Driskell

Nutrition, Physical Activity, and Health in Early Life:
Studies in Preschool Children,
Jana Pařízková

Exercise and Immune Function,
Laurie Hoffman-Goetz

Body Fluid Balance: Exercise and Sport,
E.R. Buskirk and S. Puhl

Nutrition and the Female Athlete,
Jaime S. Ruud

Sports Nutrition: Vitamins and Trace Elements,
Ira Wolinsky and Judy A. Driskell

Amino Acids and Proteins for the Athlete—The Anabolic Edge,
Mauro G. DiPasquale

Nutrition in Exercise and Sport, Third Edition,
Ira Wolinsky

Published Titles Continued

Nutritional Assessment of Athletes

Edited by

Judy A. Driskell, Ph.D., R.D.
University of Nebraska

Ira Wolinsky, Ph.D.
University of Houston

CRC PRESS

Boca Raton   London   New York   Washington, D.C.

Library of Congress Cataloging-in-Publication Data

Nutritional assessment of athletes / Judy A. Driskell, Ira Wolinsky.
    p.   cm. (Nutrition in exercise and sport)
ISBN 0-8493-0927-1 (alk. paper)
    1. Athletes--Nutrition. I. Driskell, Judy A. (Judy Anne) II. Wolinsky, Ira. III. Series
TX361.A8 N893 2002
613.2′024796—dc21   2002019232
                                                                                          CIP

Visit the CRC Press Web site at www.crcpress.com

No claim to original U.S. Government works
International Standard Book Number 0-8493-0927-1
Library of Congress Card Number 2002019232
Printed in the United States of America   2 3 4 5 6 7 8 9 0
Printed on acid-free paper

Series Preface

The CRC Series on Nutrition in Exercise and Sport provides a setting for in-depth exploration of the many and varied aspects of nutrition and exercise, including sports. The topic of exercise and sports nutrition has been a focus of research among scientists since the 1960s, and the healthful benefits of good nutrition and exercise have been appreciated. As our knowledge expands, it will be necessary to remember that there must be a range of diets and exercise regimes that will support excellent physical condition and performance. There is no single diet-exercise treatment that can be the common denominator, or the one formula for health, or a panacea for performance.

This Series is dedicated to providing a stage upon which to explore these issues. Each volume provides a detailed and scholarly examination of some aspect of the topic. Contributors from bona fide areas of nutrition and physical activity, including sports and the controversial, have participated in the Series.

Ira Wolinsky, Ph.D.
University of Houston
Series Editor

Preface

This volume is part of a miniseries within the CRC Series on Nutrition and Sport, which comprises comprehensive books on subjects of timely interest for sports nutritionists of all walks in the expanding field of sports nutrition, written by competent editors and authors who are well known in their fields. The series includes monographs, edited volumes, and textbooks. This volume focuses on assessment of athletes, with an emphasis on nutrition. The first section, dealing with dietary assessment, is followed by sections on anthropometric, physical activity needs, biochemical and clinical. We have been gratified at the response to our books — it is difficult to find such a trove of information on the subject in one place. Sports nutritionists, sports medicine and fitness professionals, researchers, students, health practitioners and the educated layman will find this book timely and useful.

Companions to this book are four other volumes in this miniseries: Sports Nutrition: Vitamins and Trace Elements; Macroelements, Water and Electrolytes in Sports Nutrition; Energy-Yielding Macronutrients and Energy Metabolism in Sports Nutrition; and Nutritional Applications in Exercise and Sport. Additionally useful will be Nutrition in Exercise and Sport, Third Edition, edited by Ira Wolinsky, and Sports Nutrition, authored by Judy Driskell.

Judy A. Driskell, Ph.D., R.D.
University of Nebraska

Ira Wolinsky, Ph.D.
University of Houston

Dedication

This book is dedicated to all of our current and former students, who continue to

stimulate our thinking and renew our dedication.

Acknowledgments

We thank and appreciate each of the individuals who so expertly wrote each of the chapters and allowed us to benefit from their expertise.

Editors

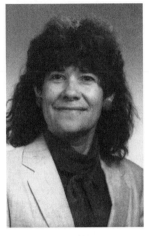

Judy Anne Driskell, Ph.D., R.D., is professor of nutritional science and dietetics at the University of Nebraska. She received her B.S. degree in biology from the University of Southern Mississippi in Hattiesburg. Her M.S. and Ph.D. degrees were obtained from Purdue University. She has served in research and teaching positions at Auburn University, Florida State University, Virginia Polytechnic Institute and State University and the University of Nebraska. She has also served as the nutrition scientist for the U.S. Department of Agriculture/Cooperative State Research Service and as a professor of nutrition and food science at Gadjah Mada and Bogor Universities in Indonesia.

Dr. Driskell is a member of numerous professional organizations including the American Society of Nutritional Sciences, the American College of Sports Medicine, the Institute of Food Technologists, and the American Dietetic Association. In 1993 she received the Professional Scientist Award from the Food Science and Human Nutrition Section of the Southern Association of Agricultural Scientists. In addition, she was the 1987 recipient of the Borden Award for Research in Applied Fundamental Knowledge of Human Nutrition. She is listed as an expert in B-complex vitamins by the Vitamin Nutrition Information Service.

Dr. Driskell coedited the CRC books *Sports Nutrition: Minerals and Electrolytes* with Constance V. Kies. In addition, she authored the textbook *Sports Nutrition* and coauthored an advanced nutrition book *Nutrition: Chemistry and Biology*, both published by CRC. With Ira Wolinsky, she coedited *Sports Nutrition: Vitamins and Trace Elements*; *Macroelements, Water, and Electrolytes in Sports Nutrition*; *Energy-Yielding Macronutrients and Energy Metabolism in Sports Nutrition*; *Nutritional Applications in Exercise and Sport* and the current book *Nutritional Assessment of Athletes*. She has published more than 100 refereed research articles and 10 book chapters, as well as several publications intended for lay audiences, and has given numerous professional and lay presentations. Her current research interests center around vitamin metabolism and requirements, including the interrelationships between exercise and water-soluble vitamin requirements.

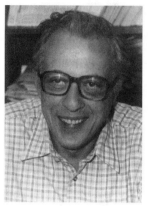

Ira Wolinsky, Ph.D., is professor of nutrition at the University of Houston. He received his B.S. degree in chemistry from the City College of New York and his M.S. and Ph.D. degrees in biochemistry from the University of Kansas. He has served in research and teaching positions at the Hebrew University, the University of Missouri and The Pennsylvania State University, as well as conducting basic research in NASA life sciences facilities and abroad.

Dr. Wolinsky is a member of the American Society of Nutritional Sciences, among other honorary and scientific organizations. He has contributed numerous nutrition research papers in the open literature. His major research interests relate to the nutrition of bone and calcium and trace elements, and to sports nutrition. He has been the recipient of research grants from both public and private sources, and of several international research fellowships and consultantships to the former Soviet Union, Bulgaria, Hungary, and India. He merited a Fulbright Senior Scholar Fellowship to Greece in 1999–2000.

Dr. Wolinsky has coauthored a book on the history of the science of nutrition, *Nutrition and Nutritional Diseases*. He coedited *Sports Nutrition: Vitamins and Trace Elements; Macroelements, Water, and Electrolytes in Sports Nutrition; Energy-Yielding Macronutrients and Energy Metabolism in Sports Nutrition; Nutritional Applications in Exercise and Sport*, and the current book *Nutritional Assessment of Athletes*, all with Judy Driskell. Additionally, he coedited *Nutritional Concerns of Women* with Dorothy Klimis-Tavantzis and *The Mediterranean Diet: Constituents and Health Promotion* with his Greek colleagues. He edited three editions of *Nutrition in Exercise and Sport*. He served also as the editor or coeditor for the CRC Series *Nutrition in Exercise and Sport; Modern Nutrition; Methods in Nutrition Research* and *Exercise Physiology*.

Contributors

Barbara E. Ainsworth, Ph.D., M.P.H.   Departments of Epidemiology and Biostatistics, and Exercise Science, University of South Carolina School of Public Health, Columbia, South Carolina

Carol Ballew, Ph.D.   Epidemiology Center, The Alaska Native Health Board, Anchorage, Alaska

Rebecca A. Battista, M.S.   Department of Kinesiology, Michigan State University, East Lansing, Michigan

Gregory P. Bondy, M.D., F.R.C.P.C.   Department of Pathology and Laboratory Medicine, University of British Columbia, Vancouver, British Columbia

Samuel N. Cheuvront, Ph.D.   U.S. Army Research, Institute of Environmental Medicine, Natick, Massachusetts

Keith C. DeRuisseau, M.S.   Department of Nutrition, Food and Exercise Sciences, Florida State University, Tallahassee, Florida

Judy A. Driskell, Ph.D., R.D.   Department of Nutritional Science and Dietetics, University of Nebraska, Lincoln, Nebraska

James R. Guest, M.D.   Pediatrician, Lincoln, Nebraska

Jean E. Guest, M.S., R.D., L.M.N.T.   Department of Nutritional Science and Dietetics, University of Nebraska, Lincoln, Nebraska

Mark D. Haub, Ph.D.   Department of Human Nutrition, Kansas State University, Manhattan, Kansas

Andrew P. Hills, Ph.D.   School of Human Movement Studies, Queensland University of Technology, Kelvin Grove, Queensland, Australia

Khursheed N. Jeejeebhoy, M.B.B.S., Ph.D., F.R.C.P., F.R.C.P.C.   Department of Medicine, St. Michael's Hospital, Toronto, Ontario

Satya S. Jonnalagadda, Ph.D.   Department of Nutrition, Georgia State University, Atlanta, Georgia

Richard E. Killingsworth, M.P.H., C.H.E.S. Division of Nutrition and Physical Activity, Centers for Disease Control and Prevention, Atlanta, Georgia

Michael J. LaMonte, Ph.D., M.P.H. Prevention Research Center, School of Public Health, University of South Carolina, Columbia, South Carolina

Scott A. Lear, Ph.D. School of Kinesiology, Simon Fraser University, Burnaby, British Columbia

Nancy M. Lewis, Ph.D., R.D., F.A.D.A. Department of Nutritional Science and Dietetics, University of Nebraska, Lincoln, Nebraska

Helena B. Löest, M.S. Department of Human Nutrition, Kansas State University, Manhattan, Kansas

Henry C. Lukaski, Ph.D. United States Department of Agriculture, Agricultural Research Service, Grand Forks Human Nutrition Research Center, Grand Forks, North Dakota

Robert Malina, Ph.D. Institute for Youth Sports, Michigan State University, East Lansing, Michigan

Michael J. LaMonte, Ph.D., M.P.H. Fitness Institute, Division of Cardiology, LDS University, Salt Lake City, Utah

Robert G. McMurray, Ph.D. Departments of Exercise and Sport Science and Nutrition, University of North Carolina, Chapel Hill, North Carolina

Robert J. Moffatt, Ph.D., M.P.H. Department of Nutrition, Food and Exercise Sciences, Florida State University, Tallahassee, Florida

Jana Pařízková, M.D., Ph.D., D.Sc. Third Department of Internal Medicine, First Medical Faculty, Charles University, Unemocnice 1, Prague, Czech Republic

Stuart M. Phillips, Ph.D. Department of Kinesiology, McMaster University, Hamilton, Ontario

Shannon R. Siegel, Ph.D. School of Sport, Physical Education and Recreation, University of Wales Institute, Cardiff, Wales, United Kingdom

Ira Wolinsky, Ph.D. Department of Human Development, University of Houston, Houston, Texas

Monika M. Woolsey, M.S., R.D. A Better Way Health Consulting, Inc., Glendale, Arizona

Contents

Section Four Physical Activity Needs Assessment of Athletes

Section Five Biochemical Assessment of Athletes

Section Six Clinical Assessment of Athletes

Section One

Introduction

1

Introduction to Nutritional Assessment of Athletes

Robert J. Moffatt and Samuel N. Cheuvront

CONTENTS

I. Introduction

Nutritional interest in special populations is the very basis of modern dietary guidelines and nutrient standards. Many of the first scientific investigations into the food requirements of man were shaped largely by the compulsion to understand his nutrient needs and to maintain the health and working capacity of soldiers, industrial workers and agricultural laborers of the late 19th and early 20th centuries.[1] Importantly, in conjunction with research-based recommendations, was the desire for rational nutrition education.[1] Ironically, the explosion of research interest in nutrition and physical activity (sports nutrition) over the past two decades is still predicated on the desire to advance health and work performance, while simultaneously opposing persistent and pervasive nutrition myth. Athlete healthcare, training, diet

0-8493-0927-1/02/$0.00+$1.50
© 2002 by CRC Press LLC

and education are accomplished best by an interdisciplinary team of sports medicine practitioners, including physicians, athletic trainers, exercise and nutrition scientists and dietitians.

II. The Practice of Sports Nutrition

A. An Emerging Field of Study

A credible "sports nutritionist" is a registered dietitian (R.D.), usually with advanced preparation in exercise sciences, particularly exercise physiology. These individuals work with recreational sports enthusiasts, high school, collegeor professional sports coaches, trainers and, of course, athletes. In the narrowest sense, their role is to optimize health and athletic performance through sound dietary intervention. Although registered dietitians are trained food and nutrition experts capable of a broad range of professional duties, specific "sports" education and training are not classical components of their education.[2] Sports nutrition is one nontraditional facet of the dietetic profession that requires a substantial working knowledge of exercise science and a sincere interest in sport. Traditionally, dietitians intent on practicing sports nutrition advanced their education in the exercise sciences and sought experience working patiently with athletes, coaches and trainers.[3] Similarly, scientists trained in the dual disciplines of exercise physiology and nutrition, public health or closely related fields, practice the science of "sports nutrition" and advance our understanding of this science through teaching, research and reliable publication.

Only recently have graduate programs evolved to meet this demand. The first American university to offer a distinguishable academic graduate degree in sports nutrition was Florida State University.[4] In 1987, its program was the first to offer a shared degree in sports nutrition through the combined efforts of the departments of Nutrition and Food Sciences and Movement Science and Physical Education. Later (1989), through a merger of those departments, Florida State became the first to offer one unique interdisciplinary program in sports nutrition (Department of Nutrition, Food and Exercise Sciences). Other universities later organized their programs in a similar manner (e.g., Virginia Tech and San Diego State), but most remain a coordinated effort between separate traditional nutrition and exercise science programs (Table 1.1). Currently, 21 universities in the United States offer interdisciplinary graduate programs in sports nutrition. In addition, 15 of the 21 universities listed (Table 1.1) also offer a coordinated dietetic internship, thus facilitating both the training and credentialing (R.D.) of sports nutrition scientists and sports nutritionists, respectively.[4] Other valid avenues of nutrition and sport enlightenment also coexist. The American Dietetic Association (ADA) fosters the communication of sports nutrition through its practice group SCAN (Sports, Cardiovascular and Wellness

TABLE 1.1

Higher Education in Sports Nutrition[4]

University	Graduate Degree	Training/ Specialization
Auburn University		×
California State Polytechnic University, Pomona	×	
Colorado State University	×	
East Carolina University		×
Florida State University	×	
Georgia State University		×
Indiana University of Pennsylvania		×
Long Island University, C.W. Post Campus		×
Marywood University		×
Pennsylvania State University		×
Saint Louis University		×
San Diego State University		×
Simmons College		×
Texas Woman's University	×	
University of Alabama, Birmingham	×	
University of Connecticut		×
University of New Mexico	×	
University of North Carolina, Chapel Hill		×
University of Texas, Austin	×	
University of Utah		×
Virginia Polytechnic Institute and State University	×	

Nutritionists). The American College of Sports Medicine (ACSM), in addition to its recognized certifications in exercise, now offers a certificate of enhanced qualification (CEQ) in nutrition and exercise as a means of providing valid information and experience to other members of the sports medicine team with typically little formal nutrition training.[2] The sports nutrition information exposure, ranging from applied certifications to graduate degrees and specializations, is an important and recognized component of the coordinated interdisciplinary approach to athlete healthcare.[5,6,7]

B. Roles and Responsibilities

The importance of nutrition in health and sport, although extremely well documented, has often met with resistance in practice. Instead, the search for a competitive edge has historically rested on highly suspect nutritional manipulations, dietary fads and ritualistic beliefs by athletes. In multiple sports, athletes from recreational, collegiate and professional ranks score poorly on nutritional knowledge surveys. Those athletes list magazines, coaches and other athletes as their primary sources of nutrition information.[2,8] Unfortunately, many coaches also rely on popular magazines and rarely consult an R.D. for dietary guidance.[2] The introduction of a reliable and sophisticated nutritional presence into the athletic arena has met with some success in hockey,[9] basketball,[10] and collegiate sports,[11] but most of all in American football.[12] According to Soliah,[12] 71% of professional American football teams employ at least the part-time services of a dietitian for menu planning, nutrition adviceor both. A survey[13] conducted with sports nutritionists in 1993 indicated that most had been working with athletes for less than 6 years, corroborating the approximate infiltration of sports nutrition into the general university curriculum in the mid 1980s. The majority also reported that 40% or less of their professional time was spent working as a sports nutritionist.[13] Clearly, athletes rely on other members of the sports medicine team for nutritional consultation. In fact, trainers and coaches reportedly provide the remaining 29% of nutrition services in the National Football League[12] and very often act in this capacity at the collegiate level too, despite little or no formal nutrition training.[2,5,8] Communication across professional disciplines within the sports medicine team is therefore crucial to maximizing athlete health and performance.

The members of the sports medicine team are responsible for integrating their individual areas of expertise with the best interest of the athlete's health and well-being as the cornerstone of safe and effective training and competition. The nutritional assessment of athletes requires detailed attention to and evaluation of, dietary adequacy, energy intake, energy expenditure, body composition and the effects of modest and extreme training on normal clinical physiology. Only a cohesive sports medicine healthcare team can properly provide these services.[7,14] Furthermore, although the need for exceptional sports medicine services between both novice and professional athletes is similar, personnel, techniques and resources vary greatly[5] and all methodologies are not created equal.

III.   Nutritional Assessment of Athletes:
A Unique Set of Challenges

A. Energy Requirements for Exercise

Regarding both health and performance, it is generally agreed that the number one priority in the nutritional care of athletes concerns the maintenance of energy balance.[15,16] The newly revised U.S. Dietary Guidelines[17] includes among its recommendations similar advice for all Americans. When putting these guidelines into practice, the USDA's Food Guide Pyramid is representative of an eating strategy that adequately helps to meet these goals as well as those of the recommended dietary allowances (RDAs) and dietary reference intakes (DRIs).[18] However, a closer look at Tables 1.2 and 1.3 shows immediately the special nature of training athletes' nutritional needs. Specifically, they must eat more. In this example, data collected on 323 Ironman Triathlon participants[19] were analyzed so that weekly training mileage in swimming, cycling and running were computed into a "daily average" of training activity. The intensities were taken directly from the same reference and appropriate

TABLE 1.2

Hypothetical Daily Energy Needs of an Ironman Triathlete[19] in Training

Activity	METS[20]	Duration (h)	Energy Expenditure (kcal)[20]
Sleep	0.9	8.0	540
Office work	1.5	8.0	900
Running (7.5 mph)*	13.5	0.8*	810
Swimming (2 mph)*	8.0	0.5*	318
Bicycling (18.6 mph)*	12.0	1.7*	1,530
Home activities (e.g. cooking, washing dishes, etc.)	2.5	3.0	563
Miscellaneous activities (reading newspaper, talking on phone, etc.)	1.3	2.0	195
			4,856

* Based on data presented in Reference 19. Energy expenditure calculated from Reference 20 as: (METS × 75 kg body weight × hours of activity = kcal)

TABLE 1.3

The Food Guide Pyramid and the Ironman Triathlete in Training

Food Groups	Recommended Servings[21]			Knowledge & Personalization*
Bread, cereal, rice & pasta	6	9	11	20 – thick crust pizza vs. thin and other simple strategies
Fruits	2	3	4	8 – add fruit juice to maximize fluid and carbohydrate intake and minimize adding too much fiber
Vegetables	3	4	5	6 – emphasize additional servings of starchy vegetables
Meat, poultry, fish, dry beans, eggs & nuts	2	2–3	3	4 – add dry beans to increase both protein and carbohydrate intake
Milk, yogurt & cheese	2	2	3	5 – add flavored milk (e.g. chocolate) to increase fluid and total energy intake
Other (fats, oils & sweets)	sparingly	sparingly	sparingly	Liberal use – includes soft drinks, sports drinks, sports bars, jelly, honey, margarine, etc.
Total kcal	~1,600	~2,200	~2,800	~4,800

* Needs of sport should not supersede balance and variety. Recommendations must include calculations for relative carbohydrate (~7g/kg)[15] and protein (~1.3g/kg)[22] requirements of endurance sport, snacking strategies, timing of meals/workouts, food preferences and much more.

MET values[20] (a single MET is equivalent to the amount of energy expended during 1 minute of rest) applied to estimate energy expenditure. The remainder of the day's calorie needs were calculated the same way, using MET values for the rest of a "normal," but largely sedentary day (Table 1.2). At the upper end of the Food Guide Pyramid serving number suggestions,[21] the athlete in question would satisfy a little more than half of his or her energy needs (Table 1.3). Furthermore, a simple doubling of the recommended portions or number of servings grossly neglects the reality of consuming 4800 kcal of energy from whole foods. The nutrition expert knows, for example, that added fat and fiber increases dietary bulk, slows gastric emptying, increases intestinal bloating and may therefore interfere with training schedules and general comfort. At the same time, there is no denying the endurance athlete's greater need for protein,[22] carbohydrates[15] and fluid.[23] Furthermore, the nutritional needs of athletes must be sport-specific and individualized.[8] Woven within this framework of dietary consultation are general, but ever-present, variables such as lifestyle (money, living situation, access to groceries and kitchen, food preparation skills, etc.), travel (especially college and professional sports), as well as simple convenience, normal food preferences and medical conditions (food allergies, lactose intolerance, eating disorders, diabetes, etc.). A more elaborate and encompassing treatise on the global nutritional needs of athletes and specific sports can be found elsewhere.[8,16] However, it is obvious that the athlete can indeed be a formidable challenge to feed.

While the concept of achieving energy balance is simple from a thermodynamic perspective, the tools with which we can estimate energy balance are at once sophisticated and rudimentary. This is especially true of estimating energy intake, which, unless observed and quantified, is usually left to the subjective recall of the athletes, who are entrusted to remember, accurately estimate and document their food intake using some form of diet record. Even when athletes practice the most conscientious recall, the usefulness of dietary surveys varies based on the dietary constituent of interest, monitoring technique (24-h recall, food frequencies, diet records) and seasonal changes in training and eating, not to mention the natural limitations imposed by estimation techniques, subject compliance and more.[8,24] In fact, the very act of measuring food intake may alter subject dietary practices, thus challenging the accuracy of the results obtained. On the opposite spectrum, energy expenditure can be very accurate when measured in a controlled laboratory by indirect calorimetry, but becomes more difficult in the field as it may be equally cumbersome (portable metabolic systems), potentially more expensive (doubly labeled water) or extremely limited by the simplicity of the technique (pedometer, accelerometer, heart rate and activity records) or the particular circumstance involved (e.g., swimming).[25] What does remain is also the definitive assessment of energy balance and control afforded by the measurement of fluctuations in body weight and body composition.

B. Anthropometry and Weight Control Issues

The relationships between diet and exercise and weight control are so closely linked that the latter is often used as a validation of balance in the former. Body weight itself is, of course, a poor indicator of the need for weight gain or loss. The desire of many athletes to alter their body weights must be evaluated on the basis of the potential for such changes to impact health and performance. This is not a simple matter. What constitutes an appropriate body weight for health and performance depends on the athlete's sport, gender, age, natural genetic predisposition and other potentially unforeseen and influential factors (social, psychological).[16] Competition in weight class (wrestling, martial arts, boxing, weight lifting) and judged (ice skating, gymnastics, diving, body building, dance) sports complicates the distinction that must be made between what is realistic and healthy versus what will bring success in "making the cut." The importance of a valid, reliable and meaningful assessment of body composition is therefore imperative as one tool in the healthcare professional's repertoire against undesirable, but common, weight change practices used by athletes.

A comprehensive index of optimal or ordinary body composition values for men and women in various sports is an excellent starting point in the assessment of athletes' desire to change their body composition for health or, more typically, performance reasons. It is imperative, however, that the limitations of the methods usually employed in measuring body composition be completely understood, lest the results do more harm than good. The range of techniques available to assess body composition vary greatly from expensive and technologically advanced devices such as dual energy x-ray absorptiometry (DEXA) that provide a sophisticated multi-compartmental analysis of body composition to inexpensive and simple instruments (skinfold calipers) that allow the differentiation of fat mass from nonfat mass only. The latter methodology is the more common two-component model of body composition assessment that relies primarily on the skill of the technician and the validity of assumptions underlying the equations used for the calculation of body fat.

Two of the most common field methods for measuring athlete body composition in mass are skinfold and bioelectrical impedance analysis (BIA). Both techniques, when done properly and under ideal circumstances, provide results that are within 3% of "gold standards" like hydrostatic weighing and DEXA.[26,27] However, even when carried out according to procedure, measurement error may exceed this acceptable range of values. For example, the Siri Equation[28] is used to derive body fat from body density measurements. This equation assumes constant values for the density of lean and fat mass within a static population (white males ages 19–55 yrs).[27] Heyward[27] has pointed out the need for adjustment in this equation based on age and ethnicity (population-specific equations). Without this adjustment, additional measurement error is introduced. More drastically, BIA requires that several conditions (hydration, posture, food intake, exercise) be controlled for accurate analysis. This can be an extremely challenging prerequisite for athletes in training. Although an athlete may follow instructions as stated, many athletes are chronically dehydrated, especially when training in hot climates or intentionally reducing body water for sport (e.g., wrestling).[29–31] Accordingly, several authors[32,33] conclude that BIA is not a valid means of body composition assessment when alterations in hydration state (hyperhydration or hypohydration) are imposed or expected. Ordinary factors such as training, acclimatization, the common mismatch between exercise fluid loss and fluid intake, intentional dehydration for weight control and menstrual cycle phase as well as less common influences like glycerol consumption[32] or creatine supplementation[34] can each uniquely affect body water content. Therefore, the choice and rationale for any given method of body composition assessment must be given careful consideration in addition to the common constraints of cost and convenience.

C. Evaluation of Biochemical and Clinical Physiology

Significant biological evidence supports the fact that athletes in particular sportsor often in general, are susceptible to changes in clinical physiology that may or may not be harmful, but are certainly abnormal with respect to more sedentary individuals. Perhaps the most widespread example of how diet and exercise may interact to confound the nutritional assessment of athletes is in the case of sports hematology. Stage III iron deficiency anemia is characterized, among other measures, by low blood hemoglobin concentrations.[35] In hemoglobin, iron is the active element that binds oxygen. Therefore, a blood hemoglobin concentration below the limits of "normal" is one index of poor iron status and negatively impacts performance due to the central role of hemoglobin in oxygen transport. Iron supplementation in this condition will improve hemoglobin values when the cause is poor dietary iron intakes, iron losses (foot strike hemolysis, gastrointestinal bleeding, menstrual losses) or both.[36] However, Shaskey and Green[37] point out that the pseudoanemia concomitant to exercise training and plasma volume expansion mimics iron deficiency anemia by diluting the concentration of hemoglobin present. In fact, this phenomenon is associated with no change or an expansion in mean red cell volume (MCV), thus having no adverse effect on performance and requiring only recognition rather than treatment.[37]

Table 1.4 is a sample summary of selected clinical and biochemical indices that may be affected by the diet and training practices of athletes. It is important to recognize that gender (females) and sport-specificity (weight-conscious sports, ultradistance endurance sports) are often hallmark correlates with potential clinical anomalies like anemia and osteopenia[36] or hyponatremia,[38] while susceptibility to other problems such as dehydration[29, 30] and compromised immunity[39] are more generalized. Finally, the ever-changing use of dietary supplements must also be investigated for the potential of some[34] to alter expected clinical laboratory results.

IV. SUMMARY

According to Tipton,[14] the influence of sports medicine as a whole on athletic achievement has been noticeable and important only since the 1970s. This is

TABLE 1.4

Selected Influences of Training and Sport on Clinical Athlete Physiology

Clinical/Biochemical Marker	Condition or Influence	Potential Sports or Athletes of Concern
Urinary Indices:[29,30] Color Specific Gravity Osmolality	Dehydration	Distance running, cycling, soccer, wrestling, (any sport practiced in the heat)
Plasma Sodium[38]	Hyponatremia	Usually ultradistance endurance exercise characterized by both copious sweating and excessive water intake
Hemoglobin[37]	Dilutional pseudo-anemia	Greatest occurrence in endurance athletes
Hemoglobin[36]	Iron deficiency anemia	Female athletes with low dietary iron intakes and potentially high iron losses (distance runners, gymnasts, ballet dancers)
Bone Mineral Density[36]	Osteopenia	Female athletes with low dietary calcium intakes (sports with weight restrictions, distance running, amenorrhea)
Immune Function Parameters[39]	Overtraining?	Any sport where training intensity and volume are excessive, especially if diet is also inadequate
Urinary Creatinine[34]	Creatine supplement use?	Most prevalent use in sports requiring strength

explained, in part, as the "… collective effects of a lack of the necessary critical mass in scientific information, a dearth of qualified and dedicated personnel, absence of professional organizations, [and] a reluctance to change social and cultural customs…."[14] Although progress toward the present and future shows undeniable growth and promise, the greatest benefit to athletes will achieve the necessary "critical mass" only when the sports medicine profession successfully integrates the knowledge and skill of a multidisciplinary athlete healthcare team. The nutritional assessment of athletes represents one significant challenge that is best accomplished by a diverse group of qualified medical, nutritional, exercise and sports oriented professionals.

References

1. Harper, A.E. Origin of recommended dietary allowances – a historic overview. *Am. J. Clin. Nutr.*, 41, 140, 1985.
2. Lewis, R.D., Massoni, J. and Crawford, K. Nutrition concerns, knowledge and recommendations of coaches and athletic trainers, in: *Nutritional Applications in Exercise and Sport*, Wolinsky, I. and Driskell, J.A., Eds., CRC, Boca Raton, 2000, chap. 17.

3. Clark, N. Developing a sports nutrition practice, *Nutrition Today*, May/June, 35, 1989.
4. Cheuvront, S.N. Sports nutrition for the next millennium: perspectives on post-baccalaureate study and practice. Alumni lecture presented at Indiana University of Pennsylvania, October 1999.
5. Gatorade Sports Science Institute, University sports medicine teams: an interdisciplinary approach, *Sports Science Exchange Roundtable*, 4, 3, 1993.
6. Storlie, J. Nutrition assessment of athletes: a model for integrating nutrition and physical performance indicators, *Int. J. Sport Nutr.*, 1, 192, 1991.
7. Lombardo, J.A. Sports medicine: a team effort, *Phys. Sportsmed.*, 13, 72, 1985.
8. Marquart, L.F., Cohen, E.A. and Short, S.H. Surveys of dietary intake and nutrition knowledge of athletes and their coaches, in: *Nutrition in Exercise and Sport*, 3rd ed., Wolinsky, I., Ed., CRC, Boca Raton, 1998, chap. 23.
9. Burns, J. and Dugan, L. Working with professional athletes in the rink: the evolution of a nutrition program for an NHL team, *Int. J. Sport Nutr.*, 4, 132, 1994.
10. Scheller, A. and Rask, B. A protocol for the health and fitness assessment of NBA players, *Clin. Sports Med.*, 12, 193, 1993.
11. Clark, K.L. Working with college athletes, coaches and trainers at a major university, *Int. J. Sport Nutr.*, 4, 135, 1994.
12. Soliah, L. Good nutrition scores with NFL players, *J. Amer. Diet. Assoc.*, 91, 1055, 1991.
13. Grandjean, A.C. Practices and recommendations of sports nutritionists, *Int. J. Sport Nutr.*, 3, 232, 1993.
14. Tipton, C.M. Sports medicine: a century of progress, *J. Nutr.*, 127, 878S, 1997.
15. Sherman, W.M. Metabolism of sugars and physical performance, *Amer. J. Clin. Nutr.*, 62, 228S, 1995.
16. American College of Sports Medicine, Joint position statement: nutrition and athletic performance, *Med. Sci. Sports Exerc.*, 32, 2130, 2000.
17. USDA, *Nutrition and Your Health: Dietary Guidelines for Americans*, 5th ed., Washington, D.C., United States Department of Agriculture and Health and Human Services, 2000.
18. Tavelli, S., Beerman, K., Shultz, J.E. and Heiss, C. Sources of error and nutritional adequacy of the food guide pyramid, *J. Am. Coll. Health*, 47, 77, 1998.
19. O'Toole, M.L. Training for ultraendurance triathlons, *Med. Sci. Sports Exerc.*, 21, S209, 1989.
20. Ainsworth, B.E., Haskell, W.L., Leon, A.S., Jacobs, D.R., Montoye, H.J., Sallies, J.F. and Paffenbarger, R.S. Compendium of physical activities: classification of energy costs of human physical activities, *Med. Sci. Sports Exerc.*, 25, 71, 1993.
21. Achterberg, C., McDonnell, E. and Bagby, R. How to put the Food Guide Pyramid into practice, *J. Amer. Diet. Assoc.*, 94, 1030, 1994.
22. Lemon, P.W. Do athletes need more dietary protein and amino acids? *Int. J. Sport Nutr.*, 5, S39, 1995.
23. Horswill, C.A. Effective fluid replacement, *Int. J. Sport Nutr.*, 8, 175, 1998.
24. Medlin, C. and Skinner, J.D. Individual dietary intake methodology: a 50-year review of progress, *J. Amer. Diet. Assoc.*, 88, 1250, 1988.
25. Montoye, H.J. Introduction: evaluation of some measurements of physical activity and energy expenditure, *Med. Sci. Sports Exerc.*, 32, S439, 2000.

26. Stewart, A.D. and Hannon, W.J. Prediction of fat and fat-free mass in male athletes using dual x-ray absorptiometry as the reference method, *J. Sports Sci.*, 18, 263, 2000.
27. Heyward, V.H. Evaluation of body composition: current issues, *Sports Med.*, 22, 146, 1996.
28. Siri, W.E. Gross composition of the body, in: *Advances in Biological and Medical Physics*, Lawrence, J.H. and Tobias, C.A., Eds., Academic, New York, 1956, Vol. 4.
29. Shirreffs, S.M. and Maughan, R.J. Urine osmolality and conductivity as indices of hydration status in athletes in the heat, *Med. Sci. Sports Exerc.*, 30, 1598, 1998.
30. Armstrong, L.E., Maresh, C.M., Castellani, J.W., Bergeron, M.F., Kenefick, R.W., LaGasse, K.E. and Riebe, D. Urinary indices of hydration status, *Int. J. Sport Nutr.*, 4, 265, 1994.
31. Zambraski, E.J., Foster, D.T., Gross, P.M. and Tipton, C.M. Iowa wrestling study: weight loss and urinary profiles of collegiate wrestlers, *Med. Sci. Sports Exerc.*, 8, 105, 1976.
32. Koulmann, N., Jimenez, C., Regal, D., Bolliet, P., Launay, J.C., Savourey, G., and Melin, B. Use of bioelectrical impedance analysis to estimate body fluid compartments after acute variations in body water, *Med. Sci. Sports Exerc.*, 32, 857, 2000.
33. Saunders, M.J., Blevins, J.E. and Broeder, C.E. Effects of hydration changes on bioelectrical impedance in endurance trained individuals, *Med. Sci. Sports Exerc.*, 30, 885, 1998.
34. Poortmans, J.R. and Francaux, M. Adverse effects of creatine supplementation: fact or fiction? *Sports Med.*, 30, 155, 2000.
35. Cook, J.D. Clinical evaluation of iron deficiency, *Semin. Hematol.*, 19, 6, 1982.
36. Haymes, E.M. and Clarkson, P.M. Minerals and trace minerals, in: *Nutrition for Sport and Exercise*, Berning, J.R. and Steen, S.N., Eds., Aspen, Gaithersburg, MD., 1998, chap. 5.
37. Shaskey, D.J. and Green, G.A. Sports haem., *Sports Med.*, 29, 27, 2000.
38. Barr, S.I. and Costill, D.L. Water: can the endurance athlete get too much of a good thing? *J. Amer. Diet. Assoc.*, 89, 1629, 1989.
39. Nieman, D.C. Is infection risk linked to exercise workload? *Med. Sci. Sports Exerc.*, 32, S406, 2000.

Section Two

Dietary Assessment of Athletes

2

Estimation of Food and Nutrient Intakes of Athletes

Carol Ballew and Richard E. Killingsworth

CONTENTS

0-8493-0927-1/02/$0.00+$1.50

I. Introduction

This chapter deals with three fundamental aspects of estimating the food and nutrient intakes of athletes:

1. General considerations in gathering food intake data
2. Special considerations in gathering food intake data from athletes
3. Converting food intake data to nutrient intake estimates

A comprehensive review of all aspects of dietary assessment methodology is beyond the scope of this chapter, but many good methodologic guides and reviews have been published.[1-4] Our goal is to provide nutritionists and other health professionals with practical guidance about the special issues they are likely to encounter in assessing the diets of athletes. We assume that the goal of estimating food and nutrient intakes of athletes is to evaluate the nutritional status of individuals. The dietary assessment methods discussed here apply to individuals who are able to record their own food intakes or recall them accurately. Generally, this includes adults and adolescents but not younger children, who may not be able to either record or recall what they eat.[5-7]

The steps in nutritional status assessment, from gathering data on food consumption to coding these data and converting them to estimates of nutrient intake, are interdependent. The accuracy of dietary assessment depends, first, on obtaining high-quality records of food consumption. Accurate and consistent coding is second only to primary data collection in determining the quality of dietary assessment. Nutrient analysis software simplify some coding and analysis tasks but the most expensive and elaborate software will not compensate for poor data or poor coding.

II. Methods of Assessing Food Intake

First, health professionals should consider the purpose of the data collection and decide what information they really need. To determine knowledge, attitudes, or beliefs about nutrition among athletes, short questionnaires may be adequate. However, clinical assessment of nutritional status, counseling about dietary practices, supporting peak performance or conducting research into the associations between nutritional status and performance require detailed and accurate food intake data. This is, unavoidably, a time-consuming and labor-intensive undertaking. Second, recognize that there is no ideal method for collecting food intake data. All methods have advantages and disadvantages and all methods require commitment and effort from professionals and their clients.

The most accurate way to determine the nutrient content of the diet is to prepare two portions of everything, one to be eaten and one to be set aside for laboratory analysis, but this is rarely done outside of metabolic ward research. In most circumstances, professionals must rely on clients to report what they eat. There are broadly three methods of collecting food intake data. The first is direct recording, usually by the person consuming the food. The second is by recall, in which a client is asked to recall each food or beverage consumed in a specified period — usually 24 hours — before the interview. The third is by gathering data on the frequency of consuming a list of foods. There is a combined method, originally called the "diet history" by Bertha Burke,[8] that includes three stages:

1. A detailed interview about usual eating patterns, sometimes centered on a 24-hour recall and how usual patterns deviate from that recall
2. A food frequency checklist
3. A 3-day diet record

Burke's diet history remains the most comprehensive method to evaluate dietary intakes but it is seldom undertaken because of the client burden and the need for substantial time investment of skilled staff to elicit and evaluate the data.

A. Diet Records

Diet records, also called food diaries, are recorded on a form with one line for each food or beverage consumed and columns for portion size, preparation method if applicable and additions of dressing or condiments at the table (Table 2.1). Additional columns are usually included for the time and place of consumption and other comments that may be useful in evaluating dietary patterns. Each item consumed can be weighed, measured with household utensils or quantified by reference to common objects (e.g., a portion of cooked meat the size of a deck of cards weighs about 3 ounces or 85 grams). Nutrient content of the diet is estimated by coding diet records and entering the data into a nutrient analysis software that links the foods and portions reported to a nutrient content database (see section IV).

Keeping diet records minimizes forgetting foods and beverages and maximizes the detail available about items, particularly if clients make entries as foods and beverages are consumed. The ability to measure portions is a major advantage of the diet record method because reconstructing portion sizes in a recall interview can be difficult. Nevertheless, there are many

TABLE 2.1

Sample Basic Diet Recording Form

Time	Place/ Source	Food: Detailed Description	Amount	Preparation Method	Condiments	Comments*
7 a.m.	Home	Frosted flakes	3/4 cup (42 g)			Reviewer get brand
		White sugar	2 tsp(8 g)			
		Milk	1 cup(244 g)			Reviewer: whole, 2%,1%, skim?
Noon	Cafeteria	Vegetarian lasagne	3″ x 3″ x 1.5″ (298 g)		Added salt and pepper	Coder ask food service for recipe
		Soft drink, regular	12 oz can (336 g)			Reviewer get brand
		Lettuce salad	1.5 cup (78 g)		Thousand Island dressing	Reviewer probe for dressing brand, amount, regular/low fat
3 p.m.	Coffee shop	Decaf latte with skim milk	x-large			Reviewer get vendor name. Coder call vendor for volume of x-large and proportion of milk
		Chocolate frosted biscotti				Coder call vendor for size and other information on biscotti
6:30 p.m.	Home	Frozen peas with butter sauce	2/3 cup (106 g)	microwaved		Reviewer get brand
		Garlic bread	2 slices (84 g)	toasted in oven	Butter and garlic	Reviewer get size of slice and amount of butter per slice
		Leftover roast beef	3″x5″x1/3″ (85 g)	microwaved	Salt, pepper, ketchup	Reviewer ask about trimming visible fat on beef, get amount of ketchup
10 p.m.	Home	Chocolate ice cream	2 cups (266 g)			Reviewer get brand and other specifics about ice cream

*Items in Comments columns indicate information to be elicited by the dietitian who reviews the food record with the client or by the coder who enters the food record into the nutritional analysis software.

Gram weight equivalents are given in parentheses.

potential sources of error in diet records. Clients must be motivated to keep detailed records and to provide all the information needed to analyze the records accurately. The food must be specified in sufficient detail to be matched unambiguously to an item in the nutrient content database, the portion sizes must be specified in units that correspond to those in the database and preparation methods that have nutritional implications must be specified. If clients prepare their own food, they should be taught to record brand names, package information, all the details of preparation methods, condiments added at the table, portion sizes consumed and plate waste (trimming of meats, removing poultry skin, etc.).[4] If clients eat in dining halls or at training tables, recipes and details about ingredients used in the kitchen are probably available.

Not all clients are sufficiently motivated, knowledgeable about the food they eat, literate, or numerically inclined enough to keep accurate and detailed records. Some detail may be recovered by reviewing diet records with clients when they are submitted (Table 2.1).[4] Investigators have tried having children and adults of low literacy keep food records with tape recorders, with uneven success.[9-11]

Clients may change their usual eating habits or misrepresent true consumption because they know someone will be evaluating their intakes. The process of keeping records may make clients conscious of what they eat and thus lead them to inadvertently change their usual consumption patterns so that even the most accurate record may not reflect typical intakes.

B. 24-Hour Diet Recall Interviews

The goal of the 24-hour recall interview is to obtain detailed information on all the foods and beverages consumed in the 24 hours before the interview. A trained interviewer, ideally a dietitian, interviews clients using a standardized protocol that incorporates systematic probes to elicit a complete list of all items consumed and a detailed description of each item. To carry out appropriate probing, the interviewer must be knowledgeable about local foods and about food preparation techniques.

In the past, recall interviews were recorded on forms similar to those used for diet records and later coded and analyzed with reference to a nutrient content database. Many dietary analysis software packages now allow recall interviews to be conducted interactively using a computer (see section IV). Some software include built-in probes to standardize the interview process and enhance completeness of recall. If consistency among several interviewers is desirable, these systems produce standardized probing. The National Health and Nutrition Examination Surveys use a computer-based, interactive, multiple-pass interview technique in which respondents are asked to make a preliminary list of foods, meal by meal, then the interviewer reviews the list with the respondent, eliciting details about each food reported (form, brand name, portion size, preparation method, added condiments and so on).[12] After the second pass, the respondent is asked, meal by meal and snack by snack, if anything else was consumed at that event or between recorded events and if so, those items are recorded and probed in detail as well. Computer-interactive recall interviews are generally preferable to paper records that must later be coded. You can probe and clarify responses immediately, with reference to food items in the nutrient database, to find the closest match and to recover as many relevant details as possible. However, a skilled interviewer who is familiar with the software and database that will be used for nutrient analysis is capable of eliciting and recording accurate data for later coding.

The dietary recall has an advantage over the food records because clients are less likely to alter eating behavior in expectation of being evaluated. Recall interviews can be conducted over the phone on a surprise basis. Disadvantages of the recall method include the possibility of forgetting items and the difficulty of reconstructing portion sizes without direct measurement. Clients can use a variety of visual aids, such as cups and bowls, serving utensils and food models, to help them estimate portion sizes.[13] Booklets of two-dimensional representations of common foods can be distributed to clients who will be interviewed over the phone. Still, clients who do not prepare their own food are particularly likely to have difficulty with portion size estimation, as well as with reporting some important details of preparation methods with nutritional impact. As with the diet record, clients may deliberately misrepresent intakes for a variety of reasons.

C. How Many Days?

A single day of food record or a single 24-hour recall is not adequate to characterize usual dietary intake and nutritional status because most people experience day-to-day variability in food intake.[9,14] Day-to-day variability may be more pronounced among athletes than among the general population because athletes often vary their diets with training and competition schedules (see section III). In the general population, the number of days required to estimate an individual's usual or long-term intake varies from nutrient to nutrient. Basiotis et al.[14] estimated that it requires approximately 30 days to estimate the usual intake of energy in the general population. Many vitamins and minerals are distributed unevenly in the food supply, requiring even more days to estimate usual intakes: approximately 60 days for protein or iron, 90 for calcium, 200 for vitamin C and more than 400 for vitamin A.[14]

It is obviously impractical to collect and analyze many days of dietary records or recalls in most situations. You must arrive at an acceptable compromise between the precision of the estimate of nutrient intakes that is acceptable and the resources available to obtain and process the data. For dietary records, it is common to collect 3 or 4 days, less often 7 days of data. This imposes a burden on the client who must keep the records and there is a tendency for the quality of the record keeping to deteriorate toward the end of a multiple-day recording period.[15]

D. Underreporting

Almost all diet records or recalls appear to be subject to some degree of underreporting.[16] The doubly labeled water technique for measuring energy expenditure over a reference period of several days now permits investigators to quantify energy underreporting.[17] Estimates of underreporting range from 15%–30% of daily energy intake.[16-18] Underreporting may be inadvertent, such as forgetting to record condiments of high nutritional density or food preparation methods of high caloric contribution (e.g., mayonnaise or butter on a sandwich; breaded and fried foods). Deliberate underreporting may be pervasive in the record, such as consistently underestimating portion sizes, or it may be limited to specific kinds of foods. Snack foods, beverages and items eaten between meals seem to be underreported more than foods eaten at meals.[19,20] Women tend to underreport more than men, overweight individuals tend to underreport more than normal weight individuals and less educated individuals tend to underreport more than more educated individuals.[16,21-24] Three independent groups of investigators have reported that preteen girls report more completely than teenage girls.[18,21,25] Among adults and adolescents, the perceived social acceptability of foods or dietary behaviors and the precepts learned from health education programs can influence the likelihood of reporting certain foods.[22,26,27] This perception of acceptability may have a greater influence on teens and adults than on preteens.

Many investigators have found that athletes of many ages and levels of competition appear to substantially underreport energy intakes relative to estimated or measured energy expenditures.[17,28-31] No entirely satisfactory explanation has been offered for this phenomenon, beyond the usual underreporting exhibited by most respondents.

E. Food Frequency Questionnaires

A food frequency questionnaire (FFQ) is a list of foods or categories of foods intended to estimate usual intakes during a specified time period such as the past month or past year. Clients are asked to indicate how often they usually ate each item on the list during the reference period. A quantitative FFQ also elicits usual portion sizes. Some quantitative FFQs include software with statistical algorithms to compute estimated nutrient intakes. Comprehensive FFQs designed to estimate the intake of many nutrients may contain more than 100 items, each with a corresponding portion size estimate. Some FFQs focus on one or a few nutrients and some provide a score for compliance with dietary recommendations such as fruit and vegetable intakes. Reviews of FFQs can be found in Thompson and Byers[3] and Sugerman et al.[4]

The FFQ is less burdensome than multiple-day food records or recalls for the client, who completes the FFQ only once. The FFQ is also less labor-intensive than diet records or recalls in terms of coding and analysis. Many are designed to be self-administered, although review of the completed form by a dietitian or interviewer-administration, either one-on-one or in a group setting such as a classroom, improves the apparent validity of the responses.[32] Some FFQs can be completed on a scanned answer sheet and some can be completed with an interactive computer program.

Proponents of the FFQ believe that it captures "usual" or long-term dietary intakes. It is difficult to document that it does so, however, because most FFQs are validated against a series of diet records.[33,34] Responses on FFQs tend to be biased by recent consumption patterns.[35] People with inconsistent eating habits may have trouble generalizing about a long reference period and may not in fact have a usual intake for many foods. Even for people with relatively consistent eating habits, the cognitive process of generalizing about usual consumption can be difficult.[35] Although quantitative FFQs produce apparently very precise estimates of nutrient intakes, it is difficult to assess the validity of these estimates and therefore their utility in clinical evaluation of nutritional status is limited.[36]

The major FFQs in wide use in epidemiologic research were developed by reviewing food records or 24-hour recall intake data for large numbers of people and determining the most common food sources of nutrients for the population as a whole.[37] This limits the applicability of FFQs for people whose eating patterns differ from those of the mainstream, for example, some ethnic or immigrant groups, vegetarians, individuals of low socioeconomic status and perhaps athletes.[38-40] Individuals may not obtain the bulk of their nutrient intake from the same foods as the general population. For example, someone who does not consume dairy products might appear to have a very low calcium intake based on an FFQ but might, in fact, have a substantial calcium intake from calcium-fortified orange juice and other less typical sources of calcium.

Another disadvantage of FFQs is that information about eating patterns that can be recovered from diet records or recalls is missed by the FFQ format. It is not apparent from FFQs that individuals skip breakfast or graze throughout the day or do not get enough fluids. For example, van Erp-Baart et al.[41] using multiple-day food records, found that one third of the daily energy intake was derived from snacks in a large sample of world-class Dutch athletes. This information would not emerge from an FFQ.

In using FFQs for dietary assessment, the health professional must be aware of two potential pitfalls. The first is taking an existing FFQ from the literature and applying it uncritically to the clients. The second is the temptation to create a new instrument. In both cases, the problem is lack of validation. No matter how widely an existing FFQ is used or how well it has been validated in previous applications, it must still be validated in any new population or demographic segment. This is particularly true when working with athletes, whose eating habits may be quite different from those of the general population or from those of the people for whom FFQs were previously validated.

It may seem desirable to develop assessment instruments specifically for a group of athletes, but the technical and logistic requirements of proper questionnaire design and validation are beyond the resources of most practitioners. The design of the FFQ and the validation process both require repeated collection of multiple days of diet records or recall interviews from a large number of representative participants.[37] Unless there is a pressing and ongoing need for FFQs or short questionnaires for a specific program or research agenda, it is rarely worthwhile to develop a new instrument. It is more cost effective and accurate to gather several days of diet records or recall interviews from clients to evaluate nutritional status.

III. Special Issues in Assessing Food Intakes of Athletes

People vary widely in age, lifestyle and health status. Athletes also vary in the sports in which they participate and their level of training and competition. Athletes usually have higher energy needs than the general population and some sports have unique physiological demands that also influence the nutritional needs of athletes.[42-46] It has been repeatedly documented that these nutritional requirements can be met by normal, well-balanced diets and there is no persuasive evidence that athletes need unusual dietary regimens or programs of supplementation.[47] Nevertheless, athletes are particularly vulnerable to promises that dietary or supplementation practices might give them an edge over their competitors or might compensate for real or perceived variation in physical endowment and technical skill. Most sports have traditions about appropriate and optimal dietary practices. Some of these traditions are based in nutritional science and some are without scientific foundation. Regardless of scientific merit, these beliefs strongly influence coaches' advice and athletes' food choices, weight management practices and supplement use.[48] Dietitians and sports nutritionists working with athletes need to be familiar with the nutrition-related beliefs of athletes and coaches.

The Heptathlete Development Project of the Nutrition, Exercise and Wellness Program at the University of Arizona is one of several college programs designed to use nutritional science to support peak athletic performance. The project Web site[49] provides several resources for the nutritional evaluation of athletes. These resources include questionnaires about many nutritional issues of special importance to athletes and the nutritionists and health professionals working with them. These resources are a good place to start in designing an individual evaluation program for athletes. We particularly recommend the extensive questionnaire eliciting information about nutrition attitudes and beliefs, feelings about weight and weight management practices, use of supplementsand dietary and fluid intakes during various stages of training and competition.

Although many special issues must be considered when evaluating the food and nutrient intake of athletes, athletes may also be relatively easy clients to work with. Elite competitors in particular are often very aware of their food intakes and able to report them accurately.

A. Periodicity

In the general population, eating patterns may differ substantially between weekdays and weekends. For this reason, multiple-day records usually include several weekdays and at least one weekend day. In addition, people experience seasonal periodicity in the availability and cost of some foods. For athletes, additional important periodicities are associated with the cycles of their sports such as the off-season, phases of training or pre- and post-competition regimens. Some athletes train and compete intensely only part of the year. The competitive season makes very different demands of energy expenditure and nutrient intake from the off-season. Some athletes train more or less year round, either competing in different sports throughout the year or training for a single sport on a nearly continuous basis. Continuous training is typical of elite competitors. Athletes who compete in different sports in different seasons may have varied nutritional regimens according to the sport. Athletes who engage in a single sport year round might engage in different training, pre-competition and post-competition regimens. Pre-competition carbohydrate loading to build muscle glycogen stores is a particularly important aspect of periodicity for many athletes, for example, including long distance runners and other endurance athletes.

Nutritionists and health professionals should be familiar with the physical demands and calendars of the various sports (Table 2.1). Because of these periodicities, it may be necessary to obtain many days of data about an athlete's dietary intakes, scheduled to capture eating patterns in different phases of activity, to accurately evaluate that athlete's overall nutritional status. At least, it is necessary to determine the appropriate time in a training cycle to gather the data. For example, a marathon runner keeping a food record in the day or two before a race might appear to have high carbohydrate intakes and low and perhaps inadequate intakes of other nutrients, largely as a result of pre-race carbohydrate loading. If the goal of dietary data collection is to support peak performance or conduct research into associations between dietary practices and performance, it may be necessary to schedule data collection to coincide with certain phases of training and competition.

B. Fluid Intake

Many athletes do not consume enough fluids before, during and after training or competition in spite of clear evidence that hydration improves performance.[50] Athletes keeping dietary records or interviewers collecting 24-hour diet recalls may not remember to record water and other fluid consumption.

TABLE 2.2

Periodicity of Selected Sports

Sport[a]	Pre-Season Training[b]	Competitive Season[c]	Active Rest[d]	Post-Season Training[e]
Baseball	November–January	February–June	3–4 weeks	August–October
Basketball	August–October	November–March	3–4 weeks	May–July
Cross country	August	September–November	Most compete in indoor/ outdoor track seasons	July–August
Football	June–August	September–December	4–6 weeks	February–May
Golf	July–August	September–May	2–3 weeks	June
Gymnastics	October–December	January–April	3–4 weeks	June–September
Ice hockey	August–September	October–March	4–6 weeks	May–July
Indoor track and field	September–November	December–February	Most compete in outdoor track season	Most compete in outdoor track season
Outdoor track and field	N/A (most have already competed during indoor track season)	March–June	3–4 weeks	July–August
Soccer	June–July	August–December	4–6 weeks	February–May
Softball	November–January	February–May	3–4 weeks	June–October
Swimming	July–September	October–March	3–4 weeks	April–June
Tennis	July–August	September–November		
	January–May	2–3 weeks	June–July	
Men's volleyball	August–September	October–May	3–4 weeks	June - August
Women's volleyball	June–August	September–December	3–4 weeks	February - May
Wrestling	September–October	November–March	4–6 weeks	June–August

[a] All sports include men and women unless specified, e.g., volleyball, where the competitive seasons are scheduled differently.

[b,e] The differences in pre- and post-season activities are associated with the training cycle and the type of conditioning that will be performed. The post-season for most athletes focuses on developing strength, power, flexibility and agility. The pre-season focuses on developing more technical abilities and specificity of movement and conditioning.

[c] Competitive seasons vary by age group and skill level. The seasons here reflect the calendars of most high school and collegiate sports in most states, governing bodiesand associations.

[d] Active rest periods vary among age groups, skill levels and whether the athlete also competes in other sports. Active rest allows the athlete to recover while engaging in other activities.

Water consumption is often especially difficult to quantify. People don't think much about water consumption; they often drink in response to thirst throughout the day and may forget many small intakes, but these add up to a substantial volume of water in the aggregate. Beverages not consumed with meals are forgotten in diet records and recalls more often than those consumed with meals.[19,20] Many athletes consume sports drinks containing carbohydrates and electrolytes that have substantial nutritional implications. During practice sessions, competition, or recovery, athletes may consume large amounts of such beverages and quantification may be difficult.

C. Snacking and Grazing

Athletes may obtain a substantial portion of their daily energy and nutrient intakes from snacks. Van Erp-Baart et al.[41] found that elite Dutch athletes competing in a variety of sports consumed about one third of their daily energy from snacks. Many other investigators have reported that grazing or snacking is a major adaptation to the high energy needs of athletes.[51] Depending on the foods eaten, snacks may also contribute substantially to nutrient intakes. Snacks tend to be underreported in diet records or recalls more often than meals.[19,20] Athletes keeping diet records should be reminded to record all snacks and interviewers should probe thoroughly.

D. Supplements

Aggressive marketing has led millions of athletes to use dietary supplements. To cite only one example, a 1993 survey of the marketplace found 624 commercial products targeted to body builders, making more than 800 unsubstantiated health and performance claims.[52] Many athletes take common vitamin and mineral supplements and may also take a wide variety of other less common supplements (Table 2.2).[53] In spite of abundant evidence that athletes' nutrient needs can be met by well-balanced diets and that most supplements have no measurable effect on performance in well-nourished athletes,[47] some athletes still take substantial quantities of supplements. Supplement abuse can cause short-term acute symptoms such as nausea or diarrhea and long-term adverse effects such as nutrient imbalances or toxicity.[54-57] Furthermore, some supplements contain substances banned by athletic governing bodies and some may contain impurities.

Many clients do not think to report various supplements in a diet record or recall interview because supplements may not be considered food and they are often not consumed with meals. Athletes may also be reluctant to disclose the use of some supplements, especially those that are prohibited by sports governing bodies. Information on the use of supplements must be elicited by educated probing. The professional should be familiar with the range of supplements used by athletes in various sports (Table 2.4) and should develop a rapport with clients that will facilitate probing about the use of supplements, both the common vitamin and mineral preparations and the more exotic products targeted to athletes.

Table 2.4 identifies common supplement categories that athletes might use. It is important to recognize that this table indicates the categories in common use in particular sports, but individuals may use a wide variety of substances, so probing should be done across all categories. It is also important

TABLE 2.4

Supplements Reported by Athletes

Sport	Anabolic	Endurance	Stimulants	Energy	Other
Baseball	×		×	×	×
Basketball	×		×	×	×
Body builders	×	×	×	×	×
Cross country		×			×
Football	×		×	×	×
Golf					×
Gymnastics			×		×
Ice hockey	×		×	×	×
Indoor track and field	×	×	×	×	×
Olympic weightlifting	×		×		×
Outdoor track & field	×	×	×	×	×
Soccer		×		×	×
Softball			×		×
Swimming	×	×	×	×	×
Tennis				×	×
Men's volleyball					×
Women's volleyball					×
Wrestling	×		×	×	×

to recognize that athletes may not equate a supplement they take with a generic category, so the interviewer should become familiar with brand names and common names of products used by athletes in a particular program. For example, anabolic compounds include creatine monohydrate, beta hydroxy beta methylbutrate, chorionic gonadotropin, human growth hormone, dihydroepiandrosterone, androstenediol and many others. Each may be marketed under a variety of common and brand names. Endurance compounds include coenzyme Q-10, medium chain tryglycerides and pyruvate. Stimulants include caffeine, ephedrine and dimethylamphetamine. Products in the energy category, consisting of sports drinks and power bars with high energy content derived mainly from simple sugars, are widely consumed and have the most direct nutritional impact. The bars may contain proteins and minerals, while the beverages typically contain high concentrations of electrolytes. The "Other" category in Table 2.4 includes herbal products that are becoming more common in the marketplace and in the athlete's pharmacopoeia. They have diverse effects ranging from diuresis to decreased perception of fatigue or pain.

E. Weight Management

Some athletes, such as football players and power lifters, try to gain weight and muscle mass. Others, like gymnasts and ice skaters, try to lose weight and body fat. And some, like wrestlers and rowers, deal with the conflicting goals of gaining muscle mass in the long term and losing weight in the short term.[48] Athletes may try a variety of idiosyncratic, unhealthy and possibly life-threatening dietary regimens to achieve their weight goals. Some sport-specific factors predispose athletes to inappropriate weight-management practices; these include the belief, common among both athletes and coaches, that there are ideal weights, body fat contents or body shapes for peak performance[58-61] Although some body shapes or body composition profiles are better adapted than others to some sports, diet or supplement-use regimens to achieve weight goals can be carried to extremes, especially by individuals who may try to achieve a standard unrealistic for their genetic endowment.

Some athletes are at risk of disordered eating patterns.[62] Eating disorders may be more common among female athletes but should not be discounted among male athletes.[59,63-66] Athletes' eating patterns may not meet the formal diagnostic criteria of anorexia nervosa or bulimia nervosa but may nevertheless lead to dangerously inadequate energy and nutrient intakes.[60,61] It can be difficult to diagnose disordered dietary practices in athletes because it is often appropriate for them to be light or slender. In fact, athletes may not be obviously underweight but may still be in negative energy balance and at risk of nutrient deficiency.[61,67] Knowledge of sport-specific body type norms and athletes' beliefs allows the professional to interview and probe effectively.

Athletes may not report their dietary practices accurately if they are aware that they are unacceptable. Reported intakes that seem, logically, to be too high or too low should be considered suspect.[68] Doubly labeled water can be used to estimate actual energy expenditure over a reference period.[69] Actual energy expenditure can be compared with reported food intakes to assess the possibility of inaccurate reporting. The method has most often been used to assess the degree of underreporting of energy intake,[17,30,31] but can also be used to assess overreporting among athletes who may try to disguise inappropriate weight management techniques. However, common sense and a close look at your client may suggest a discrepancy between reported and actual intakes that warrants further exploration.

IV.   Converting Reported Food Intakes to Nutrient Intake Estimates

In the past, coders had to match foods reported in a diet record or recall interview with entries in printed food composition tables such as those compiled by the United States Department of Agriculture (USDA) and published in the *Agricultural Handbook* series.[70] Coders had to convert the reported portion sizes to gram weight equivalents and compute the nutrient content of a portion, one nutrient at a time, then sum all the foods to obtain estimated total nutrient intakes. The advent of computerized dietary analysis software has eliminated much of the tedium but it has not made the fundamental process of coding — matching the foods and portions reported to the most appropriate corresponding items in the database — any less important.

Nutritional analysis software combines a user interface, an internal program and a nutrient content database. The user interface is where foods are entered and matched to items in the database and portion sizes are specified. Most software allows the coder to enter a brief food name and select from a number of possible corresponding foods. The internal program then maps the food entered onto the database containing nutrient content information and computes the nutrient intake corresponding to the food and portion entered.

A variety of nutrient analysis software is available. New ones come on the market frequently and those that already exist are updated periodically. We have provided general guidelines to help professionals choose software that will be most suitable for their needs (Table 2.4).[4,71-73]

Nutritional analysis software ranges in price from free (on the Internet) through a few hundred dollars to several thousand dollars. Price should not be the primary determining factor in choosing software. The most important factor is the appropriateness and accuracy of the nutrient content database the software uses, the second is the quality of the user interface. Both a good database and a good user interface can be found in the midrange of cost. In particular settings, special features may be desirable and may dictate the need for a more expensive software.

No software is perfect and none will contain all features that might be desired. Prioritize your needs. Most vendors provide a demo version to try before software is purchased and some can be tested on line. Most demos do not support all of the functions of the software so if a demo is appealing but seems to lack some desired features, the vendor can supply a full description of capabilities.

A. Hardware Considerations

Most software packages are available in versions compatible with IBM-clone computers and most offer Windows versions. Few professional-quality dietary analysis software run on MAC systems. The software should run on the purchaser's existing hardware and be compatible with the configuration and operating system of the computer to be used (Table 2.4).

B. Databases

Most dietary analysis software is packaged with an obligatory nutrient database, although a few permit the purchaser to select from one of several database options or to purchase an upgrade of the basic database. The nutrient database is used to translate reported food consumption into estimated nutrient intakes. The USDA Database for Standard Reference[74] is the most appropriate database for evaluating the diets of residents of the United

TABLE 2.4

Checklist for Choosing Dietary Software

❏ Will the software run on your computer?
   Check RAM, hard disk space, configuration (extended or expanded memory), operating
      system (DOS, Windows, version of Windows, non-IBM clone), monitor and printer
      requirements
❏ Do you need a single-user license or a multiple-user license?
❏ How much technical support does your user license entitle you to?
❏ How detailed is the documentation
   to install and manage the software?
   to run all the features of the software?
   to troubleshoot?
   to manage files?
❏ Does the documentation specify default assumptions?
❏ What is the database?
   What is the source if information for nutrients?
   How current are the data?
   Are database upgrades offered?
   Are users routinely notified of database updates?
   Does the database provide data on all the nutrients of interest?
   Are there gaps in the database for important nutrients?
   Are foods with missing data flagged and are totals including these foods also flagged?
❏ Does the software allow you to enter water/fluid consumption?
   If not, does the software include the water content of foods and can you adapt this to
      record fluid consumption?
❏ Can you add new foods to the database and is this easy to do?
   What is the maximum number of new foods that can be added?
❏ Can you add recipes to the database and is this easy to do?
   Does the recipe system include retention (cooking gains and losses) algorithm?
   What is the maximum number of recipes that can be added?
❏ Does the software produce output that meets most of your needs?
   Do you want percent of energy from macronutrients?
   Do you want intakes broken down by meal?
   Do you want intakes evaluated relative to standards (e.g., diabetic exchanges, dietary
      reference intakes)?
   Are the reference standards used current and correct?
   Do you need weight management algorithms?
   Are the algorithms appropriate for athletes?
❏ Ease of file management
   Can the software produce multiple-day averages for individuals?
   Can data be output for use in statistical software for research purposes if you need this
      feature?

States but would not be appropriate for people living elsewhere.[75,76] This
applies especially to the evaluation of micronutrient intakes because many
foods in the United States are both highly processed and highly fortified;
the extent of processing and fortification varies greatly in other countries.
Most nutritional analysis software packages sold in the United States use
part or all of the USDA database. When this chapter was written, the current
version of the USDA Database for Standard Reference was 13 (SR13),

released in 1999. The food supply changes constantly and databases keep abreast of these changes with periodic updates. Updates to the USDA database are published on the USDA Web site.[74] A software user support contract should include updates to the database as they become available, or at least notification that updates have occurred.

No database contains complete data on all nutrients. Data for selenium and soluble fiber are often missing from many foods in a database, for example, but these nutrients may not be of particular concern when working with athletes. On the other hand, it may be important to evaluate athletes' vitamin D intakes but the USDA database did not include values for vitamin D in foods until SR13. Some software offers data on the fatty acid or amino acid composition of foods or other specialized micronutrients.

The software should flag foods for which the nutrient content data are not complete and should flag daily nutrient totals and multiple-day nutrient averages that include missing data. Missing data for a nutrient in a food should be clearly distinguished from the absence of that nutrient. It should be clear whether a blank means "none" or "missing data." Missing data on the nutrient content of a given food will result in an underestimate of intake. This is not often problematic, except in the case of an estimated low intake of a nutrient for an individual whose record includes many foods with missing data for that nutrient. This may be an issue in dealing with the diets of athletes because they may eat a number of foods not in the database. The software should allow the addition of new foods and nutrient content information to a database.

C. New Foods

New foods enter the market constantly and specialized foods and nutritional products targeted to athletes are common. Even if a database is updated periodically, clients will report foods not in the database. If a food not in the database composes a substantial portion of a client's diet or appears in the records of many clients, it is important to obtain detailed nutrient content information. The first resource to check is the USDA Web site,[74] where the most recent updates are posted. If the food is not in the USDA updates, some information can be obtained from the product label. Current Food and Drug Administration (FDA) and USDA regulations require listing the amount of energy, total and saturated fat, cholesterol, sodium, total carbohydrate, dietary fiber, sugars and protein per serving and a specification of serving size.[77] The regulations also require listing vitamins A and C, calcium and iron contents as a percent of daily value, but the actual content of these nutrients in μg or mg need not be specified. Listing other vitamins and minerals on the label is optional.

The nutritional information available on food labels is therefore limited. Ideally, complete nutrient information on foods you add to the database should be available. Many food manufacturers will provide nutrient information to professional practitioners on request and many food packages list a phone number to call to request this information. Some manufacturers consider nutritional information proprietary, although this is more likely to be true of purveyors of nutritional supplements than of foods. If all other avenues fail, the nutrient content of a new food can be approximated by comparing the label nutrient information and ingredient list with those of foods already in the database and finding one that appears to be the most similar.[78]

The buyer should choose software that permits the addition of new foods and their nutrient contents and that makes this process user friendly. How many new foods can the software accommodate? There will be some upper limit but this should be in the hundreds. When working with athletes, you may need to add many foods, beverages and other products with nutritional implications.

D. Recipes

Combination dishes are problematic for any database because of the wide variety of recipes and preparation methods people use. Most databases have generic recipes for common homemade foods, but these are based on averages from national surveys[75,79] and may not accurately reflect a client's own recipe. It is preferable to elicit specific ingredients and preparation methods if clients can provide this information. Dormitory food services and training table kitchens are usually willing to share their recipes. A word of caution is in order here, however. Food service recipes are explicit about the number of portions a recipe yields but some athletes consume far more than the standard portion; it is not safe to assume that an athlete's reported serving is the same as the recipe portion.

Recipes should be easy to add to whatever software is chosen. It should also, ideally, offer the option of saving added recipes in a general file or in the file of an individual who reports a recipe. Some recipes apply to only one client, but if a number of clients are using the same recommended recipes or eating in the same dormitory or at the same training table, it is inconvenient to have to enter a common recipe repeatedly. Ask about the upper limit to the number of recipes that can be added to the database. As with new foods, when working with athletes it may be necessary to add many new recipes.

The best software incorporates information about retention factors — the nutrient gains and losses associated with the cooking process — into the recipe algorithm. Alternately, retention factors are published in the USDA website[74] and can be used to calculate the nutrient content of the prepared recipe from the raw ingredients, adjusting for cooking gains and losses.[78] The nutrient content of a recipe computed in this fashion can be added to the database, treating the recipe as a new food.

Some nutritional software applications are part of integrated food-service management packages that can maintain inventory, generate menus and recipes and provide point-of-purchase nutritional analysis, all through a single computer system. For athletic programs with training tables or other food service operations that are considering automation or upgrade, an integrated system that includes nutritional analysis may be an attractive option.

E. Water and Sports Drinks

Fluid balance is an important issue for athletes but many nutrient analysis software have no mechanism for recording water consumption as such. However, some have a column for the water content of foods, treating it like any other nutrient. The water content column can be adapted to record fluid intake. Add water to the database as a new food, with zeroes in the columns for the other nutrients and an amount of water consumed, usually in grams, in the column set aside for the water content of the food. Some databases include a few popular sports beverages, but none are up to date on all the sports drinks on the market, particularly the specialized beverages targeted to athletes. These should also be added as new foods, including an entry for their water content. Entering sports drinks into the database should be fairly straightforward because the carbohydrate and electrolyte content is generally detailed on the label.

F. Supplements

Common vitamin and mineral preparations are generally well labeled. If athletes report taking these products, the interviewer should ask to see the bottle. The information can be transcribed and added to the nutrient totals or the supplement product can be added to the database as a new food. Some products targeted to athletes may be less well labeled and it may be difficult to obtain nutritional information about them. FDA regulations about labeling these products are limited and manufacturers may consider the details of formulation to be proprietary information.[80]

G. Default Assumptions

Most software has default assumptions that can be invoked if a food is not described in detail in the diet record. The default assumptions are based on typical food use patterns reported by participants in large national surveys and may not accurately reflect the intakes of a given individual.[81] For example, "fried chicken, leg, NFS" (not further specified) may assume batter-dipped, with skin and fried in hydrogenated vegetable shortening, because this is the most common preparation method for fried chicken. The fried chicken leg a client actually consumed may have been breaded rather than battered, skinless and fried in canola oil. If the default assumptions systematically depart from what respondents consume, reliance on default assumptions will bias the results of the nutrient analysis. The default assumptions should be used only as a last resort, not as the path of least resistance. More importantly, clients should be taught to record as much detail about foods as possible.

H. Special Features

i. *Interactive Interface*

Many applications have an interactive user interface, where the screen displays the nutrient content of foods as they are entered, maintains a running total of all the foods entered so far and displays instantaneous changes to show the effects of adding, deleting, or substituting foods. An interactive interface is very useful in counseling and educating clients. Software that requires multiple file management steps to enter, analyze and output nutritional information is tedious to use and is not particularly useful in client interactions.

ii. *Output Options*

Buyers must decide what kind of printed output they need. Is it important to have detailed reports to file with clinical records? Are client-friendly outputs for education and counseling necessary? Many applications offer both options. Should the output include comparisons of the client's intake with standards such as the Food Pyramid Guidelines, Dietary Reference Intakes, or Diabetic Exchanges?[82-84] If comparisons with standards are important, does the software include the most current standards? It may be equally important to be able to evaluate clients against individualized recommendations or those of a sports program. If so, can individual goals be added to the software?

Some software now contains information on the calculated glycemic index of foods. This is of interest to practitioners dealing with athletes as well as to those dealing with patients with diabetes or hyperlipidemia, although much research remains to be done in all areas of application.[85] If this option is important to the purchaser, the accompanying documentation should be searched for the source of the data on the glycemic index. Calculations should be based on standardized methods.[86]

Some dietary assessment software has weight management algorithms linked to body size, reported energy intakes and physical activity estimates. The algorithms were probably developed from the general population and may not be accurate for athletes, who typically train and compete well beyond the maximum level of physical activity assumed by the software. There should be adequate documentation to determine how the weight management algorithms were derived. Some dietary assessment software also purports to estimate percent body fat from height, weight, sex and age. These estimates are imprecise, even for the general population from whom they were developed. Their applicability to athletes, who usually have greater lean body mass and less body fat for a given height and weight than nonathletes, is questionable. There are more accurate ways to estimate body fat content and, if this is important in evaluating the nutritional status of an athlete, the client should be referred for appropriate measurement.

iii. File Management

Will the software be expected to analyze client data one day at a time or will multiple-day average intakes be examined? Not all software will produce multiple-day averages and some that does is rather inflexible about what can be included in the average. Dietary analysis software that is exemplary in other respects may not export nutrient intake data in a form that is readily imported into statistical software for further analysis. If this is an application that will be important, a conversation with the software vendor's technical support staff should reveal the details of export file management. If this is necessary only rarely and for few clients, the data can be transcribed from the output and entered into a spreadsheet or statistical program.

I. Technical support

A software contract should entitle the purchaser to technical support services. Inquire about how much service is available and what kind. Round-the-clock service is probably not available and where technical support staff is located relative to your time zone may be important. Working around a several-hour time difference could be limiting if the technical support office has restricted hours. Try to check out the quality of the technical support. How long does it take for them to answer the phone? How many layers of menus must be traversed before talking to someone? Calling the technical support and asking questions that might arise in the process of choosing software will give a good sense of how competent and customer friendly technical support is.

J. Licensing Considerations

Decide whether you need a single-user license (less expensive) or a multiple-user or network license. If only one person will be using the software, a single-user license would be adequate. If, however, you work on different computers in different locations, the license issue becomes problematic and this must be negotiated with the vendor. In purchasing software for group use, it is important to inquire about restrictions on how many people may have simultaneous access. You should also ask what a license buys in the way of technical support and updates and ask whether annual renewal fees must be paid. If annual fees are required, regular database updates should be included.

V. Summary

Food and nutrient intake assessment is a difficult and time-consuming process for both the clients and the professionals who work with them. The most accurate technique is usually a food record kept by clients as they consume foods, measuring portions as accurately as possible. Estimation of overall nutritional status requires collecting multiple days of records. For athletes, dietary habits may vary substantially with their training and competition seasons. To assess overall nutritional status, it may be necessary to obtain multiple days of records at several periods throughout the year. To support peak performance, records should be obtained during appropriate training and competition periods. Athletes often take a variety of supplements and other products that they might not think to report on a diet record, so the interviewer should become familiar with the wide range of products and probe for them during interviews. Translating food records to nutrient intakes is much easier now than it used to be, with the advent of user-friendly interactive dietary assessment software. Nevertheless, coding remains a skilled activity and the most sophisticated software will not compensate for sloppy coding. The nutrient intake estimates obtained from a software are only as good as the dietary data supplied by the client and only as good as the coding techniques used to input the dietary data into the software. There are no shortcuts for accurate food and nutrient intake assessment and there are no substitutes for knowledgeable and sympathetic professionals to gather and analyze the data.

References

1. Bingham, S.A. et al., Methods for data collection at an individual level, in *Manual on Methodology for Food Consumption Studies*, Cameron, M.E. and van Staveren, W.J., Eds., Oxford University Press, New York, 1988, pp. 53-106.
2. Gibson, R.S., *Principles of Nutritional Assessment*, Oxford University Press, New York, 1990.
3. Thompson, F.E. and Byers, T., Dietary assessment resource manual. *J. Nutr.*, 124(suppl.), 2245S, 1994.
4. Sugerman, S.B., Eissenstat, B. and Srinith, U., Dietary assessment for cardiovascular disease risk determination and treatment, in *Cardiovascular Nutrition. Strategies and Tools for Disease Management and Prevention* , Kris-Etherton, P. and Burns, J.H., Eds., The American Dietetic Association, Chicago, 1998, pp. 39-71.
5. Peterson, L.A. and Carlgren, G., Measuring children's diets: evaluation of dietary assessment techniques in infancy and childhood, *Int. J. Epidemiol.*, 13, 506, 1984.
6. Baranowski, T. et al., The accuracy of children's self-reports of diet: Family Health Project, *J. Am. Diet. Assoc.*, 86, 1381, 1986.

7. Baranowski, T. and Simons-Morton, B.G., Dietary and physical activity assessment in school-aged children: measurement issues, *J. Sch. Health*, 61, 195, 1991.
8. Burke, B.S., The dietary history as a tool in research, *J. Am. Diet. Assoc.*, 23, 1041, 1947.
9. Todd, K.S., Hudes, M. and Calloway, D.H., Food intake measurement: problems and approaches, *Am. J. Clin. Nutr.*, 37, 139, 1983.
10. Van Horn, L. et al., Dietary assessment in children using electronic methods: telephones and tape recorders, *J. Am. Diet. Assoc.*, 90, 412, 1990.
11. Lindquist, C.H., Cummings, T. and Goran, M.I., Use of tape-recorded food records in assessing children's dietary intake. *Obesity Res.*, 8, 2, 2000.
12. McDowell, M.A. et al., The dietary collection system — an automated interview and coding system for NHANES III, in *Proc. 14th Nat. Nutrient Databank Conference in Iowa City, Iowa, June 19-21, 1989*, Stumbo, P.J., Ed., The CBORD Group, Inc., Ithaca, NY, 1989.
13. Chambers, E., Godwin, S.L. and Vecchio, F.A., Cognitive strategies for reporting portion sizes using dietary procedures, *J. Am. Diet. Assoc.*, 100, 891, 2000.
14. Basiotis, P.B. et al., Number of days of food intake records required to estimate individual and group nutrient intakes with defined confidence. *J. Nutr.*, 117, 1638, 1987.
15. Gershovitz, M., Madden, J.P. and Smiciklas-Wright, H., Validity of the 24-hour dietary recall and seven-day record for group comparisons, *J. Am. Diet. Assoc.*, 73, 48, 1978.
16. Black, A.E. et al., Critical evaluation of energy intake data using fundamental principles of energy physiology: 2. Evaluating the results of published surveys, *Eur. J. Clin. Nutr.*, 45, 583, 1991.
17. Schoeller, D.A., Limitations in the assessment of dietary energy intake by self-report, *Metabol. Clin. Exper.*, 44(suppl. 2), 18, 1995.
18. Champagne, C.M. et al., Assessment of energy intake underreporting by doubly labeled water and observations on reported nutrient intakes in children, *J. Am. Diet. Assoc.*, 98, 426, 1998.
19. Heitmann, B.L. and Lissner, L., Dietary underreporting by obese individuals — is it specific or nonspecific? *Brit. Med. J.*, 14, 986, 1995.
20. Poppitt, S.D. et al., Assessment of selective underreporting of food intake by both obese and non-obese women in a metabolic facility, *Int. J. Obes. Relat. Metab. Disord.*, 22, 303, 1998.
21. Black, A.E. et al., Measurements of total energy expenditure provide insights into the validity of dietary measurements of energy intake, *J. Am. Diet. Assoc.*, 93, 572, 1983.
22. Hebert, J.R. et al., Social desirability bias in dietary self-report may compromise validity of dietary intake measures, *Int. J. Epidemiol.*, 24, 389, 1995.
23. Klesges, R.C., Eck, L. H. and Ray, J.W., Who underreports dietary intake in a dietary recall? Evidence from the Second National Health and Nutrition Examination Survey, *J. Consult. Clin. Psychol.*, 63, 438, 1995.
24. Briefel, R.R. et al., Dietary methods research in the third National Health and Nutrition Examination Survey: underreporting of energy intake, *Am. J. Clin. Nutr.* 65(suppl. 4), 1203S, 1997.
25. Bandini, L.G. et al., Validity of reported energy intake in preadolescent girls, *Am. J. Clin. Nutr.* 65(suppl. 4), 1138S, 1997.
26. Worsley, A., Baghurst, K.I. and Leitch, D.R., Social desirability response bias and dietary inventory response. *Hum. Nutr. Appl. Nutr.*, 38, 29, 1984.

27. Kristal, A.R. et al., Dietary assessment instruments are susceptible to intervention-associated response set bias, *J. Am. Diet. Assoc.*, 98, 40, 1998.

28. Westerterp, K.R. et al., Use of the doubly labeled water technique in humans during heavy sustained exercise, *J. Appl. Physiol.*, 61, 2162, 1986.

29. Schulz, L.O. et al., Energy expenditure of elite female runners measured by respiratory chamber and doubly labeled water, *J. Appl. Physiol.*, 72, 23, 1992.

30. Edwards, J.E. et al., Energy balance in highly trained female endurance runners, *Med. Sci. Sports. Exer.*, 25, 1398, 1993.

31. Beidelman, B.A., Puhl, J.L. and De Souza, M.J., Energy balance in female distance runners. *Am. J. Clin. Nutr.* 61, 303, 1995.

32. Caan, B.J. et al., Does nutritionist review of a self-administered food frequency questionnaire improve data quality?, *Publ. Health Nutr.*, 2, 565, 1999.

33. Willett, W.C. et al., Validation of a semi-quantitative food frequency questionnaire: comparison with a 1-year diet record, *J. Am. Diet. Assoc.*, 87, 43, 1987.

34. Block, G. et al., Comparisons of two dietary questionnaires validated against multiple dietary records collected during a 1-year period, *J. Am. Diet. Assoc.*, 92, 686, 1992.

35. Joachim, G., Sources of variability in the reproducibility of food frequency questionnaires, *Nutr. Health*, 12, 181, 1998.

36. Willett, W., N*utritional Epidemiology*, Oxford University Press, New York, 1990.

37. Block, G. et al., A data-based approach to diet questionnaire design and testing, *Am. J. Epidemiol.*, 14, 453, 1986.

38. Serdula, M. et al., Evaluation of a brief telephone questionnaire to estimate fruit and vegetable consumption in diverse study populations, *Epidemiology*, 4, 455, 1993.

39. Coates, R.J. and Monteilh, C.P., Assessments of food-frequency questionnaires in minority populations, *Am. J. Clin. Nutr.*, 65(suppl. 4), 1108S, 1997.

40. Tucker, K.L. et al., Adaptation of a food frequency questionnaire to assess diets of Puerto Rican and non-Hispanic adults, *Am. J. Epidemiol.*, 148, 507, 1998.

41. van Erp-Baart, A.M.J. et al., Nationwide survey on nutritional habits in elite athletes. Part 1. Energy, carbohydrate, protein and fat intake, *Int. J. Sports. Med.*, 10(suppl. 1), S3, 1989.

42. Brouns, F.J.P.H., Saris, W.H.M. and Hoor, F.T., Dietary problems in the case of strenuous exertion, *J. Sports Med.*, 26, 306, 1986.

43. Burke, L.M., Dietary intakes of marathon runners, *Excel*, 4,14, 1987.

44. Burke, L.M. and Read, R.S.D., Diet patterns of elite Australian male triathletes, *Physiol. Sports Med.*, 15, 140, 1987.

45. Burke, L.M. and Read, R.S.D., A study of dietary patterns of elite Australian Rules football players, *Can. J. Sports Sci.*, 13, 15, 1988.

46. Burke, L.M. and Read, R.S.D., Sports nutrition: approaching the nineties, *Sports Med.*, 8, 80, 1989.

47. Joint Position Statement, Nutrition and athletic performance: American College of Sports Medicine, American Dietetic Association and Dietitians of Canada, *Med. Sci. Sports Exer.*, 32, 2130, 2000.

48. Burke, L.M., Gollan, R.A. and Read, R.S.D., Dietary intakes and food use of groups of elite Australian male athletes, *J. Sport Nutr.*, 1, 378, 1991.

49. www.ag.arizona.edu/nsc/new/hept/index.htm

50. Convertino, V.A. et al., American College of Sports Medicine position stand. Exercise and fluid replacement, *Med. Sci. Sports Exer.*, 28, i, 1996.

51. Hawley, J.A. and Burke, L.M., Effect of meal frequency and timing on physical performance, *Brit. J. Nutr.*, 77(suppl.), S91, 1997.
52. Butterfield, G., Ergogenic aids: Evaluating sport nutrition products, *Int. J. Sport Nutr.*, 6, 91, 1996.
53. Johnson, W.A. and Landry, G.L., Nutritional supplements: fact vs. fiction, *Adolesc. Med.*, 9, 501, 1998.
54. Harper, A.E., Benevenga, N.J. and Wohlheuter, R.M., Effects of ingestion of disproportionate amounts of amino acids, *Physiol. Rev.*, 50, 428, 1970.
55. Schaumberg, H. et al., Sensory neuropathy from pyroxidine abuse, *N. Eng. J. Med.*, 309, 445, 1983.
56. Benevenga, N.J. and Steele, R.D., Adverse effects of excessive consumption of amino acids, *Ann. Rev. Nutr.*, 4, 157, 1984.
57. Short, S.H. and Marquart, L.F., Sports nutrition fraud, *NY State J. Med.*, 93, 112, 1993.
58. Rosen, L.W. and Hough, D.O., Pathogenic weight-control behaviors of female college gymnasts, *Phys. Sports Med.*, 16, 140, 1988.
59. DePalma, M.T. et al., Weight control practices of lightweight football players, *Med. Sci. Sports Exerc.*, 25, 694, 1993.
60. Sundgot-Borgen, J., Eating disorders, energy intake, training volume and menstrual function in high-level modern rhythmic gymnasts, *Int. J. Sport Nutr.*, 6, 100, 1996.
61. Sanborn, C.F. et al., Disordered eating and the female athlete triad, *Clin. Sports Med.*, 19, 199, 2000.
62. Brownell, K.D. and Rodin, J., Prevalence of eating disorders in athletes, in *Eating, Body Weight and Performance in Athletes*, Brownell, K.D., Rodin, J. and Wilmore, J.H., Eds., Lea & Febiger, Philadelphia, 1992, pp. 128-145.
63. Sykora, C. et al., Eating, weight and dieting disturbances in male and female lightweight and heavyweight rowers, *Int. J. Eat. Disord.*, 14, 203, 1993.
64. Thiel, A., Gottfried, H. and Hesse, F.W., Subclinical eating disorders in male athletes. A study of the light weight category in rowers and wrestlers, *Acta Psychiatr. Scand.*, 88, 259, 1993.
65. Beals, K.A. and Manore, M.M., The prevalence and consequences of subclinical eating disorders in female athletes, *Int. J. Sport Nutr.*, 4, 175, 1994.
66. Fogelholm, M. and Hilloskorpi, H., Weight and diet concerns in Finnish female and male athletes, *Med. Sci. Sports Exer.*, 31, 229, 1999.
67. Moffatt, R.J., Dietary status of elite female high school gymnasts: inadequacy of vitamin and mineral intake, *J. Am. Diet. Assoc.*, 84, 1361, 1984.
68. Nowak, R.K., Knudsen, K.S. and Schulz, L.O., Body composition and nutrient intakes of college men and women basketball players, *J. Am. Diet. Assoc.*, 88, 575, 1988.
69. Schoeller, D.A. and van Santen, E., Measurement of energy expenditure in humans by doubly labeled water method, *J. Appl. Physiol.*, 53, 955, 1982.
70. www.nal.usda.gov/fnic/foodcomp/Bulletins/timeline.htm
71. Buzzard, I.M., Price, K.S. and Warren, R.A., Considerations for selecting nutrient-calculation software: evalaution of the nutrient database, *Am. J. Clin. Nutr.*, 54, 7, 1991.
72. Grossbauer, S., The number game, *Byting In*, 7, 3, 1997.
73. Sugerman, S., What makes a software package worth buying?, *Byting In*, 7, 1, 1996.

74. www.nal.usda.gov.fnic/foodcomp/data

75. Perloff, B.P. et al., Dietary intake methodology. II. USDA's Nutrient Data Base for nationwide dietary intake surveys, *J. Nutr.*, 120(suppl. 1), 1530, 1990.

76. Perloff, B. and Ahuja, J.K., Development and maintenance of nutrient data bases for national dietary surveys, *Pub. Health Rev.*, 26, 43, 1998.

77. Federal Register, Food labeling: mandatory status of nutrition label and nutrient content revision, format for nutrition label, part IV, January 6, 1993, vol. 58, no. 3, 1993.

78. Schakel, S.F., Buzzard, I.M. and Gebhardt, S.E., Procedures for estimating nutrient values for food composition databases, *J. Food Compos. Anal.*, 10, 102, 1997.

79. Pehrsson, P.R. et al., USDA's National Food and Nutrient Analysis Program: Food sampling, *J. Food Compos. Anal.* 13, 379, 2000.

80. Federal Register, Food labeling: requirements for nutrient content claims, health claims and statements of nutritional support for dietary supplements, September 23, 1997, vol. 62, no. 184, 1997.

81. Haytowitz, D.B., Pehrsson, P.R. and Holden, J.M., Adapting methods for determining priorities for the analysis of foods in diverse populations, *J. Food Compos. Anal.* 13, 425, 2000.

82. U.S. Department of Agriculture, *Dietary Guidelines for Americans*, U.S. Government Printing Office, Washington, DC, 1995.

83. Institute of Medicine, *Dietary Reference Intakes. Applications in Dietary Assessment*, Washington DC: National Academy Press, Washington, DC, 2000.

84. Franz, M.J., *Exchanges For All Occasions: Your Guide to Choosing Healthy Foods Anytime Anywhere*, 4th ed., IDC, Minneapolis, 1997.

85. Burke, L.M., Collier, G.R. and Hargreaves, M., Glycemic index — a new tool in sports nutrition? *Int. J. Sport Nutr.*, 8, 401, 1998.

86. Foster-Powell, K. and Miller, J.B., International tables of glycemic index. *Am. J. Clin. Nutr.*, 62(suppl.), 871S, 1995.

3

Evaluation of Nutrient Adequacy of Athletes' Diets Using Nutrient Intake Data

Satya S. Jonnalagadda

CONTENTS

I. Introduction

Given the increasing competitiveness of athletics, more and more athletes are eager to learn about and adapt methods for improving their performance. Recognizing the key role played by nutrition in physical performance, athletes are becoming more interested in learning about ways to improve their dietary intakes. Adequate and proper nutrition of athletes is important to meet their energy, essential nutrients and fluid needs. Thus, an assessment of dietary intakes and practices is an important first step when working with athletes with the aim of improving their dietary intakes and performance. It is also advisable to assess athletes' diets regularly to identify potential

0-8493-0927-1/02/$0.00+$1.50

problem areas and prevent seasonal deficiencies, such as those observed with iron.[1] In this chapter, the methods used to assess adequacy of the dietary intakes of athletes using nutrient intake data will be reviewed.

II. Dietary Assessment

Dietary assessment methods such as diet histories, food records, diet recalls and food frequency questionnaires, can be used to estimate dietary intake patterns and nutrient intakes of various groups of athletes and to determine relationships between diet and performance. However, these methods are not error proof and studies have shown that accuracy of reported dietary intake data is influenced by several factors such as age, gender, body weight, body composition, restrained eating habits, social class, consumption of certain food groups, etc.[2,3] This reporting bias can lead to misinterpretations of the nutrient adequacy of an individual's diet and nutritional status. Furthermore, differences in body size, levels of activity, competition and training programs can influence dietary macro- and micronutrient intakes and the variations in energy, macro- and micronutrient intakes observed between various groups of athletes and studies in the literature.[4] Self-reported energy intakes typically are underestimated, especially by adolescents and obese individuals, which can result in misinterpretation of individuals' nutritional status.[2,3] Jonnalagadda et al.[3] observed 61% of elite female gymnasts to underreport energy intakes and to have lower intakes of vitamin A, thiamin, riboflavin, iron and calcium, than those gymnasts who were classified as adequate energy reporters. Additionally, length of the dietary evaluation period also needs to be given attention due to day-to-day variations in intake. For example, Rico-Sanz et al.[5] observed a 26% between-day variation in energy intake of elite soccer players. It is thus best to evaluate macro- and micronutrient contributions of the diets of athletes over several days rather than looking at a single day's intake. Thus, it is not only important to use the appropriate dietary assessment methods, but to use methods to improve the accuracy of the dietary assessment, given its influence on the reported nutrient intake data. It is also important to use the same assessment method when attempting to determine nutrient adequacy of athletes' dietary intakes by comparing them to the dietary and nutrient intakes of individual athletes or groups.

III. Dietary Guidelines

The Dietary Guidelines for Americans[6] can serve as a baseline for an assessment of an individual's intake. With the passage of the 1990 Nutrition Monitoring Act, these dietary guidelines are being reviewed every 5 years and the recommendations are directed toward a prescription of health and fitness and prevention of particular disease states. These nonquantitative guidelines provide advice for the general healthy public with respect to diet — mainly macronutrients — and fitness. The latest guidelines[6] are as follows:

1. **Aim for fitness.**

   Aim for a healthy weight.

   Be physically active each day.

2. **Build a healthy base.**

   Let the pyramid guide food choices.

   Choose a variety of grains daily, especially whole grains.

   Choose a variety of fruits and vegetables daily.

   Keep food safe to eat.

3. **Choose sensibly.**

   Choose a diet that is low in saturated fat and cholesterol and moderate in total fat.

   Choose beverages and foods to moderate intake of sugars.

   Choose and prepare foods with less salt.

   If alcoholic beverages are drunk, they should be in moderation.

Additionally, the food guide pyramid[6] developed by the United States Department of Agriculture (USDA) and Department of Health and Human Services (DHHS) can serve as a guide for evaluating an individual's dietary intake. The food guide pyramid offers a pattern for daily food choices based on foods that are classified into five major food groups. The pyramid provides a range for the number of servings to be consumed daily from each group, with the lower end of the range for individuals on an approximately 1600 kcal/day diet and the upper end for individuals on an approximately 2800 kcal/day diet. At the very tip of the pyramid are fats, oils and sweets, with a suggestion to use these sparingly. A diet that includes a wide variety of foods from within each food group can ensure an adequate intake of nutrients. The food guide pyramid recommendations are as follows:

1. Bread, cereal, rice and pasta group: 6-11 servings
2. Vegetable group: 3-5 servings
3. Fruit group: 2-4 servings
4. Meat, poultry, fish, dry beans, eggs and nuts group: 2-3 servings
5. Milk, yogurt and cheese group: 2-3 servings
6. Fats, oils and sweets: use sparingly

Furthermore, based on research on the role of diet in health and disease conditions, the federal government and other national organizations have made more specific quantitative recommendations regarding the intake of macro- and micronutrients. Overall, these recommendations for the general public suggest that individuals obtain 60–65% of energy from carbohydrates, 10–15% from protein and the rest (< 30%) from fat. More specific recommendations have been developed for individuals participating in various sports based on the energy needs of the individual sports, the performance targets and dietary composition guidelines that the athlete is attempting to achieve.

An individual athlete's energy and nutrient needs will vary depending on age, gender, height, weight, type, frequency, intensity and duration of training and competition. Depending on their activity levels and sport, athletes will need to consume between 60% and 70% kcal from carbohydrate, 10–15% kcal from protein and 20–30% kcal from fat. For instance, for competitive weight lifters, muscle size and strength are important, while, for long-distance runners, the same may be a deterrent to performance. Therefore, the dietary intakes of these two groups of athletes will vary in their distribution of protein, fat and carbohydrate in the diet. Thus an assessment of the athlete's diet should take into consideration the requirements of the sport and performance goals of the athletes. Typically, diets providing a variety of foods can meet the macro- and micronutrient needs of these active individuals. Thus, athletes' nutrient intake and food consumption patterns can be compared with national recommendations and can be classified into various groups. For example, individuals with total fat intakes greater than 37% energy can be classified as high-fat eaters; these individuals are likely to have intake patterns different from the low-fat eaters. For example, Koenig and Elmadfa[7] observed low-fat eaters to have higher intakes than high-fat eaters of total carbohydrates, sucrose, dietary fiber, potassium, magnesium and folic acid and lower intakes of cholesterol, vitamin D, riboflavin and vitamin B_6. Likewise, food based evaluation showed low-fat eaters to consume less butter, margarine, fish, all types of meat and pulses, but more cereals, dark bread, milk and milk products, fruits and fruit juices, which, in turn, can impact their macro- and micronutrient intakes and the nutrient adequacy of their diets.

The passing of the National Nutrition Monitoring and Related Research Act has resulted in the development of comprehensive assessment of the nutritional status of the U.S. population and the nutritional quality of the U.S. food supply by the agencies of the federal government.[8] Three of the well-known surveys that fulfill the mandates of this bill are the National Health and Nutrition Examination Survey (NHANES), Nationwide Food Consumption Survey (NFCS) and Continuing Survey of Food Intake by Individuals (CSFII). The dietary components of these surveys include collection of food intake data over a period of time and analyses of their nutrient equivalents. The resulting data provide an idea of the food consumption and nutrient intake patterns of a healthy U.S. population by age, gender and race categories. This data can be used as the basis to assess whether the diets of the athletes under study are similar to that of the national intakes and to assess adequacy of nutrient intake. For instance, Ziegler et al.[9,10] observed elite figure skaters to have macro- and micronutrient intakes below that observed for adolescents in the NHANES III and 1994 CSFII surveys. Furthermore, these athletes were also observed to have intakes of certain nutrients below that of the dietary recommendations, suggesting that the nutritional status of these figure skaters needs to be further evaluated.[9,10]

The nutrient intake of athletes can be compared with national recommendations for healthy individuals, such as the recommended dietary allowances (RDAs), recommendations by professional organizations such as the American Dietetic Association or sport-specific recommendations if available.[11-17] Additionally, when assessing adequacy of nutrient intakes of athletes, comparisons can be made with intakes of other athletes in similar types of sports. Furthermore, impact of dietary intake on performance can also be used as a measure of adequacy, although some caution should be used when using performance as a measure of adequacy because athletes have been shown to adapt to low intakes without compromising performance.[18,19] In addition to all of the above mentioned comparisons, the absolute amount of intake should also be examined in relation to body weight before judgments of diet quality and nutritional status are made. Rico-Sanz et al.[5] observed that carbohydrate intake of elite soccer players (53.2% kcal) was higher than that of Swedish (47% kcal), Danish (46.3% kcal), Canadian (48% kcal) and American college players (48% kcal) but lower than that of Italian first division players (56% kcal) and the general recommendations for soccer players (55–65% kcal). However, when the intake of these players was examined on a g/kg body weight basis, the intake of these elite athletes (8.3 g/kg body weight) was within the values reported to maximize glycogen stores in muscle.

Comparisons of nutrient intakes with existing data in the literature of similar groups or the general population can also be made to assess where athletes stand with respect to their counterparts. However, caution should be exercised in the interpretation of such comparisons due to factors such as differences in training programs and intensities, activity levels, lifestyles, body weight and energy demands. Additionally, the growth stage and competition level of the athletes in the various studies should be taken into consideration when evaluating their dietary intakes. For instance, professional male cyclists have higher energy intakes than paddlers mainly because of the higher energy demands of the cycling events.[20] Garcia-Roves et al.[20] observed that diets of elite Spanish flatwater paddlers did not meet the recommended macronutrient intake for athletes training and competing (60–70% carbohydrate, 1.2–1.7 g protein/kg body weight, fat < 30% energy); however, these athletes had a protein intake similar to the average Spanish population but higher carbohydrate and lower fat intake, while maintaining the high consumption of olive oil typical of this Mediterranean population. These athletes, despite having low carbohydrate and high fat diets when compared with the dietary recommendations for athletes, had micronutrient intakes that exceeded the dietary recommendations. However, it is important to recognize that these recommendations are for the general population and do not make allowances for physical activity.

IV.   Dietary Standards

Over the past several decades in the U.S., the Recommended Dietary Allowance (RDA), which represents a level of intake sufficient to meet the needs of essentially all healthy people, was the most common measure used to determine adequacy of healthy individuals' nutrient intake.[11] Although the requirements of specific nutrients can vary widely, even among similar groups of individuals, based on the available scientific literature an estimate of the mean physiological requirements for a nutrient is made considering age, gender and condition. For instance, for adults, the amount of a nutrient consumed can depend on its ability to maintain nutrients stores in the body, maintain body functions and prevent development of deficiencies. It should be recognized that these nutrient recommendations are higher than the mean requirement of an individual because they take into account variations in individual nutrient requirements within a group and are therefore set higher than the mean requirements. More recently, the dietary reference intakes (DRIs), which include the estimated average requirements (EAR), RDA, adequate intake (AI) and tolerable upper intake level (UL) were developed by the National Academy of Science to provide a more complete set of reference values.[21]

The EAR is the intake that meets the estimated nutrient needs of 50% of the individuals within a particular age and gender group. If an individual's intake is two standard deviations below the EAR, it is quite positive that nutrient needs are not being met.

The RDA is the intake that meets the nutrient need of almost all (97–98%) of the individuals in a particular age and gender group. The RDAs are set two standard deviations above the mean requirements for a particular age and gender group to account for incomplete utilization by the body and for variations in the levels of the nutrient provided by various food sources. The RDAs are target or recommended intakes and are expressed as a single absolute value and not in relation to height or weight. Although an intake less than the RDA is not necessarily inadequate because it is set well above the mean physiological requirements, the more the intake falls below this standard, the greater the potential for inadequate intake. Although individuals' nutrient requirement cannot be known with certainty, if on the average, their intake meets or exceeds the RDA, it is safe to assume that the dietary intake is adequate based on current scientific knowledge.[8,11,21] When intake is less than the RDA, the risk of inadequate intake is present and this risk increases as the intake continues to fall. Although reported dietary intake by itself cannot be a sole measure of an individual's nutritional status, reported usual intakes well below the RDA may be indicative of the need for further assessment of nutritional status by biochemical or other clinical exams.[11,21] Nutrition assessment and intervention may become necessary when usual dietary intake is less than two thirds of the RDA for a nutrient in the diet of athletes.[23]

On the other hand, AIs are the average observed or experimentally derived intake by a defined population or subgroup that appear to sustain a defined nutritional state, such as normal circulating nutrient values, growth or other functional indicators of health. Thus, the AI is higher than the EAR and, given that it is based on group information, it cannot be used to assess adequacy of nutrient intake of individuals. However, in general, individuals with intakes at or above AI can be assumed to have a low risk of inadequate intake.[23]

The UL is the maximum daily level of intake of a nutrient that is unlikely to pose risks of adverse effects to almost all (97–98%) individuals. Although this maximum UL will vary from individual to individual and cannot be known with certainty, intakes below UL provide assurance that the intake will not cause adverse effects given current scientific knowledge. Thus, given the specific purpose of each of these measures, the purpose of the nutrient intake examination should be considered carefully when selecting a measure for comparison.[23]

V.   Dietary Indices

A healthy diet can be achieved by combining foods from the major food groups in an individual's daily dietary intake.[24] Food group intake patterns can provide an understanding of adequacy of dietary intakes because individuals typically do not consume a single food but rather a combination of foods that provide a combination of nutrients. An examination of these intake patterns can also be useful in determining nutrient adequacy.[25] Based on reported intakes of various individual foods and the adherence to national guidelines and recommendations Beaudry et al.[26] classified individual food intake patterns into high-energy density, traditional and health-conscious patterns. Individuals who were classified as health-conscious typically followed the dietary guidelines for macronutrients and this pattern was positively correlated with each of the indicators used to determine nutrient adequacy. Typically, women were observed to be most likely to follow the health-conscious dietary intake pattern, while men followed the high-energy density and traditional intake patterns. The high-energy density pattern was the least likely to be nutritionally adequate and correlated negatively with the recommended macronutrient intake recommendations while the traditional pattern was observed to be strongly correlated with the micronutrient recommendations but not the macronutrient recommendations. Such an examination to determine nutrient adequacy can serve as a powerful tool in developing nutrition education and nutrition intervention programs to meet the specific needs of the target population and in assessing health risks. Dietary energy, fat and selected micronutrient intakes can thus be used as indices of overall nutrient adequacy of the diet given the correlation between certain nutrients and health and performance status of athletes. For example, energy intake is highly correlated with intake of carbohydrate, fat and protein and to intakes of several micronutrients. Although high-energy diets may be high in quality based on protein and micronutrients, these diets are also likely to be high in fat, so their quality may not be high with respect to the athlete's performance ability and long-term health.[27] In addition to dietary and nutrient intake patterns, the overall diet quality and nutrient adequacy can be determined by using different indices such as:[28]

1. **Nutrient adequacy ratio (NAR)** is the ratio of intake of a nutrient relative to its RDA. Mean adequacy ratio is the average sum of the NARs and allows an evaluation of overall adequacy of selected nutrients in the diets of a given population group.

2. **Food quality index (FQI), nutrient quality index (NQI) and nutrient density (ND)** are based on the ability of a food item or a diet, respectively, to meet the RDAs relative to energy requirements. Nutrient density assesses the quantity of nutrients in an individual's diet per 1000 kcal, implying that, if the amount of nutrients per 1000 kcal is high enough, the nutrient needs of individuals are met when their energy needs are met. These measures allow for an assessment and comparison of nutritional quality of individual foods and diets independent of serving size. Thus, the foods selected should be both high in nutrients and low in energy to provide an adequate nutrient intake for individuals on a low-calorie diet. Ziegler et al.[9] observed that diets of elite male figure skaters were less nutrient dense, especially for micronutrients such as vitamin A, folate, magnesium, iodine and sodium despite these skaters' consuming more than 100% of RDA for all of these nutrients, suggesting that the diets of these athletes may be more energy dense than nutrient dense. Therefore, this measure can be used as a tool for assessing quality of intake and identifying appropriate foods that are nutrient dense.

3. **Index of nutritional quality (INQ)** allows for the comparison of the nutrient density of foods or diets to a nutrient standard. Based on the RDAs, the INQ first calculates single-value nutrient recommendations for individual nutrients. Then the amount of nutrient per 1000 kcal in food is compared with the recommendations per 1000 kcal of food. Foods with an INQ of greater than 1 are considered to be of good quality and could potentially be providing nutrients in excess of calories. On the other hand, foods with an INQ of less than 1 suggest that the individuals consuming these foods will have to consume excess calories to meet their nutrient needs.

4. **Sum of selected nutrients** consumed: at least at two thirds of the RDA can be used to calculate nutrient score of an individual's dietary intake. Klicka et al.[9] examined the nutritional adequacy of cadets intakes and meals offered at the U.S. Military Academy

(USMA) by comparing with military RDA (MRDA). Diets of cadets were classified as adequate if nutrient intake equaled or exceeded the standards, marginal if consumption was between 70% and 99% of standard and low if consumption was less than 70% of the standard. Folate intake was deficient (< 70% of MRDA) in all males, while the female cadets had inadequate intakes of vitamin B_6, folate, vitamin A, magnesium, iron and zinc. Males and individuals with a greater number of weekday meals consumed at the mess had more nutrient-dense diets. Moreover, female cadets who consumed fewer weekday evening meals at the USMA mess had only 88% of MRDA for protein, 96% of MRDA for magnesium and 80% of MRDA for zinc intakes. Furthermore, nutrient supplement users had higher nutrient-density diets than non-nutrient supplement users. Snacks, which provided 24–32% of energy in the female cadet's diet, were often substituted for meals, thus contributing to the inadequate intakes observed in the diets of these cadets. This study also shows that a combination of techniques can be used to determine nutrient adequacy of diets.

5. **Intake patterns of food or food groups** can also be used to determine nutrient adequacy. This is done by considering recommended number of servings of the major food groups and variety of intake within each group.[6,24] Based on the reported frequency of consumption of food groups, a diet score can be calculated to determine dietary diversity, diet quality and association with disease outcome.[25] For example, individuals reporting consumption of two or fewer food groups compared with those consuming all five (dairy, meat, grain, fruit and vegetables) were observed to have 40–50% higher risk of mortality.[28] The Healthy Eating Index (HEI)[30] developed by the USDA provides an overall measure of individuals' diet quality by evaluating intake of 10 dietary components that are thought to represent a healthy diet. The scoring system is based on the number of servings of the five food groups consumed, and the level of intake of total fat, saturated fat, cholesterol, sodium and dietary variety. An HEI score of greater than 80 implies a good diet, while a score of 51–80 implies a diet that "needs improvement," and a score of less than 51 indicates a "poor diet." The HEI has been shown to be positively associated with nutrient intake and disease risk.[28]

6. **Frequency of consumption and intake data** can also be used to identify eating patterns associated with various risk factors and risk behaviors .[31,32] Beals and Manore[32] observed female athletes with subclinical eating disorders to have intakes for energy, protein and carbohydrate below the recommended levels, along with a heavy dependence on vitamin and mineral supplements. Likewise, Janelle and Barr[33] observed differences in nutrient intake and ade-

quacy based on dietary patterns. Although relatively few differences in nutrient intake were observed between nonvegetarians and lactovegetarians, many differences were observed between vegetarians and both nonvegetarians and lactovegetarians. No differences were observed in energy intakes between nonvegetarian and vegetarian women, however, the former group consumed higher amounts of protein than the later (15% kcal vs. 11% kcal). Nonvegetarians had lower percent energy from carbohydrate and lower dietary fiber intakes than the vegetarians (54% vs. 58% and 22g vs. 28 g/d). Nonvegetarian females had nutrient intakes greater than the RDAs except for zinc (92% of RDA) whereas vegetarian females had intakes lower than RDA for vitamin B_6 (98% of RDA), calcium (96% of RDA), niacin (89% of RDA), zinc (70% of RDA) and vitamin B_{12} (70% of RDA). Vegetarian females had significantly lower mean intakes of riboflavin, niacin, vitamin B_{12}, zinc and sodium and higher intakes of vitamin C, folacin and copper than nonvegetarians. Restrained eating scores were also observed to be negatively associated with energy intake/kg body weight especially among vegetarians. This study also suggests that no assumptions should be made about nutrient intakes based on dietary practices and nature of dietary patterns can vary significantly under such broad classifications as "vegetarian," which, in turn, can influence nutrient intake.[33]

VI.   Dietary Recommendations: Basis for Judgment

A. Energy Intake

Energy intake should support athletes' training and competitive schedule to enable them to achieve their performance goals. Although estimating energy needs is difficult due to significant day-to-day, season-to-season variations in activity levels, intensity of training, etc., an analysis of one or more 3-day food records and stable body weight, which represents a balance between intake and output, can be used as tools to determine energy needs of the athletes and the adequacy of their intake.[11] Athletes unable to maintain body weight are likely not consuming sufficient energy to meet the demands of their activity levels and may be compromising their performance. To increase energy intake, athletes can either increase the portion sizes of the foods consumed or increase the number of daily meals and snacks consumed.

Comparing reported nutrient intake as percent of RDA, Witta and Stombaugh[19] observed adolescent female runners over a 3-year period to have decreased energy intakes from 2150 to 1647 kcal, both of which are lower than the RDA of 2200 kcals for healthy sedentary females. On the other hand, during the same time period, dietary energy from carbohydrate increased from 53% to 61%, but the mean carbohydrate intake actually decreased from 1134 to 1011 kcal (from 284 g to 253 g/d) due to a decrease in energy intake. Thus, on a kg/body weight basis, carbohydrate intake decreased from 5.5 to 4.7 g/kg/d. Likewise, protein intake decreased significantly from 1.6 to 1.1 g/kg body weight, which is lower than the recommendations of 1.2–1.7 g/kg body weight for endurance athletes. Furthermore, intake of micronutrients such as calcium, potassium and sodium also decreased (50–70% of RDA). An examination of food group intake revealed limited milk and cheese intake, which may have contributed to these lower intakes. These runners also decreased their fat intake from 31.7% to 26.4% energy, which could also help explain the decrease in protein and micronutrient intakes. Despite these changes in nutrient intakes, the performance times of the runners improved, suggesting that basal metabolism of these athletes is adapting to the lower energy intakes without compromising performance.[18,19] Furthermore, a greater percent of these runners (27%) were observed to have higher scores on the eating attitude test, which is used as a measure of disordered eating and 31% of the athletes reported experiencing stress fractures by the end of the 3-year period. Thus, a decrease in energy intake is associated not only with a decrease in macro- and micronutrient intakes, but also with the short- and long-term health status of these active individuals. Thus, improved athletic performance and decreased health risks could be used as nutrition education tools to further improve athletes' dietary intake and the nutrient adequacy of their diets.

Sugiura et al.[34] observed elite male and female Japanese track-and-field athletes to have mean energy intakes of 3141 kcal and 2508 kcal, respectively, with an ideal distribution of macronutrients. However, 54% of the males and 65% of the females consumed less than the Japanese RDA (JRDA) for at least one micronutrient but the intake of these Japanese athletes was observed to be similar to that of elite American and European athletes but lower than that of elite Chinese athletes. The inadequate intake of micronutrients by these athletes could be due to low intakes of dairy foods, eggs, meat, fish and fruits, consumption of small meals and personal preferences. In spite of these inadequate intakes, these athletes were able to perform well in their respective championships by winning 24 out of 43 medals in the Asian Championship Games, suggesting that the JRDA may not be appropriate standards for comparison of these athletes' intakes. On the other hand, Maughan[35] observed professional Scottish soccer players to have higher energy intake than the general U.K. population, but no differences were observed in average composition of the diet compared with national averages. Furthermore, these Scottish players had energy intakes lower than those in other published reports. Both studies demonstrate that, when comparing studies carried out in different countries, even though among similar groups of athletes, caution should be exercised in the interpretation of the data because of the differences in dietary habits, nutrition and practices of nutrition strategies to improve performance.

B. Carbohydrate Intake

Carbohydrates in athletes' diets provide energy for performance and exhibit a protein sparing effect.[14,36,37] Athletes undergoing prolonged (>60 min) intense training (65–70% VO$_2$max) require 8–10 g carbohydrate/kg body weight/d, while those training for less than 60 min/d require 5 g carbohydrate/kg body weight/d.[14,36,37] A minimum of 200 g carbohydrate/d is recommended to maintain liver glycogen stores to meet the energy needs of activity.[14,36,37] Sufficient muscle glycogen stores is important for optimum endurance performance and training adaptation because of its role as a major provider of energy. Thus, insufficient carbohydrate intake can result in chronic muscle fatigue during repeated days of intense training and during competition. Tanaka et al.[38] observed that male runners had energy intakes of 55–57 kcal/kg body weight/d similar to the RDA of 58 kcal/kg body weight/d for exceptionally active men, whereas the female runners had intakes of 36 kcal/kg body weight/d, which was similar to the RDA for females with light to moderate activity levels, despite these runners competing at similar levels. However, the male runners consumed less than the recommended carbohydrate intakes (56% vs. 60–70% kcal) on percent energy basis and the female runners consumed 65–67% kcal. Likewise, on a kg body weight basis, the female runners had an intake closer to recommendations (6 g/kg body weight/d vs. 8 g/kg body weight/d). This suggests that gender-appropriate comparisons should be made when comparing nutrient intakes and adequacy of intakes. Furthermore, simple carbohydrate intake was observed to be significantly different between training and competitive periods in both groups, suggesting that the time period (training, competition or off-season) when the dietary assessment is conducted should be kept in mind when assessing adequacy and comparisons should be made with appropriate time-specific recommendations and intakes adjusted appropriately.

C. Protein Intake

Heavy resistance exercise stimulates muscle growth, however, increasing dietary protein has not been shown to be necessary for maximum muscle development.[1,16] RDA for protein (0.8 g/kg body weight/d) has been determined using sedentary individuals.[11] An adequate energy intake can ensure the efficient use of dietary protein, but inadequate intake of energy will result in the use of protein to meet the energy needs of activity. Dietary protein intake in excess of the current RDA may be required for optimal muscle growth, especially for individuals involved in heavy resistance-training exercises, who have been observed to require 1.7–1.8 g protein/kg body weight/d.[1,16] However, benefits of high protein intake have been observed to plateau at intake levels well below those typically consumed by athletes.[1,16] Intakes greater than 2 g/kg body weight/d have not been shown to be beneficial to strength athletes and their performance benefits are unproven at the present time.[1,16] Such high intakes can also result in diuresis and dehydration. Furthermore, consumption of dietary protein in excess of the physiological needs can result in compromising the carbohydrate status of athletes and can adversely affect their performance during training and competition.

It should be recognized that inadequate energy intake is often the limiting factor for athletes attempting to increase muscle mass.[1] Although endurance athletes do not develop muscle mass to the same extent as strength athletes, studies have shown that dietary protein intake greater than the RDA may be required to meet the amino acid needs that arise due to the increased oxidation associated with the intensity and duration of endurance sports. Endurance trained individuals may need to consume 1.2–1.4 g protein/kg body weight/d to meet their needs.[16] The typical American diet provides this amount of protein as long as a mixed diet providing adequate energy is consumed. Individual athletes who restrict energy intake or high-quality protein intake, such as vegetarians, may be at risk of consuming insufficient protein.[33,39,40]

D. Fat Intake

Athletes typically believe that low fat intake results in lower body fat and better performance and thus typically consume very low-fat diets.[1,9,40] However, in physically active athletes consuming adequate calories, no correlation has been observed between fat intake and percent body fat and therefore, restricting fat intake may not be advisable.[1] Fat is an important source of energy for light- and moderate-intensity activity and during long-duration aerobic activity. At least 20% energy should be provided by fat in the diets of athletes, given the role of fat in providing energy for athletes involved in prolonged, low-intensity activity.[27,15] Restricting fat intake to less than 15% of energy intake is not advisable because it will not only limit performance by inhibiting intramuscular triglyceride storage, which is a significant source of energy during activities of all intensities, but will also affect important physiological functions.

E. Vitamin and Mineral Intake

Although vitamins and minerals are not a source of energy, they play a vital role in energy metabolism and overall health. RDAs for vitamins and minerals are defined to prevent nutrient deficiencies and are not targeted or determined based on physical activity levels.[11,21] Studies typically have shown athletes to have adequate intakes of vitamins and minerals as long as energy intake is appropriate. Adequate energy intake and variety in dietary intake typically can ensure adequate intakes of these micronutrients, however, typically iron and calcium are two main micronutrients that are often deficient in the diets of athletes.[41,42] Athletes who have been observed to have vitamin and mineral deficiencies are typically those who are on a weight loss diet, have specific body composition criteria, have restricted variety in dietary intake, limited access to food or eating disorders.[22] Rapidly growing male athletes, female athletes with heavy menstrual losses, athletes on energy-restricted diets, distance runners who may have increased gastrointestinal bleeding and those training heavily in hot climates with profuse sweating are most likely to have low iron stores and therefore, their dietary iron intake may need to be monitored and intake increased. An adequate calcium intake is important in maintaining bone strength and insufficient calcium has implications for stress fractures and osteoporosis in the future. Most female athletes need to increase their calcium intake to meet the RDAs and this can be achieved by incorporating low-fat and nonfat dairy products, calcium fortified fruit juice and soy milk and tofu with calcium sulfate.

With marginal deficiencies of thiamin, riboflavin, B_6 and vitamin C, a decrease in maximal aerobic capacity and anaerobic threshold were observed in normal healthy men, which improved with repletion.[17] Although exercise has been shown to increase free radical production, the use of antioxidant vitamins such as C, E and β-carotene have not shown a consistent effect on recovery from exercise. Excessive use of vitamin and mineral supplements, a common practice among athletes, can result in nutrient imbalances and may be harmful to the individuals. Singh et al.[43] observed that a high-potency multivitamin and mineral supplement did not enhance physical performance in individuals with normal biochemical measures of vitamin and mineral status while maintaining their normal level of physical activity and consuming an adequate diet.

Rankinen et al.[44] observed male Finnish athletes to have higher energy and micronutrient intakes than controls and higher than the age-specific RDAs except for vitamin D intake, while no differences except for niacin were observed between female athletes and controls. The high-energy intakes of the male athlete may explain the high vitamin and mineral intake, and an abundant consumption of dairy products by this group of Finnish athletes may also explain the higher calcium intakes. Furthermore, in pubescent club-level athletes, Fogelholm et al.[45] observed a positive relationship between body weight and changes in height, skinfolds, muscle girth, dietary copper (boys), iron (girls) and weight related energy intake (girls). Nutritional requirements are increased during puberty and are further affected by athletic training, however, this group of athletes had dietary intakes similar to or higher than the respective intakes of the control groups, suggesting that participation in club-level sports training is not detrimental to trace element status during puberty as long as an adequate quality diet is consumed.

Kaiserauer et al.[46] observed amenorrheic runners (AR) to have inadequate energy intakes based on RDAs with deficiencies in protein, fat, thiamin, riboflavin, calcium, iron, magnesium and zinc, probably as a result of inadequate energy intakes. These inadequate intakes were greater than in the regularly menstruating runners (RMR) and sedentary controls. Moreover, a greater percent of the AR (25%) were vegetarians, none of whom consumed any red meat, while only 11% of RMR were vegetarians with 44% consuming no red meat. Nutritional inadequacy, along with daily intense exercise and energy deficits, could be the main factors resulting in amenorrhea in this group of runners. Similarly, Steen et al.[47] observed female heavyweight collegiate rowers to consume 2633 kcal/d with 51% kcal from carbohydrate (4.9 g/kg body weight), 13% kcal from protein (1.4 g/kg body weight) and 36% kcal from fat. Although all rowers met 100% of the RDA for vitamins A and C, thiamin, riboflavin, niacin and folate, only 70% met 100% of the RDA for vitamin B_6 and only 80% met 100% of the RDA for vitamin B_{12}. Furthermore, suboptimal intakes of calcium, magnesium, iron and zinc were observed. Six percent of these athletes had calcium intakes less than two thirds of the RDA and 19% had zinc intakes less than two thirds of the RDA. Thus, in spite of an energy intake higher than the age- and gender-specific RDA of 2100 kcal, these athletes had micronutrient intakes less than recommendations. Low intakes of dairy foods, beef and poultry could have contributed to the lower micronutrient intakes, while intake of salad dressings, mayonnaise, cream sauces, cakes, cookies and chips could have contributed to the high fat intakes and thereby the higher energy intakes. Furthermore, main sources of protein were tuna fish, cheese and frozen yogurt, which could explain the lower intake of calcium. An in-depth analysis of dietary intake practices is required when assessing these micronutrient intakes to determine causes for the inadequate intakes.

VII. Summary

Adequate nutrient intakes by athletes is important to meet not only the demands of their increased physical activity and performance but also the demands of their growth and development (young athletes) and for their short- (injury risk) and long-term (chronic disease risk) health. Regular assessments of the dietary intakes of athletes are required to identify potential problem areas. A combination of methods should be used to assess adequacy of intake. National standards and guidelines are the most commonly used measures to determine adequacy of intake of athletes' diets. At the minimum, athletes should try to achieve these standards for maintenance of health and may need to further increase their intakes based on the demands of their sport and activity levels. Existing evidence suggests that performance and health of athletes can be compromised at intake levels below the national recommendations. In addition to absolute nutrient intakes, dietary intake patterns should be examined to identify potential causes of inadequate intakes. Furthermore, these measures need to be validated against biochemical, anthropometric and clinical parameters to determine the nutritional status of athletes and the adequacy of their dietary intakes.

References

1. Grandjean, A., Nutrition requirements to increase lean mass, *Clin. Sports Med.*, 18, 623, 1999.
2. Mertz, W., Tsui, J.C., Judd, J.T., Reiser, S., Hallfrisch, J., Morris, E.R., Steele, P.D. and Lashley, E., What are people really eating? The relation between energy intake derived from estimated diet records and intake determined to maintain body weight, *Am. J. Clin. Nutr.*, 54, 291, 1991.
3. Jonnalagadda, S.S., Benardot, D. and Neslon, M., Assessment of underreporting of energy intake by elite female gymnasts, *Int. J. Sport Nutr. Exerc. Metab.*, 10, 315, 2000.
4. Mullin, K., Practical nutrition education: special considerations for athletes. *Nurse Pract. Forum*, 7, 106, 1996.
5. Rico-Sanz, J., Frontera, W.R., Mole, P.A., Rivera, M.A., Rivera-Brown, A., and Meredith, C.N., Dietary and performance assessment of elite soccer players during a period of intense training, *Int. J. Sport Nutr.*, 8, 230, 1998.
6. Dietary Guidelines for Americans, www.health.gov/dietaryguidelines/dga2000, accessed 03/01.
7. Koenig, J. and Elmadfa, I., Food based dietary guidelines — the Australian perspective, *Br. J. Nutr.*, 81 (Suppl 2), S31, 1999.
8. Guthrie, H.A., Interpretation of data on dietary intake, *Nutr. Rev.*, 47, 33, 1989.
9. Ziegler, P.J., Nelson, J.A. and Jonnalagadda, S.S., Nutritional and physiological status of U.S. national figure skaters, *Int. J. Sport Nutr.*, 9, 345, 1999.
10. Ziegler, P.J., San-Khoo, C., Kris-Etherton, P. M., Jonnalagadda, S.S., Sherr, B., and Nelson, J.A., Nutritional status of nationally ranked junior U.S. figure skaters, *J. Am. Diet. Assoc.*, 98, 809, 1998.
11. Recommended Dietary Allowance, 10th ed., Food and Nutrition Board, Commission of Life Sciences, National Research Council, Washington, 1989.
12. Position of the American Dietetic Association, Dietitions of Canada and the American College of Sports Medicine, Nutrition and athletic performance, *J. Am. Diet. Assoc.*, 100, 1543, 2000.
13. American College of Sports Medicine, Exercise and fluid replacement: position stand, *Med. Sci. Sports Exerc.*, 28, i, 1996.
14. Beck, L., Carbohydrate review. Carbohydrates and endurance performance: how much should an athlete eat?, *J. Can. Diet Assoc.*, 56, insert 4, 1995.
15. Bloch, T.D. and Wheeler, K.B., Dietary examples: a practical approach to feeding athletes, *Clin. Sports Med.*, 18, 703, 1999.
16. Lemon, P.W.R., Is increased dietary protein necessary or beneficial for individuals with a physically active lifestyle?, *Nutr. Rev.*, 54, S169, 1996.
17. Manore, M.M., Effect of physical activity on thiamin, riboflavin and vitamin B_6 requirements, *Am. J. Clin. Nutr.*, 72 (Suppl 2), 5598S, 2000.
18. Mulligan, K. and Butterfield, G.E., Discrepancies between energy intake and expenditure in physically active women, *Br. J. Nutr.*, 64, 23, 1990.
19. Wiita, B.G. and Stombaugh, I.A., Nutrition knowledge, eating practices and health of adolescent female runners: a 3-year longitudinal study, *Int. J. Sport Nutr.*, 6, 414, 1996.

20. Garcia-Roves, P.M., Fernandez, S., Rodriguez, M., Perez-Landaluce, J., and Patterson, A.M.,Eating pattern and nutrition status of international elite flat-water paddlers, *Int. J Sport Nutr. Exer. Metab.*, 10, 182, 2000.

21. Standing Committee on the Scientific Evaluation of Dietary Reference Intakes, Food and Nutrition Board, Institute of Medicine, National Academy Press, Washington, D.C., www.nas.edu/iom, accessed 03/01.

22. Burke, L.M. and Read, R.S.D., Sports nutrition. Approaching the nineties. *Sports Med.*, 8, 80, 1993.

23. Anon., Uses of dietary reference intakes, *Nutr. Rev.*, 55, 327, 1997.

24. Food Guide Pyramid: A guide to daily food choices, *Home and Garden Bulletin No. 252*, Washington, D.C., U.S. Department of Agriculture and U.S. Department of Health and Human Services, 1992.

25. Randall, E., Marshall, J.R., Graham, S. and Brasure, J., Patterns in food use and their associations with nutrient intakes, *Am. J. Clin. Nutr.*, 52, 739, 1990.

26. Beaudry, M., Galibois, I. and Chaumette, P., Dietary patterns of adults in Quebec and their nutritional adequacy, *Can. J. Public Health*, 89, 347, 1998.

27. Kleiner, S.M., Eating for peak performance, *Phys. Sportsmed.*, 25, 123, 1997.

28. Kant, A.K., Indexes of overall diet quality: a review, *J. Am. Diet Assoc.*, 96, 785, 1996.

29. Klicka, M.V., King, N., Lavin, P.T. and Askew, E.W., Assessment of dietary intakes of cadets at the U.S. Military Academy at West Point, *J. Am. Coll. Nutr.*, 15, 273, 1996.

30. Kennedy, E.T., Ohls, J., Carlson, S. and Fleming, K., The Healthy Eating Index: design and applications, *J. Am. Diet. Assoc.*, 94, 57, 1994.

31. Fogelholm, M. and Hiilloskorpi, H., Weight and diet concerns in Finnish female and male athletes, *Med. Sci. Sports Exer.*, 31, 229, 1999.

32. Beals, K.A. and Manore, M.M., The prevalence and consequences of subclinical eating disorders in female athletes, *Int. J. Sport Nutr.*, 4, 175, 1994.

33. Janelle, K.C. and Barr, S.I., Nutrient intakes and eating behavior scores of vegetarian and nonvegetarian women, *J. Am. Diet Assoc.*, 95, 180, 1995.

34. Sugiura, K., Suzuki, I. and Kobayashi, K., Nutritional intake of elite Japanese track-and-field athletes, *Int. J. Sport Nutr.*, 9, 202, 1999.

35. Maughan, R.J., Energy and macronutrient intakes of professional football (soccer players), *Br. J. Sports Med.*, 31, 45, 1997.

36. Walberg-Rankin, J., Dietary carbohydrate as an ergogenic aid for prolonged and brief competitions in sport, *Int. J. Sport Nutr.*, 5, S13, 1995.

37. Jacobs, K.A. and Sherman, W.M., The efficacy of carbohydrate supplementation and chronic high-carbohydrate diets for improving endurance performance, *Int. J. Sport Nutr.*, 9, 92, 1999.

38. Tanaka, J.A., Tanaka, H. and Landis, W., An assessment of carbohydrate intake in collegiate distance runners, *Int. J. Sport Nutr.*, 5, 206, 1995.

39. Loosli, A.R. and Rudd, J.S., Meatless diets in female athletes: a red flag, *Phys. Sportsmed.*, 26, 45, 1998.

40. Ryan, Y.M., Meat avoidance and body weight concerns: nutritional implications for teenage girls, *Proc. Nutr. Soc.*, 56, 519, 1997.

41. Armstrong, L.E. and Maresh, C.M., Vitamin and mineral supplements as aids to exercise performance and health, *Nutr. Rev.*, 54, S149, 1996.

42. Stang, J. et al., Relationships between vitamin and mineral supplement use, dietary intake and dietary adequacy among adolescents, *J. Am. Diet Assoc.*, 100, 905, 2000.

43. Singh, A., Moses, F.M. and Deuster, P.A., Chronic multivitamin-mineral supplementation does not enhance physical performance, *Med. Sci. Sports Exerc.*, 24, 726, 1992.

44. Rankinen, T. et al., Dietary intake and nutritional status of athletic and nonathletic children in early puberty, *Int. J. Sport Nutr.*, 5, 136, 1995.

45. Fogelholm, M. et al., Growth, dietary intake and trace element status in pubescent athletes and schoolchildren, *Med. Sci. Sports Exerc.*, 32, 738, 2000.

46. Kaiserauer, S. et al., Nutritional, physiological and menstrual status of distance runners, *Med. Sci. Sports Exer.*, 21, 120, 1989.

47. Steen, S.N. et al., Dietary intake of female collegiate heavyweight rowers, *Int. J. Sport Nutr.*, 5, 225,1995.

4

Assessment of Possible Presence of Eating Disorders

Monika M. Woolsey

CONTENTS

0-8493-0927-1/02/$0.00+$1.50
© 2002 by CRC Press LLC

I. Introduction

In the past two decades, awareness of the importance of diet and exercise to health and well-being has grown. However, the use of dieting and exercise to extremes that can provoke injury and death has become a growing problem. Perhaps this is inevitable in cultures where the attitude, "If a little is good, a lot must be better," prevails. Unlike chemical addictions or criminal behavior, eating and exercise behaviors are often viewed as positive choices. While a commitment to a healthy diet and regular exercise do not constitute disordered behavior, there are patterns within each of these choices that do appear to be dysfunctional. These patterns have been given a variety of names; some such as anorexia nervosa are bona fide medical diagnoses. Others, such as exercise dependence, have only recently appeared in the literature and have yet to be included in the *Diagnostic and Statistical Manual of Mental Disorders* (DSM-IV).[1]

Athletes, who may be expected to maintain a low body weight as part of their sport participation, may be at particular risk for developing harmful eating and exercise habits. In the process of trying to meet the expectations of coaches, trainers, and parents, eating and exercise behaviors may drift into regimens that no longer reflect internal cues of hunger and fatigue. As nutrition intake decreases and caloric expenditure increases, these behaviors may exceed the individual's ability to replenish the energy that has been consumed in training. Mood changes may occur and performance may be impaired. The literature consistently documents that athletes in the aesthetic sports (e.g., gymnastics, figure skating, ballet) report greater body dissatisfaction and more persistent dieting than athletes in other sports (e.g., basketball, volleyball, field hockey). The inability to control weight and body shape can lead to frustration, guilt, and even despair.

Athletes with a history of low self esteem and difficulty with problem solving and handling stress independent of their training history, may turn to food as a coping mechanism. What began as a casual diet or an extra workout to shed a few pounds to please the coach or improve performance can end in a lifelong battle with food or exercise dependence. In the athletic world, it is not uncommon for athletes to be disciplined and determined, and to push the limit of physical performance. The line between normal training routines (e.g., long workouts, pre-game food rituals, skipping meals) and eating disorders is often very fine. In fact, behaviors that would be suspect in a nonathlete may be validated or encouraged on the athletic field. By the time an eating disorder is even suspected, the behaviors could be well ingrained and challenging to address.

Whether an individual is an athlete or not, the definitions for healthy eating and disordered eating remain the same. Healthy eating is defined as:

- Consuming balanced meals and snacks at regular times
- Eating enough calories to maintain a healthy weight
- Eating to maintain health
- Eating to enhance performance

Disordered eating is defined as eating — or not eating — more often in response to external cues (e.g., a diet) as opposed to internal cues (e.g., physical hunger). A person whose eating is disordered is more likely to eat to demonstrate "willpower," to follow a preplanned "diet," to manipulate weight or to eat in response to emotions, than to eat as a response to internal regulatory mechanisms. The risks of disordered eating include malnutrition, impaired athletic performance, and exacerbation of mental health issues such as depression.

Almost everyone experiences disordered eating at some time in life. It is when the time spent in external eating is greater than the time spent eating in response to internal hunger cues that the situation can develop into an eating disorder. Athletes, coaches, trainers, team physicians, and sports nutritionists need to be aware of the special needs of athletes with weight concerns and to help them safely achieve a body weight that promotes optimal health and performance. This chapter presents an overview of eating and exercise disorders in athletes, including definition and diagnostic criteria, risk factors, effects on health and performance, and the role of the sports nutritionist in treatment.

II. Definitions and Diagnostic Criteria

According to the fourth edition of the DSM-IV, eating disorders are characterized by severe disturbances in eating and exercise behaviors.[1] The term eating disorder typically refers to anorexia nervosa, bulimia nervosa, or binge eating disorder. However, eating disorders can range from anorexia nervosa to obesity, and new variations (e.g., anorexia athletica, exercise dependence) are being proposed as they are identified. Within this continuum are found a number of categories for disorders that do not meet specific DSM-IV criteria, including concerns about weight and shape, excessive dieting, and bingeing behaviors. While the criteria for a given diagnosis may be specific, the common thread that connects these diagnoses is a situation of imbalance; eating and exercise behaviors develop into a compulsive behavior that results in an inability to perform activities of daily living, to socialize, sleep on a normal schedule, to exhibit appropriate emotional and behavioral responses to daily events, and to maintain metabolic functions that sustain life.

A. Anorexia Nervosa

Anorexia nervosa is a disorder in which anxiety, compulsive tendencies, and preoccupation with food and dieting lead to excessive weight loss. With this disorder, issues related to food and weight (e.g., nutritional content of individual foods, mealtimes, weight on the scales) become highly emotional. Despite an emaciated body, anorexics see themselves as fat when they look in the mirror.

Anorexia is characterized by four primary presentations:

1. Body weight less than 85% of expected weight or body mass index (BMI) less than 17.5
2. Intense fear of weight gain
3. Inaccurate perception of own body size, weight, or shape
4. Amenorrhea

The classic anorexic is intelligent, a high achiever and willing to please. The individual may have been slightly overweight as an adolescent, and on the subtle suggestion of a coach or family member, began to diet. A low body weight was achieved either through anxiety related to an emotional stressor or restricting food. Because losing weight often encourages positive feedback from peers, family and coaches, behaviors that maintain weight loss can develop to maintain the body shape that received the compliments. These rituals can include frequent weigh-ins, skipping meals, counting fat grams and exercising excessively to burn calories developed. Anorexia commonly coexists with some psychiatric diagnosis having an anxious component (e.g., anxiety disorder, obsessive-compulsive disorder).[2] When these conditions exist, it is not uncommon to hear clients describe a recent significant life change or trauma (illness, puberty, parental divorce, moving to college) that likely raised their stress level over an extended period of time. Regardless of how the weight loss initially developed, when low body weight is maintained, the resulting malnutrition can affect central nervous system function and exacerbate the problem.

Anorexia is a potentially life-threatening disorder. Treatment is important, as evidence is emerging suggesting that brain tissue is lost with chronic caloric restriction, increasing the likelihood of permanent disability and impaired functioning in the untreated individual. Although many people undergo a single episode of anorexia and fully recover, unsuccessful treatment can result in death related to medical complications including cardiac atrophy, electrolyte imbalance and even death.[3] The consequences of anorexia nervosa cannot be minimized, as the disease has the greatest mortality rate of any psychiatric diagnosis and a suicide rate equivalent to that of schizophrenia. This places the 0.5 to 1% of adolescent and young women who have the disease at great risk if left unrecognized and untreated.

B. Bulimia Nervosa

Bulimia nervosa occurs in roughly 2 to 5% of the population. On college campuses, the incidence may be as high as 20% of all women. It is described as recurring episodes of binge eating, usually followed by purging. To meet the criteria, the binge eating and purging must occur, on average, at least twice a week for 3 months.[1] Purging is defined as a deliberate behavior designed to compensate for ingested calories. Examples of purging behaviors include dietary restriction, self-induced vomiting, misuse of laxatives or diuretics, or excessive exercise.

Bulimia is characterized by four primary presentations:

1. Recurrent binge eating
2. Recurrent purging, excessive exercise, or fasting
3. Excessive concern about body weight or shape
4. Absence of anorexia nervosa.

The typical bulimic is an 18- to 25-year-old Caucasian female who is concerned about her appearance, though she is usually of normal weight or only slightly overweight. To control her weight, the bulimic becomes entrapped in a vicious cycle: diet, starve, binge and purge. The binge–purge behavior occurs in an effort to relieve guilt and shame. Some evidence is emerging to suggest that both bingeing and purging also affect biochemical balance in the central nervous system and may serve as forms of self-medication when an imbalance of energy substrates and neurotransmitters exists.

Bulimics, by their nature, are very secretive, which is why this disorder is often difficult to diagnose. Unlike anorexia, where extreme weight loss is apparent, many physical features of bulimia do not appear until late in the course of the illness. Common signs of binge–purge behavior include swollen parotid glands (cheeks), calluses on the backs of hands and dental erosion.

C. Binge Eating Disorder

Binge eating disorder is a serious and prevalent problem among the over-weight population.[4] It is characterized by recurrent overeating episodes wherein an individual consumes a large amount of food while feeling a loss of control over eating behaviors.[1] This disorder differs from bulimia nervosa in that compensatory behaviors, such as purging, fasting, and compulsive exercise are not present. Binge eating disorder is characterized by the following criteria:[1]

1. Recurrent episodes of binge eating (consuming, within any 2-hour period, a large amount of food, being unable to control eating during the episode)

2. Eating until uncomfortably full
3. Eating large amounts of food, even when not physically hungry
4. Eating alone out of embarrassment
5. Feelings of disgust, depression, low self-esteem, lack of willpower
6. Occurs, on average, at least 2 days a week for at least 6 months
7. Not associated with the regular use of inappropriate compensatory behaviors (i.e. purging, fasting, excessive exercise).

Binge eating disorder is frequently associated with a history of depression, low self-esteem, and personality disturbances. A distorted body image and preoccupation with food are also prevalent. Although binge eating disorder is not usually an issue with athletes, it is likely to manifest in the case of a serious injury, when physical activity is eliminated or curtailed as part of the rehabilitative treatment plan. Athletes who may have been in denial about the possibility of an eating disorder as long as they could train and compensate physically for calories eaten may be forced to face the fact that their exercise and eating behaviors were not without dysfunction.

D. Muscle Dysmorphia

Muscle dysmorphia is a relatively new term used to describe individuals who are pathologically preoccupied with being fit and muscular. It is a form of body dysmorphic disorder (BDD), which is an obsession with a defect in visual appearance, usually involving the face, skin, hair or nose.[5] Muscle dysmorphia is not considered an eating disorder but rather a psychiatric disturbance involving body image.

Muscle dysmorphia affects both men and women, although it may be more common in men. Individuals with this disorder have extreme body dissatisfaction coupled with low self-esteem and depression. Despite being large and muscular, they perceive themselves as small and weak.[5] Athletes with muscle dysmorphia can become completely consumed with weightlifting and dieting in an attempt to achieve their ideal body shape. They can become extremely anxious if something interferes with their daily ritual. The individual frequently gives up important social, occupational, or recreational activities to maintain a rigorous workout and diet regimen. Abuse of anabolic steroids and other substances is common.[6]

Muscle dysmorphia parallels obsessive-compulsive disorder in that the person exhibits obsessive thoughts and behaviors, such as checking, comparing, seeking reassurance and excessive exercise.

Characteristics associated with muscle dysmorphia include:[5]

1. Preoccupation with body size
2. Long hours of lifting weights
3. Excessive attention to diet

4. Sacrifice of important social, occupational or recreational activities to maintain the desired workout and diet schedule

5. Avoidance of situations where one's body is exposed to others

6. Clinically significant distress related to preoccupation with body size

7. Fear of being too small or not muscular

8. Persistent use of harmful ergogenic substances and exercise and diet patterns despite the knowledge of associated physical and mental health consequences

E. Anorexia Athletica

This category has not yet been included in the DSM-IV, but is important to recognize. Also called a "subclinical eating disorder," this presentation may be the initial sign that an athlete is headed toward a more serious problem. Intervention at this point may prevent the development of the diagnoses described above. The proposed diagnostic criteria for anorexia athletica are:[1]

1. Preoccupation with food, calories, body shape and weight, as evidenced by a score of 20 on the Eating Attitudes Test (EAT-26)

2. Distorted body image, as evidenced by a score of ≥ 14 on the body image dissatisfaction scale of the Eating Disorder Inventory (EDI)

3. Intense fear of gaining weight or becoming fat even though moderately or extremely underweight (5% to 15% below normal weight for height) or extremely low body fat

4. Over at least a 1-year period, the athlete maintains a body weight below "normal" 9%–15%) for age and height using one or a combination of the following:

   - restricting energy intake (energy intake $\leq 80\%$ of energy expenditure)

   - severely limiting food choices or food groups, as evidenced by food frequency, a 7- to 14- day diet record, or both

   - excessive exercise (i.e., more than necessary for success in sport or as compared with athletes of similar fitness levels

   - absence of medical illness or affective disorder explaining the weight loss or maintenance of low body weight

5. Gastrointestinal complaints

6. Menstrual dysfunction (i.e., primary or seconday amenorrhea or oligomenorrhea)

7. Frequent use of purging methods (i.e., self-induced vomiting or use of laxatives or diuretics for at least 1 month)

8. Bingeing (≤ 8 episodes per month for at least 3 months)

F. Exercise Dependence

While exercise is often promoted as one of the best ways to relieve stress, control weight and improve cardiovascular health, recreational running has also been identified as a behavior on which one can become dependent.[7] Individuals with this tendency seem to have more of an inability to maintain a perspective of moderation in their running efforts. This syndrome is present if people believe they require exercise daily and if signs of withdrawal manifest when exercise is deprived for any reason. These withdrawal effects could become sufficiently severe to promote continued exercise even when it is medically unadvisable, interferes with the addict's work, or causes serious social conflicts. This syndrome is most commonly described in the literature as "obligatory running."[8]

Veale[9] noted the relationship between exercise dependence and other dependence syndromes and coined the term "exercise dependence." Veale also found similarities among the profiles of exercisers displaying compulsive behaviors. Most consistent is the tendency to develop a mood disorder when the exercisers, particularly runners, are unable to exercise. This mood disorder manifests itself as depression, irritability, impaired concentration and sleep disturbance, all of which define a withdrawal state. The withdrawal symptoms are relieved by exercise but, as exercise continues, a tolerance level is reached and the exercisers believe they must increase the amount of exercise to relieve or avoid withdrawal. Veale proposed the following set of diagnostic criteria for exercise dependence:

1. A rigid stereotyped pattern of exercise performed at least once a day
2. Prioritizing exercise over other activities
3. Developing a tolerance to the level of exercise
4. Experiencing withdrawal symptoms in the form of mood alterations when unable to exercise
5. Avoiding withdrawal or relieving it by exercising
6. Exercising against the advice of a health professional
7. Continuing the exercise pattern even though it causes work, family or social difficulties
8. Weight loss to enhance exercise performance
9. Awareness of the compulsion to exercise

G. Eating Disorders Not Otherwise Specified

Many young women and men can experience a preoccupation with food, exercise and weight, but without neatly fitting into the diagnostic categories described above. The DSM-IV refers to situations where all of the diagnostic criteria are not met, yet exercise and food behaviors are creating a problem. This diagnosis is called **eating disorders — not otherwise specified** (ED-NOS).[1] The term "subclinical eating disorder" has also been used to identify individuals who display some, but not all of the signs of an eating disorder. These individuals may restrict food intake significantly but not enough to be diagnosed as anorexic.[1] They may also binge and purge, but only occasionally. Regardless of the situation, serious eating problems and health consequences can develop if the proper education and support are not provided.

III. Prevalence of Eating Disorders in Athletes

Athletes have followed bizarre diets and rigorous training schedules since ancient times. However, not until the last 20 years have researchers really looked at actual numbers of athletes afflicted with these behaviors and the impact they can have on health and performance. Early studies on the prevalence of eating disorders in athletes focused more on pathogenic weight control behaviors than on physical symptoms.[10] More recent data have used self-reported questionnaires including the 40-item Eating Attitudes Test (EAT)[11] or the 64-item multiscale Eating Disorder Inventory (EDI)[12] to measure the wide range of psychological and behavioral traits common in individuals with eating disorders.

Sundgot-Borgen[13] evaluated the prevalence of eating disorders in 522 Norwegian elite female athletes representing 35 different sports, using the EDI as the screening instrument. Athletes were interviewed and then clinically examined. According to Sundgot-Borgen, both personal interviews (survey data) and clinical examinations are necessary to obtain reliable data on the prevalence of ED in athletes.

Results showed that 18% of the total population met the criteria for an eating disorder. When data were compared between sport groups, notable differences were observed. Eating disorders were significantly higher among athletes in aesthetic (34%) and weight-dependent (27%) sports than in endurance (20%), technical (13%), and team sports (11%). Further analysis revealed differences within sport groups. For example, within the endurance-sport group, the prevalence was significantly higher in cross-country skiers (33%) than orienteers (0%). In another large study involving 363 athletes (173 females and 190 males) representing 21 different sports, Fogelholm and Hiilloskorpi[14] reported that the prevalence of weight and diet concerns was highest among athletes in weight-class sports (judo, wrestling, boxing, and karate) and aesthetic sports (ballet, gymnastics, and figure skating).

IV.   Etiology

Many sociocultural, familial and psychological factors have been implicated in the development of eating disorders (Table 4.1).[15] Females have traditionally been at greater risk, presumably because society places greater demands on women to achieve and maintain an ideal body shape. However, in recent years, the incidence of eating disorders in males has been recognized as a growing problem.[16] Even young children who are underweight for their height are dieting to combat fears of being overweight and not being accepted by their culture.[17] For many girls, weight and dieting concerns emerge as early as 8 years of age.[18]

Dieting appears to be a major predictor of an eating disorder.[19,20] A recent study involving adolescents concluded that females who dieted (severely restricted food intake) were 18 times more likely to develop an eating disorder than those who did not diet.[20] Even subjects who dieted at a moderate level were five times more likely to develop an eating disorder than those who did not. For many athletes, weight concerns and, subsequently, dieting, becomes the focal point of their athletic existence.[21] Athletes who are strongly committed to their sport are at greatest risk of dieting to improve appearance and chances of success. Another factor implicated in the development of eating disorders in athletes relates to the emphasis some sports place on weight and appearance. Two large-scale studies involving athletes from a variety of sport groups concluded that aesthetic and weight-dependent sports have a higher percentage of athletes with eating disorders.[22, 23] In sports where athletes are judged on appearance, presentation, and performance, there is enormous pressure to achieve an ideal body shape. Many athletes fall victim to eating disorders in a desperate attempt to be thin to please coaches and judges.

Some athletes do not have the genetic makeup to attain the "ideal body" for their particular sport.[24] There are three basic body types:

- **Ectomorph,** or lean and slightly muscular
- **Mesomorph**, or naturally muscular and strong
- **Endomorph,** or stocky in build with wide chest and hips and short bones.

Most individuals exhibit a predominance of one body type with aspects of the other two. For the endomorph, weight gain is easy and fat loss is difficult. This body type may not be as naturally inclined to excel in certain sports; in frustration, it can be easier to blame performance on the visually obvious difference (weight) than it is to consider genetically programmed differences in bone and muscle structure and center of gravity.

Do athletics cause an eating disorder? Personality characteristics that can be of benefit in sport participation (e.g., high self-expectation, perfectionism,

TABLE 4.1

Common Behavioral Self-Report Inventories Used in Eating Disorder Assessment

Test	Acronym	Number of Items	Eating Disorders Assessed	Free/Pay for Use	Uses	Special Notes
Eating Disorder Inventory[61]	EDI	64	A, Bu	P	Screening	Contains 8 subscales: Drive for Thinness, Bulimia, Body Dissatisfaction, Ineffectiveness, Perfectionism, Interpersonal Distrust, Interoceptive Awareness, and Maturity Fears.
Eating Disorder Inventory 2[62]	EDI-2	91	A, Bu	P	Assess	Contains 64 original EDI symptoms, Questions plus 27 new treatment items and three additional planning subscales: Asceticism, Impulse Regulation, and Social Insecurity.
Eating Attitudes Test[63]	EAT	40	A, B	F	Group	Test distinguishes outcomes, anorexics from controls screening and bulimics from control, but has not been shown to distinguish between anorexia and bulimia.
Bulimia Test-Revised[64]	BULIT-R	36	B	F	Screening	
Questionnaire for Eating Disorder Diagnosis[65]	Q-EDD	50	A, B		Diagnosis	Can distinguish: women who have and who have not been diagnosed with an eating disorder, anorexia vs. bulimia, women with eating disorders with symptoms vs. women with eating disorders without symptoms
Mizes Anorectic Cognitions[66]	MAC	33	A, B	F	Research, screening	Not recommended for clinical decision making

competitiveness) may become a problem when combined with pressures from coaches and parents to meet certain weight and performance expectations. One study found that athletes at risk for an eating disorder are those who are experiencing considerable distress achieving self-identity, who are conflictually dependent on their parents and who engage in destructive forms of self-restraint.[25]

A. Warning Signs

Detection of eating disorders among athletes can be very difficult because many pathogenic weight control behaviors are secretive in nature. Athletes may avoid treatment or underreport disordered eating behaviors for fear of being discovered and losing their position on the team. Preoccupation with weight and dieting do not automatically signal an eating disorder. Some athletes may show signs of disordered eating during the season but resume normal eating habits when the season is over. Coaches and trainers must recognize when healthy training routines become an obsession and when an athlete is using pathogenic weight control behaviors to become thin. An assessment is warranted if the athlete displays any of the following warning signs:

- Negative comments about food
- Omission of entire food groups such as meat or dairy
- Dramatic decrease in performance
- Excessive concerns about weight
- Dramatic weight loss
- Mood swings
- Depression
- Wearing baggy and layered clothing
- Social withdrawal from teammates
- Visits to the bathroom following meals.

V. Primary or Secondary Disorder?

There is accumulating evidence that eating disorders may present both as primary and secondary behavioral disorders. Some researchers suggest that the most substantial physiology indicating eating disorders relates to mood alteration.[26-31] Correlations between nutrition and exercise habits and mood, cognitive functioning, occupational performance, and sleep patterns are well-documented in the literature. In addition, exercise is often prescribed as a means of reducing stress; the "runner's high" is a commonly accepted phenomenon associated with regular running.

The greatest difficulty in defining eating disorders is the lack of a specific physiological or biochemical marker. Numerous attempts have been made to measure changes in plasma or urinary catecholamines, corticosteroids and endorphins, but no specific, sensitive test has yet been identified. Empirical evidence for the existence of these disorders has been largely based on self-report of behaviors, a very subjective measurement. Perhaps the best "marker" to distinguish between nonabusive and healthful food and exercise choices is the refusal to change behaviors in the face of medical, occupational, social, or familial contraindications. Some researchers have proposed that eating disorders may actually be a form of obsessive-compulsive behavior, which is a common comorbid condition in anorexia nervosa, bulimia nervosa, and binge eating disorder.[32] The connection has been proposed with the other diagnoses, but has yet to be formalized. Based on the literature, there appear to be four models of disease etiology currently in favor:

1. Eating disorders and exercise dependence are separate syndromes.
2. Exercise dependence overlaps with and leads to eating disorders.
3. Both eating disorders and exercise dependence are aspects of another disorder.
4. Exercise dependence is a variant of eating disorders.

A. Separate Syndromes

Veale[9] separates primary exercise dependence from exercise dependence that is secondary to an eating disorder. He argues that "a diagnosis of primary exercise dependence can be differentiated from an eating disorder by clarifying the ultimate aim of the exercise." When performance of the exercise itself is the end point, with dieting and weight loss used as a means to improve performance, then the behavior should be classified as primary exercise dependence. In anorexia nervosa, the aim of excessive exercise is for achieving weight loss or preventing fatness, making the exercise a secondary behavior.

Bamber, Cockerill, and Carroll[33] made a somewhat finer distinction between exercise dependence and eating disorders, finding distinctive psychological differences between the following groups:

1. Primary exercise dependence without evidence of a comorbid eating disorder
2. Secondary exercise dependence occurring in conjunction with an eating disorder
3. Eating disorder without evidence of exercise dependence

In a sample of female exercisers given the Reasons for Exercise Inventory, Appearance/Motive was the only reason associated with a negative body image. The authors suggest that female exercisers who specifically cite weight control, muscle tone or attractiveness as reasons for exercising should be examined for eating disorders but that excessive exercising in males is not related to disordered eating.

In contrast, a well-designed study of females showed that obligatory exercisers did not demonstrate disordered eating tendencies compared with symptomatic bulimics and controls[34] bulimics who exhibited excessive exercise were excluded from this study, and the groups, while equal, were small (n = 25 in each). The researchers used a number of reliable, valid instruments to measure disordered eating behaviors, one being the EAT-26. While the obligatory exercisers in this study had significantly lower scores than the bulimics, the mean score was positive for an eating disorder (24) with a relatively large standard deviation ($\pm$ 11.8). The authors expressed concern that some of the obligatory exercisers in this sample may have shown signs of disordered eating, or may have had a prior history of eating disorder. However, the subscale scores and the scores on the remaining scales did not indicate an overlap of exercise dependence and eating disorders.

B.   Exercise Dependence Leads to Eating Disorders

In this model, normal, healthy exercise would progress to an excessive pattern. Accompanying diet manipulations would lead to the development of an eating disorder. While Veale[9] maintains that the goal of the exercise differentiates the two, Dewsnap[35] points out that "exercise aims" are abstractions and individuals with anorexia may not provide an honest answer to their aims. Another possibility is that while individuals with anorexia may be aware of their drive to exercise, they may not understand the core reason for its existence. In an attempt to make sense of it, they may explain it with behaviors that make sense to them (i.e., I must be doing this to lose weight.) Finally, a person with a compulsive exercise habit who says that the aim of his exercise is to develop higher levels of fitness may be equating fitness with lower levels of body fat. Thus, while in theory "exercise aim" may be important to identify, defining this feature may not be possible in practice.

Because excessive exercise is a diagnostic criterion for anorexia nervosa and bulimia nervosa,[1] several researchers have studied the role that exercise plays in these disorders. Richert and Hummers[36] found that, among the 345 college students participating in their survey, duration of jogging related to higher scores on the EAT-26. These authors thought that hours of jogging among college students could be a predictor for eating disorders. However, the correlation coefficient, while statistically significant, was small (r = 0.20), data from males and females were not analyzed separately, and the "at risk" comparison group consisted of 29 students who scored higher than 30 on the EAT-26. In a more comprehensive study, 60 female college students were recruited into three equal categories: (1) distance runners who had lost at least 4.5 kg without diet manipulation, (2) individuals with bulimia, and (3) non-dieter non-exerciser controls. No differences were found between the runners and the controls using valid measures of depression, bulimic symptoms and body image disturbance. However, the individuals with bulimia had significantly higher scores on all measures. The mean scores for these individuals were all indicative of disorder. The authors stated that their findings could not support the notion that distance runners are at risk for eating disorders.

Contrary to the previous study, Davis et al[37] found that excessive exercise preceded the onset of eating disorders. When hospitalized eating disorder patients and age-matched controls were interviewed regarding both their physical activity history and their eating disorder history, 78% engaged in excessive exercise, 60% were competitive athletes prior to the onset of their disorder, 60% reported that sport or exercise predated dieting, and 75% claimed that physical activity levels steadily increased during the period when food intake and weight loss decreased the most. The authors concluded that, "Sport/exercise is an integral part of the pathogenesis and progression of self-starvation." Brewerton et al[38] found excessive exercise to be more common among anorexic patients than bulimic patients, but 28% of their sample were compulsive exercisers. These researchers suggested that coaches and family members need to be alert to excessive exercising as an indicator of anorexia nervosa.

C. Another Disorder Underlies Both

Some researchers and clinicians have suggested that both eating disorders and exercise dependence are manifestations of another psychiatric disorder. Veale[9] likened exercise dependence to a compulsive behavior and stated that the proposed diagnostic criteria were based on "the core features of a dependence syndrome." Rudy and Estok[7] also defined exercise dependence as an addictive behavior. Davis and Claridge[39] discuss the possibility that anorexia nervosa is an addiction to the body's own opioids. Despite the many possibilities presented, the most common root disorder discussed in the research as underlying both eating disorders and exercise dependence remains obsessive-compulsive disorder. Matsunaga et al[40] found strong evidence of obsessive-compulsive behaviors that were beyond those related to the disorder itself among patients suffering from anorexia nervosa. The findings of Davis et al[41] suggest that among women with anorexia, obsessional personality characteristics are linked to high-level exercising, and that exercising is associated with a greater degree of obsessive-compulsive symptomatology.

The relationship between serotonin imbalance, obsessive-compulsive disorder and eating disorders is well documented in the literature. Both obsessive-compulsive disorder and eating disorders respond to selective serotonin uptake inhibitor (SSRI) therapy. Currently, there are no reports of the response of exercise dependence to these medications. However, Dwyer and Browning[42] have reported that, in rats, endurance training decreases receptor sensitivity to a serotonin agonist. Whether this relationship exists in humans remains to be seen, but it may explain how exercise dependence develops; initial bouts of exercise provided a sense of well-being related to increased serotonin levels, but with training, increased the dose of exercise required to achieve a serotonin-enhancing benefit. Standardized methods of research and a clearer definition of exercise dependence are needed before this model can be tested.

D. Exercise Dependence is a Variant of Eating Disorders

When exercise dependence first began to appear in the literature, this model was considered perhaps the most difficult model in terms of evaluation and acceptance.[9] However, Bamber et al.[43] suggest that exercise dependence always manifests in the context of an eating disorder. They designed a study in which female exercisers, four in each case, were allocated *a priori* to four groups:

1. Primary exercise dependent
2. Secondary exercise dependent, where there was a coincidence of exercise dependence and an eating disorder
3. Eating disordered
4. Control, where there was no evidence of either exercise dependence or eating disorder

Subjects were interviewed regarding their exercise and eating attitudes and behavior, and psychological history. Participants initially classified as primary exercise dependent turned out to exhibit features of exercise dependence only if they also displayed symptoms of an eating disorder. All of those with positive histories of exercise dependency and eating disorder also reported a history of psychological distress. These results support the concept of secondary (with eating disorder), but not primary (independent of eating disorder), exercise dependence.

VI. Nutritional Status

A. Nutrient Intake

Beals and Manore[44,45] have examined the energy intake and nutritional status of athletes with subclinical eating disorder. These researchers[46] studied 48 female athletes between the ages of 16 and 36 who trained at least 6 hours a week. Subjects were screened for subclinical eating disorders using a health and diet history questionnaire, the EDI and the Body Shape Questionnaire. Twenty-four athletes met the criteria for subclinical eating disorder and 24 served as the control group. Energy and nutrient intakes and energy expenditure were determined by weighed food records and 7-day activity logs. Results showed that energy intakes of athletes with subclinical eating disorders were significantly lower than in the control athletes, 1989 kcal/day vs. 2293 kcal/day, respectively. The athletes with subclinical eating disorders also consumed significantly less fat (43g/day or 19% of total calories) than the control athletes (61g/day or 23% of total calories). In another study that assessed the nutrient intake of female athletes with eating disorders, Sundgot-Borgen reported diets low in energy and essential vitamins and minerals, particularly calcium, vitamin D and iron. Mean carbohydrate intakes were significantly lower than the 8 to 10 g/kg body wt/day recommended for optimal performance.[46] The anorexics averaged 1.7 g/kg body wt/day with a range of 1.0 to 2.3 g/kg.

Chronic energy deprivation coupled with high levels of physical activity can lead to serious health consequences including chronic fatigue, compromised immune function, poor or delayed healing, electrolyte imbalances, cardiovascular alterations and reduced bone density.[47] Roemmich and Sinning[48] assessed the influence of energy restriction on growth, maturation, body composition, protein nutrition and muscular strength in adolescent wrestlers and a control group. Subjects were evaluated before, at the end (late season) and 3 to 4 months after a wrestling season. Wrestlers consumed a high-carbohydrate, low-fat diet during the season but did not consume adequate energy or protein intake. Although dietary restriction and wrestling training had little effect on growth or maturation, it did produce significant reductions in protein nutritional status, body protein and fat stores, and muscular strength and power.

B. Female Athlete Triad

Female athletes with eating disorders are at risk of developing amenorrhea and premature osteoporosis; the three issues together compose the female athlete triad.[49] Each component of this triad increases the chance of morbidity and mortality. Amenorrhea is characterized by low levels of circulating estrogen. Two major categories of amenorrhea exist; primary amenorrhea is the absence of menarche by the age of 16, and secondary amenorrhea is the absence of three to six consecutive menstrual periods after normal menses have begun.

Many nutritional and physiological factors have been associated with amenorrhea. Frequently cited are weight loss, low body-fat levels, excessive exercise, and nutritional inadequacy.[50] Research has failed to consistently show that one single factor causes amenorrhea; in all likelihood, it results from a combination of factors. The prevalence of amenorrhea in athletes varies between and within sport groups. In a study of 226 elite female athletes, gymnasts had the highest incidence of amenorrhea (71%), followed by lightweight rowers (46%) and runners (45%).[51]

A primary concern of amenorrheic athletes is reduced bone mineral density.[52] Compared with regularly menstruating athletes, amenorrheic athletes have significantly lower bone mineral density and this can occur at multiple skeletal sites including the femoral neck, lumbar spine, and lower leg.[53] Goebel et al.[54] found that low bone mineral density was significantly correlated to present and past minimum weights in patients with eating disorders.

The primary cause of reduced bone mineral density in amenorrheic athletes is low circulating levels of estrogen. The major health consequences of decreased bone mineral density are higher chances of stress fractures and premature osteoporosis.

In managing athletic amenorrhea, treatment goals include:[55]

- Reestablish normal weight and menstrual cycle
- Reduce training level
- Increase caloric intake

Although an increase in bone density may occur before the return of normal menses, this increase may still be significantly below the normal range for optimal bone health. If female athletes are not willing to change their training routine or diet, estrogen replacement therapy and calcium supplementation may be necessary to preserve and protect bone mass.[56]

VII. Identification and Assessment

If an athlete is suspected of having an eating disorder, it is important to intervene. Many colleges and universities have developed policies and procedures addressing the identification, intervention and treatment of eating disorders. A multidisciplinary team of professionals who have knowledge in the different areas of recovery offers the best approach. The team includes a physician, psychologist, psychiatrist, nutrition therapist and coach or athletic trainer.

Members of the treatment team work closely together so that messages communicated to the athlete are consistent. The team should have experience working with athletes and have an appreciation for the particular sport. Athletes can be afraid to talk about eating disorders because they are fearful of losing a financial scholarship or their place on the team. If athletes' eating disorders put them at risk for medical complications and they are not willing to comply, a written contract signed by the coach, treatment team and the athlete may be necessary. To stay on the team, the athlete is required to show up for counseling and medical appointments.

Because eating disorders are biopsychosocial in nature, thorough assessment of medical parameters as well as beliefs and behaviors is necessary to fully understand the impact of the eating disorder on the individual's well-being.

A. Medical Nutritional Evaluation

The medical nutritional evaluation should center around five categories of information:

1. *Food eaten*: amount, variety, timing of eating, presence of other individuals vs. eating alone, eating location, amount of time spent thinking about, preparing and eating.

2. *Exercise behavior*: type, frequency, duration, intensity, variety of exercises performed, purpose of exercise, what triggers exercise cessation, time of day and where exercise is performed.

3. *Compensatory behaviors used*: restrictive eating, skipping meals, self-induced vomiting (need to distinguish if vomiting is induced or is spontaneous upon eating), diet pills, laxatives, ergogenic metabolic enhancers.

4. *Supplements*: vitamins, minerals, meal replacements, ergogenic aids, herbs.

5. *Feelings about food and body*: thoughts and feelings that influence choices made in the above categories, rules that are used to eliminate foods or food groups (including vegetarian practices).

If a food journal is used to obtain information, keep in mind the strong likelihood of overreporting intake in anorexia and underreporting intake in bulimia. It is important to accept the information provided by the client without judgment (be sure that facial expressions, body language, and tone of voice do not create the impression that the clinician disapproves or believes the client is lying about what was eaten). Eating disorders are often accompanied with cognitive distraction. It is important to understand that this distraction serves a purpose. Completion of a food journal requires a cognitive movement away from distraction to being aware of the present moment. If that awareness is painful or anxiety producing, the client may not be able to complete food records. If a client comes to sessions without food records, discussing what happened that prevented their completion can be equally as therapeutic as discussing what was recorded. It is important to individualize nutrition assessments to accommodate the ability of the client to provide information.

Height, weight, and body composition are important to determine as well. It is important to obtain this information in a compassionate manner, as the numbers needed for clinical assessment contain emotional meaning to the person being evaluated. Because many of the behaviors included in the eating disorder affect hydration status, weight is highly likely to be variable and may not be the most reliable indicator of nutrition status. It is important to work with the client toward comfort with numbers that may feel threatening, while, at the same time, not putting so much emphasis on weight as a marker of progress that the client is encouraged to manipulate it to gain the "approval" of the treatment team. Many practitioners prefer to weigh the client facing backward on the scale to reduce the anxiety surrounding weight. This method needs to be explained to clients prior to weigh-in so they understand the purpose of the method.

Body composition can be a useful measurement. However, it is important to use body fat percentages in conjunction with information about lean body mass and midarm muscle circumference to avoid promoting an obsession with body fat as a substitution for an obsession with weight. It is also important, when calculating weight goals for recovery, to base these calculations on what a healthy amount of lean tissue would be.[58] Most body fat formulas only manipulate the weight in the fat compartment; in an individual whose eating disorder has compromised muscle and lean tissue, using body fat formulas as they were designed to be used in healthy individuals may result in significantly underestimating a healthy goal weight.

Because individuals with eating disorders tend to be dehydrated, any body composition measurement based on total body water is likely to be inaccurate, and to overestimate body fat percentage. Standard calipers are the preferred measurement tool for this population. When using calipers, it is important to perform assessment measurements in a comfortable environment. When possible, choose a quiet, private location, away from mirrors. Be sure to talk the client through the measurements you will be taking before touching any body part. If clients feel uncomfortable with any measurement, or having the body composition measurement taken at all, honor their feelings and delay this measurement until they consent to participation.

Psychological evaluation indicates that eating disorders very frequently occur with other psychological and psychiatric diagnoses, including:

- Anxiety disorder[57]
- Depression,[31] bipolar disorder[58]
- Obsessive-compulsive disorder[59]
- Post-traumatic stress disorder[59]
- Substance abuse[59]
- Schizophrenia[59]

The eating disorder is often secondary to these diagnoses and cannot respond to intervention until the core diagnosis is addressed. For some individuals, recovery may be impossible without the inclusion of psychotropic medications. It is important to ask athletes if they have ever been treated for any problems by a psychologist, therapist, social worker, or psychiatrist, or if there is any family member with any of the above diagnoses, and, if there is a positive history, to refer clients for evaluation. Even if no history is reported, it is important that athletes receive a thorough psychological or psychiatric evaluation in addition to nutrition therapy to have a complete understanding of the thought patterns and influences that shape their attitudes and behavior toward food and exercise.

Mental health diagnoses tend to be feared or rejected, as they may imply "craziness." Oftentimes, people with eating disorders will seek the help of a nutrition therapist hoping that a nutritional answer will allow them to avoid psychological treatment. It is crucial that the nutrition therapist not allow the reluctant client to receive nutrition therapy without collaboration from qualified mental health practitioners. Eating disorders are complex syndromes with neuroendocrine, nutritional and emotional components, and they require input from specialists in each of these disciplines to respond to any intervention.

Behavioral evaluation is just as important to recovery as restoration of a healthy weight and nutrition status are attitudes about self, body and food. If focus is placed on restoring food and weight but the thoughts and behaviors that created unhealthy eating and weight behaviors are not addressed, the client is likely to relapse as a result of those untreated core thoughts and behaviors. Many validated inventories are available to measure an individual's progress in the behavioral realm. Most inventories are self-reported. While they are relatively cheap and easy to administer, it is important to keep in mind that individuals who are in denial about the severity of their illness can defend this position by not answering the inventory questions honestly. An athlete may be motivated to minimize the existence of a problem if there is a concern that an athletic scholarship may be lost if an eating disorder is revealed. Therefore, these surveys may work better in anonymous screenings and surveys where the individual's identity is not revealed. The most frequently used self-report inventories are summarized in Table 4.1. Structured interviews, in which the clinician interviews the client using a predetermined sequence of questions, is another method of gathering information that can be used to make a diagnosis. While the client may still not be completely forthcoming in providing information, in situations where there is time to utilize such interviews, they may provide information pertinent to diagnosis and treatment planning. Two popular structured interviews are the Eating Disorder Examination (EDE)[67] and the Structured Clinical Interview for Axis I DSM-IV Disorders (SCID).[68]

VIII. The Role of the Sports Nutritionist in Treating Eating Disorders

The sports nutritionist is often the person in an athlete's life with the ability to identify and intervene when a potential eating disorder exists. It is not uncommon for an athlete to arrive at a consultation with complaints of fatigue, poor performance, the inability to gain weight with strength training, feeling cold, and extreme mood changes. In the early stages of an eating disorder, the athlete may present with a strong sense of denial. The goal is to establish a trusting relationship so that the athlete will return for further counseling. Assessment will not occur in a single session, but will evolve as rapport strengthens between the athlete and the sports nutritionist. The role of the sports nutritionist is to assist with the normalization of the athlete's weight and eating behavior. The responsibilities of the sports nutritionist include:[57]

- Evaluating the athlete's current food intake
- Estimating and determine the athlete's appropriate weight goal
- Supporting athletes as they try new eating behaviors
- Educating the athlete about normal and abnormal food intake patterns
- Helping the athlete understand weight and performance issues dispel myths and misconceptions about diet, health, and exercise (i.e., eating meat will make you fat; eating after 8 p.m. will result in weight gain)
- Teaching principles of good nutrition and planning
- Working with the multidisciplinary team in treating the athlete

When counseling the athlete with an eating disorder, remember that each athlete's recovery process is unique and treatment plans and goals should be individualized.[57] For the underweight athlete, the most important goal is to establish 95% of normal body weight. Weight gain is a priority because many of the existing symptoms of an eating disorder are secondary to starvation.[69] A weight gain of 0.5 kg (1 lb) per week is advised until the athlete achieves the desired goal weight.[57]

Physicians, trainers, coaches and athletes should be informed about eating disorders and what to do if a problem is suspected. Early detection and intervention are important to the athlete's health and performance. The preparticipation exam provides an opportunity to screen for disordered eating behaviors. Athletes should be questioned about weight and performance goals. If the athlete displays any of the warning signs of a possible eating disorder, nutrition counseling should be provided. If a nutrition intervention is implemented, it is important for all personnel providing guidance to the athlete (including coaches, trainers, strength coaches, etc.) to agree on who will discuss weight and nutrition and who will not. It is important to minimize the chance of giving conflicting information, and to avoid overwhelming the athlete with too much focus on food and weight gain. This kind of focus could result in intensifying the symptoms instead of promoting recovery.

Emphasizing the role of good nutrition and weight control in optimizing athletic performance can reduce the risk of triggering an eating disorder. If an athlete's performance is declining, it is important to not suggest weight loss to improve speed, strength or appearance without ruling out other factors. Many times, body fat or body weight is not the issue, and the attempt to lose weight by dieting or purging only predisposes the athlete to — or exacerbates — the depression that was the root of the problem to begin with.

Education is a primary tool for reducing the risk of eating disorders in athletes. Because coaches, trainers, and parents have the ability to negatively or positively influence the athlete, it is essential that they be included in educational programs regarding healthy weight, body image and performance. Results of a recent study found that fewer than half of 258 NCAA Division I coaches from five universities (44.5%) reported ever having attended an educational program about eating disorders.[70] This is surprising, considering that, in 1989, the NCAA provided NCAA schools with educational videos and materials on eating disorders. Furthermore, a number of colleges and universities have implemented prevention, education and intervention programs. Perhaps these programs are sponsored by campus recreation centers instead of athletic departments, making resources more available to students than athletes and coaches.

Programs aimed at reducing the cultural obsession with thinness and society's distorted meaning of gender identity are needed. Eating Disorders Awareness and Prevention, Inc. (EDAP), is a national nonprofit organization dedicated to prevention of eating disorders. It provides information to health-care professionals, educators, families, friends, and sufferers. One of the programs sponsored by EDAP is *Eating Disorders Awareness Week (EDAW)*. During a week in February, volunteer coordinators -- health professionals and educators -- organize educational outreach programs and presentations in schools and communities. EDAP also provides videos, curricula, a newsletter, conferences, workshops, and a national speaker's bureau.

IX. Summary

Eating disorders, in their many presentations, are a risk of athletic participation. Whether the symptoms fit the DSM-IV diagnostic criteria, (e.g., anorexia nervosa, bulimia nervosa and binge eating disorder), or present in symptom combinations not yet formally recognized (e.g., muscle dysmorphia, anorexia athletica and exercise dependence), these syndromes reflect internal neuroendocrine imbalance that can affect performance, health and even ability to sustain life.

Some sports seem to have more eating disorders than others. Those sports most susceptible include the aesthetic sports, which emphasize weight and appearance, and individual sports, such as running, which may appeal to individuals with compulsive personality characteristics.

Athletes looking to dietary changes to enhance performance may become susceptible to eating disorders, particularly if these changes focus on significant calorie reduction. Athletes with body types (endomorphic) not traditionally seen in successful athletes may turn to diets as a way to gain an edge that was not given to them genetically. It is important to be aware of food habits and mealtime behaviors exhibited by athletes; these might be clues that intervention and counseling are needed.

Many theories as to the etiology of eating disorders have been proposed. Currently, there is no evidence to support any one theory over any other. What *is* known is that these diagnoses contain imbalances in medical, nutritional, psychological and neuroendocrine functioning that require the intervention of a team of specialists who understand the complexity of the interactions of each of these areas of functioning. Assessment should consider nutritional needs, psychological factors and behavioral or attitudinal issues that affect athletes' ability to perceive and respond to their environment. Treatment planning should include interventions in each of these areas, even if the athlete insists the problem is purely nutritional.

Sports nutritionists are an important part of screening and treatment of eating disorders. In addition, they can be a source of accurate information regarding nutrition and supplements that the athlete can use when working toward recovery. When possible, the sports nutritionist can be most effective in the area of prevention, minimizing the possibility that an eating disorder has fertile ground in which to grow.

References

1. American Psychiatric Association. *Diagnostic and Statistical Manual of Mental Disorders,* 4th ed., Washington, D.C., 1994.
2. Bulik, C.M., Sullivan, P.F., Fear, J.L.and Joyce, P.R. Eating disorders and antecedent anxiety disorders: a controlled study. *Acta Psychiatr Scand,* 96, 101, 1997.
3. Neumarker, K.J. Mortality and sudden death in anorexia nervosa. *Int J Eat Disord,* 21, 205, 1997.
4. Kinzl J.F., Traweger, C., Trefalt, E., Mangweth, B.and Biebl, W. Binge eating disorder in females: a population-based investigation. *Int J Eat Disord,* 25, 287, 1999.
5. Pope, H.G. Jr, Gruber, A.J., Choi, P., Olivardia, R., Phillips, K.A. Muscle dysmorphia. An underrecognized form of body dysmorphic disorder. *Psychosomatics,* 38, 548, 1997.
6. Olivardia, R., Pope, H.G. Jr. and Hudson, J.I. Muscle dysmorphia in male weightlifters: a case-control study. *Am J Psych,* 157, 1291, 2000.
7. Rudy, E.B. and Estok, P.J. Running addiction and dyadic adjustment. *Res Nurs Health,* 13, 219, 1990.
8. Yates, A., Shisslak, C.M., Allender, J., Crago, M.and Leehey, K. Comparing obligatory to nonobligatory runners. *Psychosomatics,* 33, 180, 1992.
9. Veale, D.M. Psychological aspects of staleness and dependence on exercise. *Int J Sports Med,* 12, S19, 1991.
10. Taub, D.E. and Blinde, E.M. Eating disorders among adolescent female athletes: influence of athletic participation and sport team membership. *Adolescence,* 27, 833, 1992.
11. Ziegler, P., Hensley, S., Roepke, J.B., Whitaker, S.H., Craig, B.W and Drewnowski, A. Eating attitudes and energy intakes of female skaters. *Med Sci Sports Exerc,* 30:583J, 1998.

12. McNulty, K.Y., Adams, C.H., Anderson, J.M.and Affenito, S.G. Development and validation of a screening tool to identify eating disorders in female athletes. *J Am Diet Assoc*, 101, 886, 2001.
13. Sundgot-Borgen, J. Prevalence of eating disorders in elite female athletes. *Int J Sport Nutr*, 3, 29,1993.
14. Fogelholm, M. and Hiilloskorpi, H. Weight and diet concerns in Finnish female and male athletes. *Med Sci Sports Exerc*, 31, 229, 1999.
15. Gardner, R.M., Stark, K., Friedman, B.N.and Jackson, N.A. Predictors of eating disorder scores in children ages 6 through 14: a longitudinal study. *J Psychosom Res*, 49(3):199, 2000.
16. Braun, D.L., Sunday, S.R., Huang, A. and Halmi, K.A. More males seek treatment for eating disorders. *Int J Eat Disord*, 25, 415, 1999.
17. Shapiro, S., Newcomb, M. and Loeb, T.B. Fear of fat, disregulated-restrained eating, and body-esteem: prevalence and gender differences among 8- to 10-year-old children. *J Clin Child Psychol*, 26, 358, 1997.
18. Huon, G., Lim, J., and Gunewardene, A. Social influences and female adolescent dieting. *J Adolesc*, 23, 229, 2000.
19. Krowchuk, D.P., Kreiter, S.R., Woods, C.R., Sinal, S.H and DuRant, R.H. Problem dieting behaviors among young adolescents. *Arch Pediatr Adolesc Med*, 152, 884, 1998.
20. Patton, G.C., Selzer, R., Coffey, C., Carlin, J.B and Wolfe, R. Onset of adolescent eating disorders: population based cohort study over 3 years. *BMJ*, 318, 765, 1999.
21. Selby, R., Weinstein, H.M. and Bird, T.S. The health of university athletes: attitudes, behaviors, and stressors. *J Am Coll Health*, 39, 11, 1990.
22. Karlson, K.A., Becker, C.B. and Merkur, A. Prevalence of eating disordered behavior in collegiate lightweight women rowers and distance runners. *Clin J Sport Med*, 11, 32, 2001.
23. Sundgot-Borgen, J. Risk and trigger factors for the development of eating disorders in female elite athletes. *Med Sci Sports Exerc*, 26, 414, 1994.
24. Claessens, A.L., Lefevre, J., Beunen, G. and Malina, R.M. The contribution of anthropometric characteristics to performance scores in elite female gymnasts. *J Sports Med Phys Fitness*, 39, 355, 1999.
25. Rickarby, G.A. Psychosocial dynamics in anorexia nervosa. *Med J Aust*, 30, 587, 1979.
26. Marcus, M.D., Loucks, T.L. and Berga, S.L. Psychological correlates of functional hypothalamic amenorrhea. *Fertil Steril*, 76, 310, 2001.
27. Ivarsson, T., Rastam, M., Wentz, E., Gillberg, I.C., and Gillberg, C. Depressive disorders in teenage-onset anorexia nervosa: a controlled longitudinal, partly community-based study. *Compr Psychiatry*, 41, 398, 2000.
28. Koo-Loeb, J.H., Costello, N., Light, K.C. and Girdler, S.S. Women with eating disorder tendencies display altered cardiovascular, neuroendocrine, and psychosocial profiles. *Psychosom Med*, 62, 539, 2000.
29. Zaider, T.I., Johnson, J.G. and Cockell, S.J. Psychiatric comorbidity associated with eating disorder symptomatology among adolescents in the community. *Int J Eat Disord*, 28, 58, 2000.
30. Podar, I., Hannus, A. and Allik, J. Personality and affectivity characteristics associated with eating disorders: a comparison of eating disordered, weight-preoccupied, and normal samples. *J Pers Assess*, 73, 133, 1999.

31. Striegel-Moore, R.H., Garvin, V., Dohm, F.A. and Rosenheck, R.A. Eating disorders in a national sample of hospitalized female and male veterans: detection rates and psychiatric comorbidity. *Int J Eat Disord*, 25, 405, 1999.
32. Lennkh, C., Strnad, A., Bailer, U., Biener, D., Fodor, G and de Zwaan, M. Comorbidity of obsessive compulsive disorder in patients with eating disorders. *Eat Weight Disord*, 3, 37, 1998.
33. Bamber, D., Cockerill, I.M. and Carroll, D. The pathological status of exercise dependence. *Br J Sports Med*, 34, 125, 2000.
34. Cash, T.F., Novy, P.L. and Grant, J.R. Why do women exercise? Factor analysis and further validation of the Reasons for Exercise Inventory. *Percept Mot Skills*, 78, 539, 1994.
35. Dewsnap, P.A .Exercise dependence. *Br J Addict*, 83, 446, 1988.
36. Richert, A.J. and Hummers, J.A. Patterns of physical activity in college students at possible risk for eating disorder. *Int J. Eating Disord*, 5(4), 757, 1986.
37. Davis, C., Kennedy, S.H., Ravelski, E., and Dionne, M. The role of physical activity in the development and maintenance of eating disorders. *Psychol Med*, 24, 957, 1994.
38. Brewerton, T.D., Stellefson, E.J., Hibbs, N., Hodges, E.L. and Cochrane, C.E. Comparison of eating disorder patients with and without compulsive exercising. *Int J Eat Disord*, 17, 413, 1995.
39. Davis, C. and Claridge, G. The eating disorders as addiction: a psychobiological perspective. *Addict Behav*, 23, 463, 1998.
40. Matsunaga, H., Kiriike, N., Iwasaki, Y., Miyata, A., Yamagami, S. and Kaye, W.H. Clinical characteristics in patients with anorexia nervosa and obsessive-compulsive disorder. *Psychol Med*, 29, 407, 1999.
41. Davis, C., Kaptein, S., Kaplan, A.S., Olmsted, M.P. and Woodside, D.B. Obsessionality in anorexia nervosa: the moderating influence of exercise. *Psychosom Med*, 60, 192, 1998.
42. Dwyer, D. and Browning, J. Endurance training in Wistar rats decreases receptor sensitivity to a serotonin agonist. *Acta Physiol Scand*, 170, 211, 2000.
43. Bamber, D., Cockerill, I.M., Rodgers, S. and Carroll, D. "It's exercise or nothing": a qualitative analysis of exercise dependence. *Br J Sports Med*, 34, 423, 2000.
44. Beals, K.A. and Manore, M.M. Behavioral, psychological, and physical characteristics of female athletes with subclinical eating disorders. *Int J Sport Nutr Exerc Metab*, 10, 128, 2000.
45. Beals, K.A. and Manore, M.M. Nutritional status of female athletes with subclinical eating disorders. *J Am Diet Assoc*, 98, 419, 1998.
46. Sundgot-Borgen, J. Nutrient intake of female elite athletes suffering from eating disorders. *Int J Sport Nutr* 3, 431, 1993.
47. Shephard, R.J. Chronic fatigue syndrome: an update. *Sports Med*, 31, 167, 2001.
48. Roemmich, J.N. and Sinning, W.E. Weight loss and wrestling training: effects on nutrition, growth, maturation, body composition, and strength. *J Appl Physiol*, 82, 1751, 1997.
49. Yeager, K.K, Agostini, R., Nattiv, A. and Drinkwater, B. The female athlete triad: disordered eating, amenorrhea, osteoporosis. *Med Sci Sports Exerc* 25, 775, 1993.
50. Manore, M.M. Nutritional needs of the female athlete. *Clin Sports Med*, 18, 549, 1999.
51. Larsen, H.M. and Hansen, I.L. Effect of specific training on menstruation and bone strength. *Ugeskr Laeger*, 160, 4762, 1998.

52. Nattiv, A. Stress fractures and bone health in track and field athletes. *J Sci Med Sport*, 3, 268, 2000.

53. Pettersson, U., Stalnacke, B., Ahlenius, G., Henriksson-Larsen, K. and Lorentzon, R. Low bone mass density at multiple skeletal sites, including the appendicular skeleton in amenorrheic runners. *Calcif Tissue Int* 64, 117, 1999.

54. Goebel, G., Schweiger, U., Kruger, R. and Fichter, M.M. Predictors of bone mineral density in patients with eating disorders. *Int J Eat Disord* 25, 143, 1999.

55. Dueck, C.A., Matt, K.S. and Manore M.M.and Skinner, J.S. Treatment of athletic amenorrhea with a diet and training intervention program. *Int J Sport Nutr*, 6, 24, 1996.

56. Fagan, K.M. Pharmacologic management of athletic amenorrhea. *Clin Sports Med*, 17, 327, 1998.

57. Ruud, J.S., Woolsey, M.M. and Dorfman, L. Eating disorders in athletes, In *Sports Nutrition: A Guide for the Professional Working With Active People*, Rosenbloom, C.A., The American Dietetic Association, Chicago, IL, 1999, chap. 28.

58. Striegel-Moore, R.H., Garvin, V., Dohm, F.A. and Rosenheck, R.A. Eating disorders in a national sample of hospitalized female and male veterans: detection rates and psychiatric comorbidity. *Int J Eat Disord* 25, 405, 1999.

59. McElroy, S.L., Altshuler, Suppes, T., Keck, P.E., Jr, Frye, M.A, Denicoff, K.D., Nolen, W.A., Kupka, R.W., Leverich, G.S., Rochussen, J.R., Rush, A.J. and Post, R.M. Axis I psychiatric comorbidity and its relationship to historical illness variables in 288 patients with bipolar disorder. *Am J Psychiatry*, 158, 420, 2001.

60. Lennkh, C., Strnad, A., Bailer, U., Biener, D., Fodor, G. and de Zwaan, M. Comorbidity of obsessive compulsive disorder in patients with eating disorders. *Eat Weight Disord*, 3, 37, 1998.

61. Garner, D.M. and Olmsted, M.P. *The Eating Disorder Inventory Manual*. Psychological Assessment Resources, Odessa, TX, 1984.

62. Garner, D.M. *Eating Disorder Inventory-2 Professional Manual*, Psychological Assessment Resources, Inc., Odessa, TX, 1991.

63. Garner, D.M. and Garfinkel, P.E. The Eating Attitudes Test: an index of the symptoms of anorexia nervosa. *Psychol Med*, 9, 273, 1979.

64. Thelen, M.H., Farmer, J., Wonderlich, S and Smith, M. A revision of the Bulimia Test: the BULIT-R, *Psychological Assessment*, 3, 119, 1991.

65. Mintz, L.B., O'Halloran, M.S., Mulholland, A.M and Schneider, P.A. Questionnaire for eating disorder diagnoses: reliability and validity of operationalizing DSM-IV criteria into a self-report format. *J Counseling Psychol*, 44, 63, 1997.

66. Mizes, J.S. and Klesges, R.C. Validity, reliability, and factor structure of the anorectic cognitions questionnaire. *Addictive Behaviors*, 14, 589, 1989.

67. Cooper, Z. and Fairburn, C. The Eating Disorder Examination: a semi-structured interview for the assessment of the specific psychopathology of eating disorders. *Int J Eating Disorders*, 6, 1, 1997.

68. *First, M.B, Spitzer, R.L., Gibbon, R.L, Gibbon, M. and Williams, J.B.W. Structured Clinical Interview for Axis I DSM-IV Disorders, Patient Edition (SCID-L, Version 2.0)*, Biometrics Research Department, New York, 1994.

69. Mehler, P.S., Gray, M.C., and Schulte, M. Medical complications of anorexia nervosa. *J Women's Health* 6, 533, 1997.

Section Three

Anthropometric Assessment of Athletes

5

Assessment of Growth in Child Athletes

Jean E. Guest, Nancy L. Lewis and James R. Guest

CONTENTS

I. Introduction

Children are not just little adults. This pediatric mantra refers to the unique medical, nutritional, psychological and physical requirements of childhood. These requirements are associated with the dynamic process of growth. Children between 5 and 12 years of age experience constant height (HT), weight (WT), and body mass increases.[1] Routine assessment of physical growth to assure maintenance of a normal growth pattern is central to good health and well-being during childhood. It is particularly important for child athletes whose nutritional status and physical activity are heavily influenced by training programs.

Anthropometry is the scientific study of human body measurement.[2] Various anthropometric measurements (Z scores) have been identified for use in assessing body composition in children. In this chapter HT, WT, body mass index (BMI), triceps skinfold thickness (TSF), midarm muscle circumference (MAC), midarm muscle area (MAMA), and bioelectric impedance (BIA), will be discussed. Anthropometric information included in this chapter is focused on healthy prepubescent children (Tanner[3] stage I), and may not be valid in children experiencing early maturation.

II. Assessment of Growth

Children grow at constant and predictable rates. However, individual growth patterns may vary. Standardized growth charts provide an easy and effective tool to monitor individual growth in children. Deviation from established growth norms alert physicians and other health care professionals to potential health problems associated with alterations in growth patterns.[4]

School-age children experience steady physical growth with a mean WT increase of 3 kilograms (kg) to 3.5 kg per year (6.6 pounds (lbs) to 7.7 lbs), and a mean HT increase of 6.0 cm per year (2.4 inches). This period of steady increase in HT and WT ends in a prepubescent growth spurt at about age 10 years in females and 12 years in males.[1]

Physiological growth is influenced by four factors: genetic, neurohumoral, nutritional, and mechanical force. Influence of genetic transmissibility on growth is estimated to range from 41% to 71%.[4,5] Neurohumoral influence depends on energy balance,[6] and specific growth factors.[7,8] Stimulation and release of growth hormone, thyroid hormones (T3 and T4), and sex steroid (gonadal and adrenal) hormones for the express purpose of facilitating growth is dependent on positive nutritional status.[9-12] Mechanical force promotes muscle development[13] and bone mineralization.[14,15] Childhood sets the stage for the significant growth maturation associated with adolescence and signaled by the onset of puberty.

A. Growth Charts

H.P. Bowditch,[16] dean of Harvard Medical School, developed the first growth charts in the United States in 1877. These represented the average HT and WT of American schoolchildren, and were based on school-age children in Boston. Growth patterns in school-age children were well described by Boas[17] and others,[18-21] resulting in development of many age- and gender-specific growth charts. Those developed prior to 1977 were limited in clinical application due to a lack of ethnic, genetic, geographical and statistical representation. They also lacked expert agreement on reference data.[18-22] In 1977, the National Center for Health Statistics (NCHS) published the first growth charts incorporating large, nationally representative samples of children (NCHS Health Education Survey [HES][23] and Health and Nutrition

Education Survey [HANES][24]) with expert agreement of reference data.[22] The 1977 NCHS growth charts, which were adopted for worldwide use by the World Health Organization,[25-27]included age-specific weight-for-height (WT/HT) percentiles.[23,24]

Secular population changes as well as improved curve smoothing statistical and transformation[28] techniques require periodic updating of growth charts. The Centers for Disease Control (CDC) collaborated with the National Center for Chronic Disease Prevention and Health Promotion (NCCDPHP) and the NCHS to develop updated growth charts (Tables 5.1–5.6). These were published by CDC in May 2000.[29] The 2000 CDC/NCHS growth charts include data from NCHS surveys conducted between 1963 and 1994 (two cycles of the National Health Examination Survey [NHES II and III] and three cycles of the National Health and Nutrition Examination Surveys [NHANES I, II, and III]).

The 2000 CDC/NCHS growth charts were developed to provide a more useful growth assessment tool for clinicians and other health care providers. Clinically relevant changes provided in the 2000 CDC/NCHS growth charts include extending HT and WT percentile ranges from 5th and 95th percentiles to 3rd and 97th percentiles, and the upper age limit from 18 years to 20 years. Additionally, age-specific WT/HT percentiles were replaced with age-specific BMI percentiles. BMI is a more specific indicator of relative WT.[21] Concerns regarding increasing rates of obesity in children in the United States prompted inclusion of BMI percentiles in the updated growth charts.

Appropriate use and interpretation of growth charts includes accuracy of measurement techniques, devices, and recording. Longitudinal tracking of growth data is essential to providing adequate data for monitoring of growth. Single plot data is of little value. Measurement and recording of growth data over time is the only method by which valid assessment of growth can be made during childhood.

B. Height

Height (linear growth) provides insight into individual health and nutritional status. Tanner[3] has suggested that accurate monitoring of linear growth in children identifies medical or physiologic anomalies that influence linear growth. Appropriate linear growth reflects adequacy of energy intake for a particular training regimen in child athletes.

Normal linear growth is considered to be encompassed by the 95th percentile confidence interval for a specific population. Children with a linear growth pattern that remains below the lower 2.5 percentile (approximately –2.0 standard deviation [SD]), and who are otherwise normal should reach genetically determined height potential. However, children whose linear growth falls below –2.0 SD are more likely to have a condition preventing the attainment of genetically determined HT potential.[30]

TABLE 5.1

Males 2–20 Height-for-Age Growth Chart

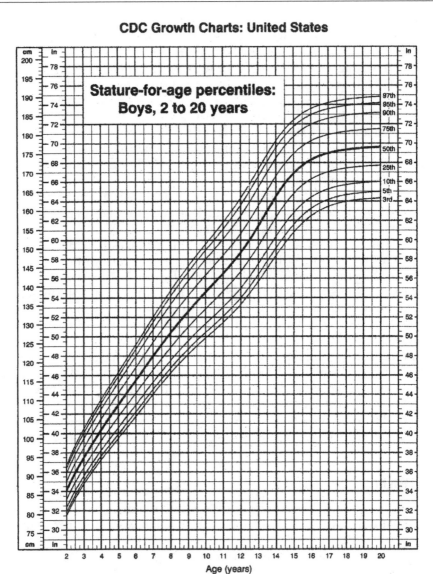

Conflicting reports of linear growth status in young male[31] and female[32] athletes in the early 1960s have resulted in continuing concern about linear growth in child athletes. Malina and Bielicki[33] in 1966 reported that 25 males aged 10 years to 12 years did not differ significantly from chronological age (CA) references until adolescence, when skeletal age (SA) progressed significantly (p < 0.01) relative to CA. In this same study, Malina and Bielicki[33]

TABLE 5.2

Females 2–20 Years Height-for-Age Growth Chart

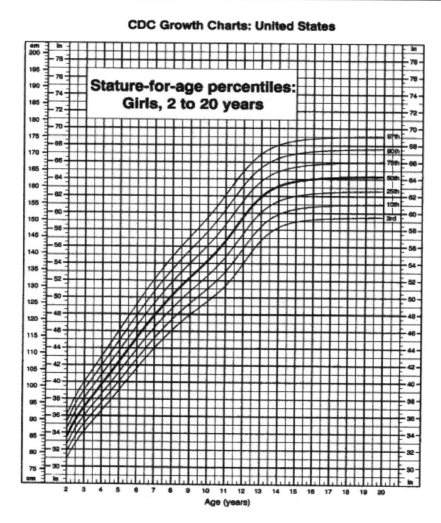

reported that 13 female athletes aged 8 years to 18 years had significant (p < 0.05 and 0.01) differences in HT, but not body WT compared with references.

Studies in children participating in specific sports such as gymnastics (male and female), ballet dancing (female), figure skating (female), and diving (male) have demonstrated shorter stature compared with reference data.[34] The relationship between sports activity and linear growth may be related specifically to the type and intensity of athletic competition and training.

The question of whether short stature results from selection bias or intensive physical training involved in some sports was explored by Daly et al.[35] Competitive prepubertal and early pubertal (Tanner[3] stage ≤ 2) male

TABLE 5.3

Males 2–20 Years Weight-for-Age Growth Chart

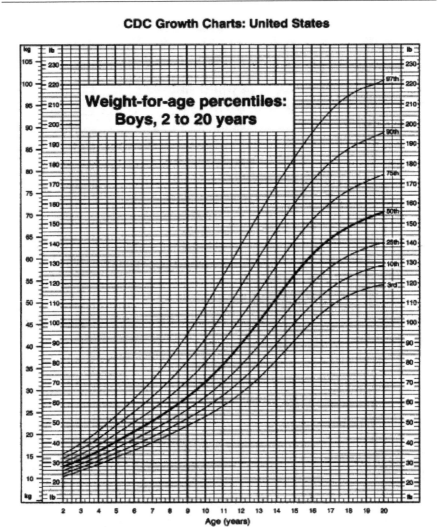

gymnasts (n = 31) were studied along with a normo-active control group (n = 35). Serial HT, sitting HT, leg length, and segmental lengths (humerus, radius, femur, and tibia) and breadths (bi-acromial and bi-iliac), diet, serum insulin-like growth factor-I (IGF-I), testosterone, and cortisol measurements were collected every 3 months to 4 months over an 18-month period. Results indicated that, although at baseline gymnasts were a mean 0.7 years older than the control group (p < 0.05); n = 50), there were no differences in maturity (Tanner[3] stage) levels. Age-adjusted Z scores showed that the gymnasts were shorter than controls (–0.5 ± –0.2 SD; p < 0.05) because of reduced

TABLE 5.4

Females 2–20 Years Weight-for-Age Growth Chart

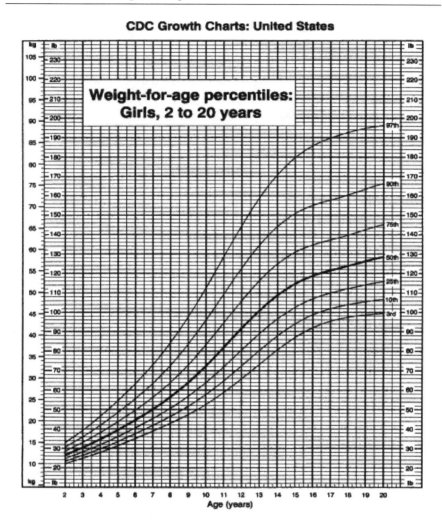

leg length (–0.8 ± –0.2 SD; p < 0.001), but not sitting height. Age-adjusted Z scores for segmental lengths and bi-iliac breadth were also reduced in the gymnasts (p range < 0.05 to < 0.001). No significant differences were detected for serum IGF-I or cortisol. After 18 months of follow-up, there were no differences in rate of change in HT, sitting HT or leg lengths, segmental lengths, IGF-I, or cortisol between gymnasts and control subjects who remained prepubertal and early pubertal (gymnasts n = 18; controls n = 35). However, the magnitude of baseline differences in Z scores persisted throughout the study. These authors concluded that short stature, but not sitting HT, in these competitive male gymnasts was due to a reduced leg

TABLE 5.5

Males 2–20 Years Body Mass Index-for-Age Growth Chart

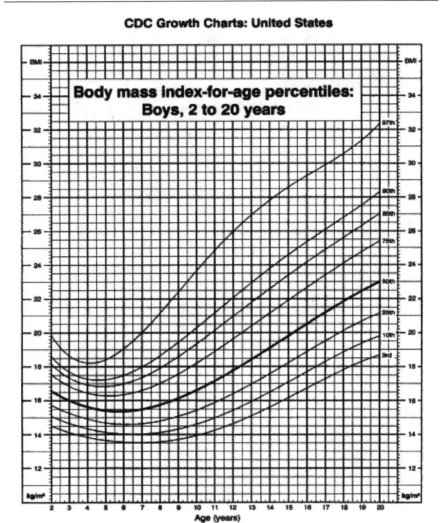

length. Lack of difference in growth rates, IGF-I, and diet over the 18-month period indicated that short stature reported in male gymnasts was due to selection bias rather than gymnastics training.

Another study assessing body composition in female junior elite gymnasts (n = 146) was conducted by Benardot and Czerwinski.[36] In this study, selected body composition measurements were performed cross sectionally. The gymnasts were divided into a younger age group (7 years to 10 years) and an older age group (11 years to 14 years). Their results indicated gymnasts in this study were in the 50th percentile for WT/HT ratio, regardless of age.

TABLE 5.6

Females 2-20 Years Body Mass Index-for-Age Growth Chart

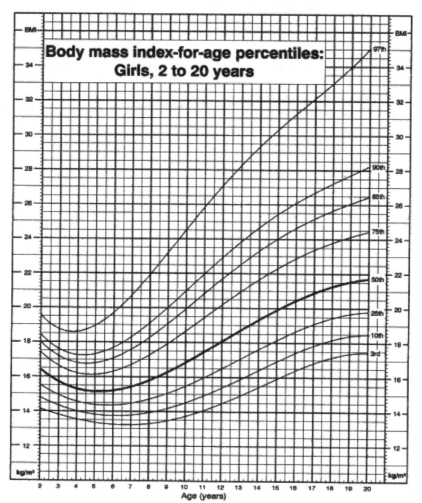

However, WT/age and HT/age percentiles progressively dropped from 48th percentile to 20th percentile as age increased. Body fat percentage did not differ significantly between the two age groups. Triceps and subscapular skinfolds decreased when compared with age-related standards with the 7-year-old and 10-year-old groups at 63rd percentile and 56th percentile, respectively, while the 11-year-old and 14-year-old groups were 52nd percentile and 39th percentile, respectively. Arm muscle circumference and calculated arm muscle area were about 75th percentile regardless of the gymnasts' age grouping. In general, as they grew older, gymnasts became progressively smaller in HT and WT for age but were highly muscled for size. These authors concluded the steady age-related drop in HT/age and WT/age percentiles may be attributable to nutritional deficits, a sport-specific selection favoring retention of small but powerful gymnasts, or a combination of these two factors. Furthermore, these authors recommend that young gymnasts should be carefully monitored longitudinally by trained professionals for any signs of growth disruption.

Ideally, linear growth measurement in children is accomplished by use of a stadiometer. Use of movable measuring rods on platform scales is not recommended. Stadiometers should be wall mounted and leveled to assure accuracy of measurements. Linear growth measurements should be performed while the child stands erect on an uncarpeted floor, shoulder blades and buttocks flush against the measurement surface, heels almost together, feet bare or in very thin stockings. The child's shoulders should be relaxed with arms hanging on either side of the body, legs straight, knees almost touching, and head positioned such that the child is looking straight ahead (Frankfurt plane).[37,38] The mean of three serial HT measurements should be recorded on an age- and gender-specific growth chart.

C. Weight

Weight is a crude measurement of body mass. The terms "desirable" or "ideal" are often used to characterize body WT. However, these terms define body WT only in relation to body HT. Body WT measurement alone is not a reliable indicator of lean or fat tissue body mass. Body WT changes in childhood are associated with age and maturational stage.[4]

Currently, assessment of WT status in children is focused on preventive screening of overnutrition (overweight or obesity) due to the increasing incidence of obesity in the United States.[39,40] However, children's concerns about their own body image also suggests a need for vigilance regarding undernutrition or disordered eating, which has been associated mainly with adolescent females,[41] but may now be occurring in prepubescent children.

A community-based intervention program aimed at the primary prevention of disordered eating in preadolescent females was studied by Neumark-Sztainer et al.[42] Girl Scouts (n = 226) with a mean age of 10.6 ± HT 0.7 years were randomized into control and intervention groups. Six 90-minute sessions focusing on media literacy and advocacy skills were presented as the intervention. Attitudes toward body image, media knowledge, dieting behaviors and habits were evaluated pre-intervention, post-intervention and at a 3-month follow-up.

Results in this study indicated that 29% of females (control and intervention) were trying to lose WT at the time of the pre-intervention evaluation. Short-term positive effects on body-related knowledge and attitudes (i.e., on body size acceptance, puberty knowledge, and perceived weight status) were observed post-intervention in the intervention group, but not in the control group. However, at the 3-month follow-up, these effects were no longer present and no significant dieting behavior changes were noted between the two groups.

WT concerns and body dissatisfaction are not limited to females. Robinson et al.[43] examined the prevalence of overweight concerns and body dissatisfaction among 969 third-grade males and females with a mean age of 8.5 years. These schoolchildren represented diverse ethnic (44% Caucasian, 21% Latino, 19% non-Filipino Asian American, 8% Filipino, and 5% African-American), and socioeconomic backgrounds. Assessment of overweight concerns, body dissatisfaction, and desired shape, HT, and WT were collected. Results demonstrated a desire to lose WT in 26% of males and 35% of females while 17% of males and 24% of females reported dieting to lose weight. In this study, body dissatisfaction and overweight concerns were highly prevalent among third-grade males and females regardless of ethnicity or socioeconomic status.

There are few WT or body satisfaction studies in child athletes. However, it is reasonable to assume that they share the concerns of their non-athletic child counterparts over WT and body satisfaction. Furthermore, as increasing numbers of children participate in "elite" sports or sports specialization requiring year-round intensive training, WT and body satisfaction issues are becoming the concern of individuals involved with these children. To address these concerns, the Committee on Sports Medicine and Fitness of the American Academy of Pediatrics[44] published recommendations for young athletes (Table 5.7). These recommendations include all areas of concern, but their emphasis on monitoring of WT status and body composition in child athletes should be noted.

TABLE 5.7

Intensive Training and Sports Specialization Recommendations for Child Athletes

Child athletes should:
- Participate in sports at a level consistent with their abilities and interests. Single-sport participation in prepubescent children should be discouraged.
- Participate in sports where coaches are properly trained and knowledgeable about child athlete needs and characteristics.
- Be monitored routinely for:
  - Early recognition and treatment of stress injuries, emotional stress, and overtraining (i.e., WT loss, anorexia, and sleep disturbances).
  - Nutritional status with serial anthropometric measurements assessing body composition (HT, WT, and TSF/MAC) to ensure adequacy of caloric intake and early identification of pathological eating behaviors.
- Be educated, along with family members and coaching personnel, about risks of heat injury and its prevention.

From American Academy of Pediatrics Committee on Sports Medicine and Fitness, Intensive training and sports specialization in young athletes, *Pediatrics,* 106, 154, 2000.

Ideally, WT measurement is accomplished by use of a beam balance scale. The beam balance scale should be calibrated (with standard weights) routinely, and zeroed prior to each use. Calibration and zeroing should also be performed after any movement or relocation of the scale. While spring balance scales are less reliable, they are less bulky and lighter for use in nonclinical settings. Use of digital scales in nonclinical settings is becoming more common, but the reliability of digital scales for use in children is unclear. Scales should be located on hard flat surfaces without carpeting.

Children should be weighed after emptying the bladder and prior to consuming any food or liquids. Ideally, children should be weighed naked, but this is not always practical. Therefore, light clothing or paper gowns can be worn without shoes or stockings. Standard corrections for clothing should not be used. WT measurement(s) should be recorded serially on an age- and gender-specific growth chart.[38]

D. Body Mass Index

Body type or physique results from genetic growth potential and environmental influences,[30] and may be helpful in assessing body composition. Body somatotypes include endomorphic, ectomorphic, and mesomorphic. Endomorphs are stocky, with excessive soft body tissue. Ectomorphs are lean, with a relatively small bone structure and small body mass. Mesomorphs are muscular, with relatively proportionate body mass. Somatotyping is useful for indicating body configuration, but not body mass.

A more useful indicator of body mass in assessment of weight-for-height is BMI. BMI is a better indicator of relative WT than WT/HT.[45] BMI is expressed as WT in kilograms (kg) divided by HT in meters (m) squared (kg/m^2). Mean BMI levels increase during the first year of life $(\sim 5 kg/m^2)$, decrease during early childhood, reach a nadir between 4 years and 8 years of age $(\sim 15 kg/m^2)$, and subsequently increase again until adulthood $(\sim 20–25 kg/m^2)$.[46] Application of BMI in children is limited by the varying growth and maturity levels associated with childhood.[47,48] Despite these inherent limitations, BMI has been selected by an expert committee on childhood obesity as the index of adiposity in children in the United States.[49]

Annual BMI increases in children, unlike adults, cannot be automatically attributed to concurrent increases in fat tissue body mass. To describe body composition changes in relation to BMI during childhood, Maynard et al.[50] evaluated 387 (201 males and 186 females) healthy Caucasian children, who were measured one to 11 times annually from ages 8 years to 18 years. Data collection for each child included HT, WT, BMI, total body fat (TBF), fat-free mass (FFM), and percent body fat (%BF). TBF and FFM were determined from hydrodensitometry, while BMI and %BF were calculated. Longitudinal data containing both cross-sectional and serial measurements totaling 1748 observations were analyzed. Annual changes in BMI, TBF/HT^2, FFM/HT^2,

WT, TBF and FFM were determined by analyzing an additional 1150 observations from a subset (n = 291) of children in this study.

Results in this study indicated that BMI values increased with age in both males and females. However, BMI was significantly (p < 0.005) higher in females than males at ages 12 years to 13 years. BMI and HT were positively and significantly (p < 0.005) correlated at ages 10 years to 14 years in males, and at age 9 years in females. BMI and WT were positively and significantly (p < 0.005) correlated at all ages in males and females. BMI correlations with %BF and TBF were generally stronger than BMI and FFM except in females aged 8 years and 13 years. Mean annual increases in BMI in males between ages 8 years and 9 years and between 12 years and 17 years resulted exclusively from increases in FFM/HT^2 with TBF/HT^2 decreasing. Corresponding mean BMI annual increases in females demonstrated both FFM/HT^2 and TBF/HT^2 were responsible at ages 8 years to 9 years and 10 years to 16 years, while FFM/HT^2 alone accounted for mean increase of BMI from ages 10 years to 14 years.

These authors concluded that BMI is a suitable measure of adiposity in children. Furthermore, BMI can be an effective clinical tool in assessing body composition changes over time during childhood. However, these authors caution that a few individuals with large BMI values may have greater FFM than TBF. Therefore, BMI interpretation must include consideration of both fat and lean compartments of body mass, which change annually and are associated with growth.

In another study, Pietrobelli et al.[51] tested BMI as a valid measure of fatness that is independent of age in both males and females in a healthy pediatric population. In this study, TBF (kg) and %BF were estimated by dual energy x-ray absorptiometry (DXA) in 188 (90 males and 98 females) Italian children and adolescents aged 5 years to 19 years. HT, WT, and DXA measurements were collected with standardized methods by the same technician on the same day. Statistical analysis included zero-order correlations to assess unadjusted associations among BMI, TBF, and %BF. Two sets of multiple regression analyses were performed where TBF and %BF were each used as the criterion-dependent variable. Also, separate gender analyses were conducted for each dependent variable.

Results in this study indicated a significant association between BMI and TBF (p < 0.0001) in males (R^2 = 0.85) and females (R^2 = 0.89). BMI explained 85% of between-subject TBF variance in males and 89% in females with an additional variance of 2% in males and 3% in females being observed with increasing age. BMI and %BF (p < 0.0001) were also significantly associated in both males (R^2 = 0.63) and females (R^2 = 0.69). BMI explained 63% of between-subject %BF variance in males and 69% in females. After adjusting for BMI in this study, increasing age was associated with significantly greater TBF and %BF in both males and females, which, these authors point out, is consistent with changes in body composition as children age.

These authors support the use of BMI as a fatness measure in groups of children and adolescents. However, they suggest cautious interpretation when comparing BMI across age groups or when predicting a specific individual's TBF or %BF.

In a similar analysis, Daniels et al.[47] demonstrated a correlation between BMI and %BF in 89 African-American and 103 Caucasian children (100 males and 92 females). BMI and %BF were highly correlated in African-American and Caucasian females ($R^2 = 0.83$) while BMI and %BF were less strongly correlated in African-American ($R^2 = 0.54$) and Caucasian ($R^2 = 0.50$) males. However, in this study, a multiple regression analysis indicated BMI, gender, ethnicity, Tanner[3] stage, and fat distribution (waist:hip ratio) were all highly significant independent correlates of %BF (multiple $R^2 = 0.77$). Additionally, BMI and %BF were dependent on sexual maturity, gender (females have greater %BF than males at equivalent BMI), ethnicity (Caucasians have higher %BF than African-Americans at equivalent BMI and waist:hip ratio, where Caucasian males had higher waist:hip ratios than African-American males at an equivalent BMI (individuals with central obesity have greater %BF than those with peripheral obesity).

An interesting characteristic of BMI is that, in addition to being highly correlated with TBF[47,51–53] and %BF, it is also correlated with FFM.[54] In children, BMI has a high specificity as an indicator of fat mass, but variable sensitivity.[55,56] Validity studies in children focus primarily on BMI as an index of overnutrition (obesity). Few, if any, studies address the validity of BMI as an index of undernutrition. BMI is limited in scope as a body composition assessment tool, especially in lean children such as child athletes.

Child athletes may have more lean tissue body mass than their non-athletic counterparts. Child athletes with high lean tissue body mass may at different stages of maturation have high BMI values while not being overweight or obese. Use of BMI as an assessment tool in child athletes or in very physically active children should be done with caution.

E. Other Anthropometric Measurements

All athletes are interested in the relationship between body composition and performance. The practice of modifying body composition to enhance physical performance is not uncommon. However, this practice may result in serious negative health outcomes in child athletes. Monitoring and assessing changes in specific lean- and fat-tissue body mass utilizing other anthropometric (TSF, MAC, MAMA, and BIA) measurements assists in assuring positive health outcomes in child athletes.

Reliability of anthropometric measurements (HT, WT, BMI, TSF, MAC, MAMA, and BIA) has been studied in varying clinical and nonclinical settings as well as among different ethnic groups.[57,58] The primary focus of anthropometric measurement studies in child athletes has been in relation to growth and physical performance.

Frequency of anthropometric data collection depends on the intensity of physical activity or training regimen. Serial measurement and recording of anthropometric measurements over time best represent changes in body composition. Interpretation of this data should utilize age- and gender-specific standardized reference norms.

1. Triceps Skinfold Thickness

TSF thickness is an index of body fatness.[59] Measurement of TSF thickness provides an indirect estimate of body fat percentage based on the size of the subcutaneous fat depot.[60] Triceps are the most common site of skinfold thickness measurements due to easy accessibility and close correlation with total body fat.[53] TSF measurement is thickest when compared with three other skinfold sites (subscapular, iliac, and abdominal) in 90% of children.[61]

Reliability of skinfold thickness measurements varies with age, size, hydration, examiner technique, and skinfold caliper precision. Examiner reliability requires training and experience in skinfold thickness collection methods. TSF thickness measurements are most reliable when obtained by the same examiner. Intra-examiner reliability has been demonstrated in adults,[62] though not in children.

Many types of skinfold thickness calipers are commercially available. These include spring-type (metal or plastic) and computerized digital models. Selection of type and model of skinfold thickness caliper should be determined by setting and utilization. Routine calibration is necessary to obtain valid data. Skinfold thickness calipers should exert a constant pressure of 10 g/mm, provide a range of at least 2mm to 40 mm, a contact surface of 20 mm to 40 mm, and be accurate to 0.1 mm.[59]

TSF thickness measurements should be obtained at the midpoint mark (see MAC section below for recommended midpoint arm measurement technique) on the posterior aspect of the nondominant arm. Use of the nondominant arm in collecting TSF thickness measurement is believed to provide a more accurate estimate of fat tissue body mass, although recommendations regarding the use of the right[59] or left[37] arm vary.

TSF thickness measurements should be performed on an uncovered arm with the subject standing, the arm hanging freely at the side of the body, and the palm of the hand facing forward. The skinfold parallel to the long axis of the arm at approximately 1 cm above the midpoint mark should be grasped between the examiner's thumb and forefinger while lifting slightly to separate fat and muscle tissue. Care should be taken to avoid tissue compression by not pinching too tightly. While holding the caliper in a horizontal position, its jaws should be applied to the midpoint mark. After waiting 3 to 4 seconds, the measurement nearest 0.1 mm on the scale should be read. The mean of three TSF thickness measurement readings should be recorded.[37,59,63] TSF thickness measurement recordings should be maintained with other anthropometric measurement records.

Interpretation of TSF thickness measurements should utilize gender- and age-specific reference standards developed by Frisancho.[64] These reference standards are based on NHANES I (1971–1974) and NHANES II (1976–1980) survey data, which are valid for use in children.

TSF thickness measurement may be a better indicator of fat tissue body mass than BMI. Use of BMI in child athletes with increased lean tissue body mass may result in falsely elevated BMI percentages. Therefore, TSF thickness measurements may best represent fat tissue body mass in child athletes.

2. Midarm Muscle Circumference

MAC is an index of lean tissue body mass. MAC represents the circumference of muscle mass surrounding a central core of bone.[65] MAC is a sensitive indicator of large — but not small — shifts in total lean tissue body mass.[66]

MAC measurements should be accomplished with the subject standing, arm uncovered and bent at a 90° angle, with the palm of the hand facing up. The midpoint between the lateral tip of the acromial process of the scapula and the olecranon process of the ulna should be located. A non-stretch measuring tape and a soft-tipped pen should be utilized in measuring and marking the midpoint between these two landmarks on the posterior aspect of the arm over the triceps muscle. The circumference of the arm should then be measured by drawing the nonstretch tape measure firmly around the arm at the midpoint mark, taking care to avoid compression of soft tissue. The MAC measurement reading should be taken to the nearest centimeter and recorded along with the TSF thickness measurement. Some authors[43,59,65] suggest MAC measurements should be collected on the non-dominant arm.

Interpretation of MAC measurements should incorporate gender- and age-specific reference standards developed by Frisancho.[64] In general, MAC has been suggested to be a sensitive indicator of morbidity and mortality risk in children.[67] However, MAC measurement in child athletes serves as an marker of current lean tissue body status.

3. Midarm Muscle Area

MAMA is an index of lean tissue body mass. [37,59,68] It is derived from TSF thickness and MAC measurements. MAMA reflects the true magnitude of any shifts in lean tissue body mass. However, MAMA overestimates lean tissue body mass in obese individuals and those with TSF thicknesses above the 85th percentile ranking for age and gender.[66]

Jelliffe and Jelliffe,[69] Gurney and Jelliffe,[70] Frisancho[64] and others[71] have developed regression equations using MAC and TSF thickness measurements to predict MAMA. MAMA can also be estimated by use of a nomogram developed by Gurney and Jelliffe.[70] Age- and gender-specific percentiles developed by Frisancho[64] should be utilized for MAMA interpretation.

4. Bioelectrical Impedance

BIA is an indirect, noninvasive method for assessing human body composition. It is based on the principle of human body impedance to a frequency-dependent flow of an administered alternating electrical current.

BIA measures a relationship among impedance, resistance, reactance and phase angle when an alternating electrical current is introduced into the body. Impedance is composed of resistance and reactance. Resistance is the opposition of the conductor (mainly ions in aqueous solutions) to the flow of electrical current. Reactance is the storage of voltage for a short period of time. Reactance in the human body is associated with polarization of electrical current by cell membranes and tissue interfaces.[72] Phase angle occurs when an administered current lags behind voltage, resulting in a phase shift.[73] The impedance plot created from the geometric relationship among impedance, resistance, reactance and phase angle is dependent on the frequency of the administered electrical current. Conduction cannot occur at too low a frequency, while only resistance occurs at too high a frequency.

Application of impedance theory in assessment of human body composition relies on various models. These include simple electrical circuit resistance[74] (based on extracellular fluid volume and composition) that encompasses single (50 kilohertz [kHz]) and multiple[75,76] (5 kHz and 1 kHz) signal frequencies as well as impedance spectroscopy[77-79] (scans from a few kHz up to megahertz [mKz]) and a parallel[80] model (predicts regional muscle mass).

Validity of BIA measurements may be limited by examiner reliability, environmental factors, and prediction equations utilized. Factors influencing examiner reliability include use of a nonconductive testing surface, appropriate subject position (supine), dominant-side application of electrodes (generally right side), analyzer calibration, and constant state timing of data collection. Environmental factors affecting BIA measurement accuracy include exposure to heat or acute exercise (increases peripheral blood flow), as well as cold exposure or restricted fluid intake (decreases peripheral blood flow).[81-83]

BIA measurement limitations discussed above apply to both adults and children. However, the application of BIA measurement in children is limited by the absence of a gold standard prediction equation. Several authors[24,84-86] have developed BIA prediction equations for use in children. However, a BIA prediction equation of choice for use in children has yet to be identified.

Is BIA a better predictor of body fatness than TSF or BMI? Bandini et al.[87] addressed this question while also attempting to cross-validate selected published equations for determination of FFM from BIA. In this study, HT, WT, BMI, TSF, and BIA were collected in 132 pre-menarcheal, non-obese females aged 8 years to 10 years. Correlation analysis was utilized to determine the relationship of %BF to TSF and BMI. Results demonstrated that the explained variance in the prediction of %BF was 70% by BIA, 68% by TSF, and only 38% by BMI. The predictive ability of published equations differed by

Tanner[3] stage. Kushner's equation (Kushner et al.,[86] 1992), based solely on HT^2/resistance was the only equation that provided estimates that did not differ significantly from measured values among all Tanner[3] stages. These authors concluded that BIA appeared to be a valid and reliable measure of FFM, but was no better than TSF in predictions of body fat.

The limitation presented by the absence of a BIA gold standard prediction equation for use in children prompted Nagano et al.[88] to explore BIA by use of phase angle without prediction equations. Phase angle has been reported to be a parameter reflecting body cell mass[89] and can be obtained from the measured values of electrical resistance and reactance.

Nagano et al.[88] included 71 well-nourished and 10 malnourished children aged 1 month to 12 years in their study. Anthropometric measurements collected in this study included HT, WT, % ideal body WT, TSF, MAC, %MAC, total protein, and serum albumin. A single-frequency (50 mKz) analyzer was used to collect BIA data. Results indicated a significant correlation between BIA and WT ($r = 0.818$; $p < 0.001$) as well as BIA and MAC ($r = 0.901$; $p < 0.001$). Malnourished subjects had lower phase angles that increased parallel to WT, MAC, and nutritional repletion. These authors concluded BIA phase angle was a useful tool in assessing body cell mass (nutritional) status in children. This study suggests that BIA phase angle may be a useful tool in monitoring body composition in child athletes who restrict their energy intake.

General application of BIA measurement as a body composition assessment tool in child athletes should be done only after limitations discussed above have been considered. Further study regarding effects of environmental and body temperatures, hydration status, and validity of prediction equations on BIA in child athletes is needed.

III. Summary and Recommendations

Traditional body composition assessment tools such as densitometry (underwater weighing), isotope dilution (total body water), neutron activation, and total body potassium (^{40}K) are useful in research settings. However, these assessment tools are not practical in clinical or field settings. In contrast, simple anthropometric measurements discussed in this chapter are inexpensive, noninvasive, and reliable in all settings where child athletes might best be served.

Concerns regarding body composition are becoming more common in children. Child athletes may be at increased risk for physical consequences of intensive training programs or competition than their nonathletic child counterparts. Routine growth assessment is essential in assuring maintenance of an appropriate growth pattern, assessing effects of training and competition, and identifying child athletes at risk for disordered eating.

Utilizing body composition data to design training programs intended to enhance physical performance in child athletes is not recommended.

The goal for child athletes is to enjoy sports/physical activity while maintaining a healthy lifestyle. Recommendations to assure appropriate and reliable assessment of growth in child athletes are as follows:

1. Monitor and assess HT and WT measurements at least annually.
   a. Plot HT, WT, and BMI percentiles on age- and gender-specific growth charts (updated 2000 CDC/NCHS).
   b. Plot growth data in a longitudinal fashion.
   c. Multiple data plots required for meaningful assessment.
2. Interpretation of appropriate growth pattern includes:
   a. HT and WT encompassed by 5th and 95th percentiles.
   b. HT and WT percentiles < 5th or > 95th indicates need for medical or nutritional evaluation.
   c. HT and WT percentiles should track parallel to established growth channels over time. Crossing (upward or downward) of two or more percentile rankings indicates need for medical/ nutritional evaluation.
   d. BMI best utilized as a marker of overnutrition. Exercise extra caution when interpreting BMI in highly muscled or lean child athletes.
      i. BMI < 85th percentile indicates normal range.
      ii. BMI ≥ 85th but < 95th percentiles indicates risk of overweight.
      iii. BMI ≥ 95th percentile indicates overweight.
3. Monitor body composition to evaluate/track effects of training/ competition:
   a. TSF — estimates percent body fat; especially in lean child athletes.
   b. MAC — estimates large shifts in lean tissue body mass.
   c. MAMA — estimates magnitude of shifts in lean tissue body mass; not sensitive in obese children.
   d. BIA — estimates percent body fat; limited application in child athletes.
4. Interpretation of TSF, MAC, and MAMA measurements include:
   a. Utilization of age- and gender-specific standardized reference data to estimate percentile rankings.
   b. Normal range encompassed by 5th and 95th percentiles.
   c. Percentile rankings < 5th or > 95th indicates need for medical/ nutritional evaluation.

    d. Coordination with other growth chart data.

  5. Reliable anthropometric data collection should include:

    a. Collection of data by trained personnel.

    b. Appropriate measurement tools routinely maintained and calibrated.

  6. Individual application of growth assessment data in child athletes.

References

1. Committee on Nutrition, American Academy of Pediatrics, *Pediatric Nutrition Handbook*, 4th ed., Kleinman, R.E., Ed., American Academy of Pediatrics, Elk Grove Village, IL, 1998, p.141.
2. *Stedman's Medical Dictionary*, 25th ed., Hensyl, W.R., Ed., Williams and Wilkins, Baltimore, MD, 1990, p.93.
3. Tanner, J.M., *Growth at Adolescence*, 2nd ed., Blackwell Scientific, Oxford, 1962.
4. Tanner, J.M., *Fetus into Man: Physical Growth from Conception to Maturity*, Harvard University Press, Cambridge, MA, 1989.
5. Sinclar, D., *Human Growth After Birth*, Oxford University Press, London, 1978.
6. Young, V.R., Steffe, W.P., Pencharz, P.B., Winterer, J.C. and Scrimshaw, N.S., Total human body protein synthesis in relation to protein requirements at various ages, *Nature*, 253, 192, 1975.
7. Heyner, S., Smith R.M. and Schultz, G.A., Temporally regulated expression of insulin and insulin-like growth factors and their receptors in early mammalian development, *Bioessays*, 11, 171, 1989.
8. Hill, D.L. and Han, V.K., Paracrinology of growth regulation, *J. Dev. Physiol.*, 15, 91, 1991.
9. Brook, C.G.D. and Hindmarsh, P.C., The somatotropic axis in puberty, *Endocrinol. Metab. Clin. North Am.*, 21, 767, 1992.
10. Holly, J.M.P. and Wass, J.A.H., Insulin-like growth factors: autocrine, paracrine, or endocrine? New perspectives of the somatomedin hypothesis in the light of recent developments, *J. Endocrinol.*, 122, 611, 1989.
11. Green, H., Morikawa, M. and Nixon, T., A dual effector theory of growth hormone action, *Differentiation*, 29, 195, 1985.
12. Schwartz, H.L., Effect of thyroid hormone on growth and development, in *Molecular Basis of Thyroid Hormone Action*, Oppenheimer, H., and Samuels, H. H., Eds., Academic Press, New York, 1983, pp. 413-444.
13. McDonough, M.J.N. and Davies, C.T.M., Adaptive response of mammalian skeletal muscle to exercise with high loads, *Eur. J. Appl. Physiol.*, 52, 139, 1984.
14. Aloia, J.F., Cohn, S.H., Ostini, R.H., Cane, R., and Ellis, K., Prevention of involutional bone loss by exercise, *Ann. Int. Med.*, 89, 356, 1978.
15. Morey, E.R. and Baylink, D.J., Inhibition of bone formation during space flight, *Science*, 201, 1138, 1978.
16. Roberts, L.J., Nutrition Work with Children, University of Chicago Press, 1935.
17. Boas, F., The growth of children, *Science*, 19, 256, Chicago, 1892.

18. Wetzel, N.C., Physical fitness in terms of physique, development and basal metabolism, with a guide to individual progress from infancy to maturity: a new method for evaluation, *J. Am. Med. Assoc.*, 116, 1187, 1941.

19. Jackson, R.L. and Kelly, H.G., Growth charts for use in pediatric practice, *J. Pediat.*, 27, 215, 1945.

20. Stuart, H.C. and Meredith, H.V., Use of body measurements in the school health program, *Am. J. Public Health*, 36, 1365, 1946.

21. Reed, R.B. and Stuart, H.C., Patterns of growth in height and weight from birth to 18 years of age, *Pediatrics*, 24, 904, 1959.

22. Hamill, P.V.V., Drizd, T.A., Johnson, C.L., Reed, R.B., Roche, A.F. and Moore, W.M., Physical growth: National Center for Health Statistics Percentiles, *Am. J. Clin. Nutr.*, 32, 607, 1979.

23. National Center for Health Statistics, Height and weight for youth 6–11 years, United States, *Vital and Health Statistics,* Series 11, no.124, Health Services and Mental Health Administration, Washington, D.C., United States Government Printing Office, 1970.

24. National Center for Health Statistics, Height and weight for youth 12–17 years, United States, *Vital and Health Statistics*, Series 11, no.124, Health Services and Mental Health Administration, Washington, D.C., United States Government Printing Office, 1973.

25. World Health Organization, A growth chart for international use in maternal and child health care: guidelines for primary health care personnel, Geneva, World Health Organization, 1978.

26. DeOnis, M. and Yip, R., The WHO growth chart: historical considerations and current scientific issues, *Bibl Nutr Dieta*, 53, 74, 1996.

27. Dibley, M.J., Staehling, N., Bieburg, P. and Trowbridge, F.L., Interpretation of Z-score anthropometric indicators derived from the international growth reference, *Am. J. Clin. Nutr.* 46, 749, 1987.

28. Flegal, K.M., Curve smoothing and transformations in the development of growth curves, *Am. J. Clin. Nutr.*, 70, S163, 1999.

29. Kuczmarski, R.J., Ogden, C.L., Grummer-Strawn, L.M., Flegal, K.M., Guo, S.S., Wei, R., Mei, Z., Curtin, L.R., Roche, A.F. and Johnson, C.L., CDC growth charts: United States, *Advance data from vital and health statistics*, National Center for Health Statistics, 314, 1, Hyattsville, MD, 2000.

30. Behrman, R.E. and Vaughan, V.C., Developmental pediatrics: growth and development, in *Textbook of Pediatrics*, 13th ed., Nelson, W.E., Ed., W.B. Saunders, Philadelphia, 1987, pp.26-30.

31. Schuck, G.R., Effects of athletic competition on the growth and development of junior high school boys, *Res. Q.*, 33, 288, 1962.

32. Astrand, P.O., Engstrom, L., Eriksson, B.O., Karlberg, P., Nylander, I., Saltin, B. and Thoren, C., Girl swimmers with special reference to respiratory and circulatory adaptation and gynecological and psychiatric aspects, *Acta. Paediatr,* S147, 1, 1963.

33. Malina, R.M. and Bielicki, T., Retrospective longitudinal growth study of boys and girls active in sport, *Acta. Paediatr.*, 85, 570, 1996.

34. Malina, R.M., Physical growth and biological maturation of young athletes, *Exerc. Sports Sci. Rev.*, 22, 389, 1994.

35. Daly, R.M., Rich, P.A., Klein, R. and Bass, S.L., Short stature in competitive prepubertal and early pubertal male gymnasts: the result of selection bias or intense training? *J. Pediatr.*, 137, 510, 2000.

36. Benardot, D. and Czerwinski, C., Selected body composition and growth measures of junior elite gymnasts, *J. Am. Diet. Assoc.* 91, 29, 1991.

37. Robbins, G.E. and Trowbridge, F.L., Anthropometric techniques and their application, in *Nutrition Assessment: A Comprehensive Guide for Planning Intervention*, Simko, M.D., Cowell, C. and Gilbride, J.A., Eds., Aspen Publishers, Inc., 1984, pp.69-92.

38. Gibson, R.S., Assessment of growth: recumbent length and stature, in *Nutritional Assessment: A Laboratory Manual*, Oxford University Press, 1993, pp. 45-55.

39. Troiano, R.P., Flegal, K.M., Kuczmarski, R.J., Campbell, S.M. and Johnson, C.L., Overweight prevalence and trends for children and adolescents, The National Health and Nutrition Examination Surveys, 1963 to 1991, *Arch. Pediatr. Adolesc. Med.*, 149, 1085, 1995.

40. Barlow, S.E. and Dietz, W.H., Obesity evaluation and treatment: expert committee recommendations, *Pediatrics*, 102, 1998.

41. Rhea, D.J., Eating disorder behaviors of ethnically diverse urban female adolescent athletes and nonathletes, *J. Adolesc.*, 22, 379, 1999.

42. Neumark-Sztainer, D., Sherwood, N.E., Coller.T. and Hannan, P.J., Primary prevention of disordered eating among preadolescent girls: feasibility and short-term effect of a community-based intervention, *J. Am. Diet. Assoc.*, 100, 1466, 2000.

43. Robinson, T.N., Chang, J.Y., Haydel, K.F. and Killen, J.D., Overweight concerns and body dissatisfaction among third-grade children: the impacts of ethnicity and socioeconomic status, *J. Pediatr.*, 138,181, 2001.

44. American Academy of Pediatrics Committee on Sports Medicine and Fitness, Intensive training and sports specialization in young athletes, *Pediatrics*, 106, 154, 2000.

45. Himes, J.H. and Dietz, W.H., Guidelines for overweight in adolescent preventive services: recommendations from an expert committee, *Am. J. Clin. Nutr.*, 70, 123S, 1994.

46. Rolland-Cachera, M.F., Deheeger, M., Bellisle, F., Sempe, M., Guilloud-Bataille, M. and Patois, E., Adiposity rebound in children: a simple indicator for predicting obesity, *Am. J. Clin. Nutr.*, 39, 129, 1984.

47. Daniels, S.R., Khoury, P.R. and Morrison, J.A., The utility of body mass index as a measure of body fatness in children and adolescents: differences by race and gender, *Pediatrics*, 99, 804, 1997.

48. Guo, S.S., Chumlea, W.C., Roche, A.F. and Siervogel, R.M., Age- and maturity-related changes in body composition during adolescence into adulthood: the Fels Longitudinal Study, *Int. J. Obes.*, 21, 1167, 1997.

49. Bellizzi, M.C. and Dietz, W.H., Workshop on childhood obesity: summary of the discussion, *Am. J. Clin. Nutr.*, 70, S173, 1999.

50. Maynard, L.M., Wisemandle, W., Roche, A.F., Chumlea, W.C., Guo, S.S. and Siervogel, R.M., Childhood body composition in relation to body mass index, *Pediatrics*, 107, 344, 2001.

51. Pietrobelli, A., Faith, M.S., Allison, D.B., Gallagher, D., Chiumello, G. and Heymesfield, S.B., Body mass index as a measure of adiposity among children and adolescents: a validation study, *J. Pediatr.*, 132, 204, 1998.

52. Goran, M.I., Driscoll, P., Johnson, R., Nagy, R.R. and Hunter, G., Cross-calibration of body-composition techniques against dual-energy radiograph absorptiometry in young children, *Am. J. Clin. Nutr.*, 63, 299, 1996.

53. Roche, A., Siervogel, R., Chumlea, W. and Webb, P., Grading body fatness from limited anthropometric data, *Am. J. Clin. Nutr.*, 34, 2831, 1981.
54. Garn, S., Leonard, W. and Hawthorne, V., Three limitations of body mass index, *Am. J. Clin. Nutr.*, 44, 996, 1986.
55. Himes, J.H. and Bouchard, C., Validity of anthropometry in classifying youths as obese, *Int. J. Obes.*, 13, 183, 1989.
56. Marshall, J.D., Hazlett, C.B., Spady, D.W., Conger, P.R. and Quinney, H.A., Validity of convenient indicators of obesity, *Hum. Biol.*, 63, 137, 1991.
57. Lohman, T.G., Caballero, B., Himes, J.H., Hunsberger, S., Reid, R., Stewart, D. and Skipper, B., Body composition assessment in American Indian children, *Am. J. Clin. Nutr.*, 69, S764, 1999.
58. Wong, W.W., Stuff, J.E., Butte, N.F., Smith, E.O. and Ellis, K.J., Estimating body fat in African American and white adolescent girls: a comparison of skinfold-thickness equations with a four-compartment criterion model, *Am. J. Clin. Nutr.*, 72, 348, 2000.
59. Grant, A. and DeHoog, S., Anthropometric assessment, in *Nutritional Assessment and Support*, Grant and DeHoog, Seattle, WA, 1991. pp. 9-98.
60. Durin, J.V.G.A. and Rahaman, M.M., The assessment of the amount of fat in the human body from measurements of skinfold thickness, *Br. J. Nutr.*, 21, 681, 1967.
61. Garn, S.M., Sullivan, T.B. and Hawthorne, V.M., Evidence against functional differences between "central" and "peripheral" fat, *Am. J. Clin. Nutr.*, 47, 836, 1988.
62. Klipstein-Grobusch K., Georg, T. and Boeing, H., Interviewer variability in anthropometric measurements and estimates of body composition, *Int. J. Epidemiol.*, 26, S174, 1997.
63. Owen, G., Measurement, recording and assessment of skinfold thickness in childhood and adolescence: report of a small meeting, *Am. J. Clin. Nutr.*, 35, 629, 1982.
64. Frisancho, A.R., New norms of upper limb fat and muscle areas for assessment of nutritional status, *Am. J. Clin. Nutr.*, 34, 2540, 1981.
65. Gurney, J.M. and Jelliffe, D.B., Arm anthropometry in nutrition assessment: nomogram for rapid calculation of muscle circumference and cross-sectional muscle and fat areas, *Am. J. Clin. Nutr.*, 26, 912, 1973.
66. Gibson, R.S., Assessment of growth: recumbent length and stature, in *Nutritional Assessment: A Laboratory Manual*, Oxford University Press, 1993, pp. 67–101.
67. Chen, L.C., Chowdhury, A. and Huffman, S.L., Anthropometric assessment of energy-protein malnutrition and subsequent risk of mortality among preschool aged children, *Am. J. Clin. Nutr.*, 33, 1836, 1980.
68. Trowbridge, F.L., Hiney, C.D. and Robertson, A.D., Arm muscle indicators and creatinine excretion in children, *Am. J. Clin. Nutr.*, 36, 691, 1982.
69. Jelliffe, E.F.P. and Jelliffe, D.B., The arm circumference as a public health index of protein-calorie malnutrition of early childhood, *J. Trop. Pediatr.*, 32, 1527, 1969.
70. Gurney, J.M. and Jelliffe, D.B., Arm anthropometry in nutritional assessment: nomogram for rapid calculation of muscle circumference and cross sectional muscle and fat areas, *Am. J. Clin. Nutr.*, 26, 912, 1973.
71. Heymsfield, S.B., McManus C., Smith, J., Stevens, V. and Nixon, D.W., Anthropometric measurements of muscle mass: revised equations for calculating bone-free arm muscle area, *Am. J. Clin. Nutr.*, 36, 680, 1982.

72. Ackman, J.J. and Seitz, M.A., Methods of complex impedance measurements in biological tissue, *Crit. Rev. Biomed. Eng.*, 11, 281, 1984.

73. Barnett, A. and Bango, S., The physiological mechanisms involved in the clinical measure of phase angle, *Am. J. Physiol.*, 129, 306, 1936.

74. Hoffer, E.C. and Meadow, C.K., Correlation of whole-body impedance with total body water volume, *J. Appl. Physiol.*, 27, 531, 1969.

75. Thomasset, A.L. and Beruard, M., Body composition assessment by electrical impedancemetry, *Age Nutr.*, 5, 76, 1994.

76. Segal, K.R., Use of bioelectrical impedance measurement for estimation of extracellular water in normal adult males, *Age Nutr.*, 5, 97, 1994.

77. Cole, K.S., Membranes, ions, and impulses: a chapter of classical biophysics, UCLA Press, Los Angeles, 1972.

78. Lofgren B., The electrical impedance of a complex tissue and its relation to changes in volume and fluid distribution, *Acta. Physiol. Scand.*, 23(S81), 2, 1951.

79. Jebb, S.A. and Elia, M., Assessment of changes in total body water in patients undergoing renal dialysis using bioelectrical impedance analysis, *Clin. Nutr.*, 10, 81, 1990.

80. Brown, B.H., Karatzas, T., Nakielny, R. and Clarke, R.G., Determination of upper arm muscle mass and fat areas using electrical impedance analysis, *Clin. Phys. Physiol. Meas.*, 9, 47, 1988.

81. Webster, B.L. and Barr, S.I., Body composition analysis of female adolescent athletes: comparing six regression equations, *Med. Sci. Sports Exerc.*, 25, 648, 1992.

82. Liang, M.T. and Norris, S., Effects of skin blood flow and temperature on bioelectrical impedance after exercise, *Med. Sci. Sports Exerc.*, 25, 1231, 1993.

83. Lukaski, H.C., Bolonshuk, W.W., Siders, W.A. and Hall, C.B., Body composition assessment of athletes using bioelectrical impedance measurements, *J. Sports Med. Phys. Fitness*, 30, 434, 1990.

84. Deurenberg, P., Kusters, C.S.L. and Smit, H.E., Assessment of body composition by bioelectrical impedance in children and young adults is strongly age-dependent, *Eur. J. Clin. Nutr.*, 44, 261, 1990.

85. Houtkooper, L.B., Going, S.B. and Lohman, T.G., Bioelectrical impedance estimation of fat-free body mass in children and youth: a cross-validation study, *J. Appl. Physiol.*, 72, 366, 1992.

86. Kushner, R.F., Schoeller, D.A., Fjeld, K.R. and Danford, L., Is the impedance index (ht^2/R) significant in predicting total body water? *Am. J. Clin. Nutr.*, 56, 835, 1992.

87. Bandini, L.G., Vu, D.M., Must, A. and Dietz, W.H., Body fatness and bioelectrical impedance in non-obese pre-menarcheal girls: comparison to anthropometry and evaluation of predictive equations, *Nutrition*, 14, 105, 1998.

88. Nagano, M., Suita, S. and Yamanouchi, T., The validity of bioelectrical impedance phase angle for nutritional assessment in children, *J. Ped. Surg.*, 35, 1035, 2000.

89. Richard, N.B., Chumlea, W.C. and Alex, F.R., Bioelectrical impedance phase angle and body composition, *Am. J. Clin. Nutr.*, 48, 16, 1988.

6

Assessment of Growth in Adolescent Athletes

Andrew P. Hills and Jana Pařízková

CONTENTS

I. Introduction

The average layperson considers the process of growth an uncomplicated and uniform affair whereby a young person simply becomes taller and heavier. However, the process of growth is far more complicated. Although individuals follow similar general growth trends, certain important differences are specific to each individual. The two primary indicators of growth status and the most common anthropometric measurements are stature (standing height) and body mass (body weight). The accurate measurement of these physical characteristics tells us a great deal about maturation and nutritional status and enables a basis of comparison between individuals of the same chronological age. The variability in the timing of puberty also has important physical, social and psychological consequences. Implications for

0-8493-0927-1/02/$0.00+$1.50
© 2002 by CRC Press LLC

physical growth include differences in size and shape as reflected in stature, body mass, body proportions and body composition. In adolescent athletes, linear growth may provide an indication of general health and nutrition and adequacy of energy intake in relation to training volume.[1]

The aim of this chapter is to provide an overview of the main options available for the assessment of physical growth in adolescent athletes. A related aim is to consider the relative strengths and limitations of each of the assessment techniques presented. Decisions regarding the choice of assessment technique must also take account of the specific features of the growth process, particularly pubertal growth. Anthropometry, the systematized measurement of size and shape of the human body, represents the most prominent group of techniques used in the quantification of growth and development. As a consequence, the chapter is dominated by reference to anthropometry and kinanthropometry. Kinanthropometry has gained widespread acceptance in relation to measurement and evaluation of different aspects of human movement[2] and individual variability in body size, shape, proportions and composition.[3] Other field methods used for the assessment of body composition in athletes are also discussed and, finally, reference is made to laboratory methods that may form part of an assessment profile for some adolescent athletes.

II.   Growth Process

Growth refers to an increase in physical size of the whole body or any of its component parts. An important feature of the increase in physical size of adolescents is the considerable intra- and interindividual variability. Individual body parts do not grow at the same rate nor does growth of these parts cease when physical maturity is attained. The character and degree of synchronic or asynchronic growth can also show marked individual variability, that is, some individuals develop in a more harmonious way than others. Therefore, the proportionality of the organism is also changing and this feature of physical growth has important implications for the involvement of adolescents in sport and physical activity.

III.   Adolescence

Adolescence is the period of growth and development during which a child grows to adulthood. Chronologically, adolescence may extend from about 12–13 years of age to the early 20s. A wide individual variation is influenced by environmental and cultural conditions. The upper developmental limit of adolescence is not clear because no objective physiological traits can be used to define an end point. Physiological and psychological changes during adolescence prepare the individual for mature adult biological and emotional functioning. All changes concern both morphological and physical performance characteristics. Adolescence tends to start earlier in girls than in boys. Puberty is a more restrictive term for the biological and physiological changes associated with physical and sexual maturation. While some changes due to puberty may not be manifest clinically until the second decade, subtle physiological changes may occur as early as 8 years of age. Pubescence is the time during which the reproductive functions mature. This includes the appearance of secondary sexual characteristics and physiological maturation of the primary sex organs. Puberty is reached when full reproductive maturity has been achieved.[4]

IV. Hormonal Changes During Adolescence

The specific trigger —or triggers — of adolescence and puberty is not known, although it appears to be the response of the anterior pituitary to a stimulus from the hypothalamus. There is evidence that, with maturation, sensitivity to the inhibition by gonadal sex hormones of the hypothalamus and other central nervous system centers decreases. This causes an increase in hypothalamic releasing factors and subsequent increase in pituitary tropic hormones. This, in turn, results in an increase in gonadal and sex hormones. In the middle of puberty in girls, there is also a stimulating effect of requisite amounts of estrogens on the hypothalamus, causing an increase in luteinizing hormone. The gonadotropic hormones, follicle-stimulating hormone (FSH), luteinizing hormone (LH) and prolactin are the major hormones involved. Serum gonadotropin levels during early childhood are low in both sexes and increase during adolescence in association with pubertal genital staging.

The female hormones, the estrogens, are produced in the ovaries, testes and adrenals. Estrogens produced before puberty are probably of adrenal origin and start to increase at approximately 11 years of age. The secretion of estrogens assumes a cyclic pattern that appears approximately 2 years before menarche. Gradually, the secondary sex characteristics appear and, during this period, morphological characteristics and the level of performance can change in a characteristic way along with other changes.

In boys, the adrenal cortex and the testes produce the androgenic hormones, the former contributing approximately two thirds. Some of the earliest changes in adolescence are a by-product of androgen stimulation. The androgens are responsible for the development of sex organs, growth of pubic hair, and enlargement of the larynx that results in the deepening of the voice. The androgens are also believed to be responsible for the growth spurt during adolescence and for the increase in muscular development.[4] Serum testosterone levels in males are related to pubertal stage.

The adrenal corticoids are excreted in gradual increments from birth to maturity. In adults they correlate with body size and appear to have no relation to age or sex. Thyroid hormones may decline slightly during puberty, reaching the lowest level in the period of greatest sexual maturation. Parathyroid hormone is believed to increase slightly during adolescence.

V. Changes of Growth

One of the most obvious features of the adolescent period is the acceleration of growth. Therefore, it is logical to use the growth spurt to assess the stage of development of the individual. The start of the growth spurt varies considerably, consistent with the above mentioned hormonal changes.

The growth spurt commonly occurs earlier in girls than in boys, usually between 11 and 14 years of age. In boys, the growth spurt generally appears between 12 and 16 years. In recent decades, considerable secular changes have resulted in taller and heavier adolescents and the earlier appearance of menarche. This trend has been seen in more developed countries. In contrast, the acceleration of growth commonly appears later in the countries of the Third World. The trend has been explained by different diet, especially the amount of energy and proteins, which significantly influence the final level of somatic development (height, weight, body mass index, and lean body mass including musculature). Differences in developmental changes are reflected in measurements such as height and weight. BMI reveals considerable variability in different parts of the world.[5,6] The age of maximum velocity of growth acceleration may occur anywhere between the ages of 11 and 17 years. The growth spurt in girls is usually slower and less extensive than in boys. Body composition evaluation in boys during adolescence has shown that the period of maximal height and weight increases corresponds to the period of maximal lean body mass development. At the same time, the absolute and relative amount of depot fat fluctuated, and does not show consistent changes and relationship to peak height velocity.[7]

The adolescent growth spurt proceeds in a consistent order. Leg length usually begins to increase first and is the first measure to reach the adult value. After several months there is an increase in chest breadth and hip width. Shoulder width increases later and is followed by an increase in trunk length and chest depth. Most of the changes in weight and musculature tend to occur after the bone growth spurt of the long bones.

VI. Psychological Changes

During adolescence there are significant changes in cognitive development, the development of ego, and the emergence of personal and sexual identity.

At this time, the adolescent begins to break away from parental influence and the peer group attains increasing importance and may even dominate the adolescent's thinking and behavior. In a group setting, the adolescent finds the sense of security is a source of comfort in dealing with conflict. This may cause, in the case of negative stimuli of a particular group, great problems concerning behavior and the learning discipline. The regular participation of youth in organized sport has a major positive impact from both the short- and longer-term perspective. Psychological factors can also determine whether an adolescent participates or avoids such activities, with all the associated consequences.

VII.   Pubertal Growth

Numerous changes during the growing years are obvious, yet arguably, the most definitive encompass the time of puberty. This dynamic period is marked by rapid changes in body size, shape and composition, all of which are sexually dimorphic.[1] The comprehensive nature of the physical changes at puberty has been classified in a variety of ways. The following representation, adapted from Marshall,[8] provides a useful introduction to the various considerations that may influence the assessment of the most apparent changes in growth during adolescence:

- An acceleration followed by deceleration of skeletal growth (the adolescent growth spurt)
- Changes in body composition affecting the distribution of subcutaneous fat and alterations in lean tissue with growth in skeletal and muscular tissue
- A refinement in the cardiorespiratory system, contributing to an increase in strength and endurance, particularly in boys.
- Development of the reproductive organs and associated secondary sexual characteristics
- A compendium of neuroendocrine elements that modulate these changes

As mentioned previously, the age of onset of puberty equates to a biological (skeletal) age of approximately 11 years in girls and 2 years later at 13 years in boys.[9] While the pubertal events are generally orderly and predictable, the timing and tempo of puberty are quite variable. Normal biological variability may be increased as a function of adjustments in energy intake and energy expenditure. For some adolescents, sport and physical activity that requires a high training volume and also stresses weight control, for example champion gymnasts, can be potentially hazardous in terms of short- and longer-term health status.[10] For many groups in society, including adolescent athletes, issues related to body size, shape, weight and fatness are extremely important.[11] The most common strategies used by adolescents who wish to alter their body size and weight are diet and exercise.[11] However, diet and exercise are commonly abused by such individuals[10] and the primary motivation for change is cosmetic or appearance related rather than to improve health.[11] In relation to sports performance, inappropriate diet and exercise behaviors are often mediated by the desire to attain a low level of body fat, which is widely considered a desirable physical characteristic. Many athletes work hard to attain a lean and perceived "ideal" body size and shape for their sport.

During the adolescent growth spurt, girls, on average, attain a peak height velocity of 9 cm. per year at 12 years of age with a total increment in stature during this growth period of approximately 25 cm. In contrast, boys attain a peak height velocity of 10.3 cm. per year on average 2 years later than girls. Overall, an increase of 28 cm. in stature can be expected. The later appearance and greater peak height velocity in boys provides a longer time period for linear growth in boys and, in combination, these factors contribute to the biological gender difference in stature of adults of approximately 13 cm.

VIII.   Changes in Body Composition

Marked changes in body mass and composition also occur during puberty. During the adolescent period, both genders show significant body mass increases, in the order of 50% of adult weight. Peak weight velocity in girls occurs approximately 6 months later than peak height velocity, whereas in boys it occurs at approximately the same time. The preferential deposition of body fat in girls and skeletal muscle in boys represents the profound and obvious body composition changes during adolescence. In relation to skeletal growth, the characteristic increases in shoulder breadth as opposed to pelvic breadth in girls also become pronounced at this time. From the perspective of body shape, the combined effects of body fat increase or change in deposition, and skeletal changes result in the characteristic android and gynoid shapes in males and females, respectively.

The increase in testosterone release causes an enhanced development of skeletal musculature and an increase in total lean body mass, given concurrent changes in all internal organs. The same appears in girls but the increase in musculature is significantly smaller. The ratio and absolute amount of lean body mass in boys increases significantly, often at the expense of depot fat, however, this depends directly on the status of energy balance or diet and physical activity.[7,10] In girls, the ratio of depot fat increases more significantly and this results in a decrease in the percentage of lean body mass. However, energy intake and expenditure and the resulting balance also influence the changes in body composition in girls.[12] When comparing different age categories, the differences in lean body mass and depot fat ratio are most apparent at the time of puberty, later these differences are much smaller.[7]

In addition to the changes in depot fat, the distribution of subcutaneous fat is altered significantly with the characteristic android and gynoid fat distributions evident at later stages of puberty. In obese adolescents, the percentage of lean body mass and depot fat is often the same, with little difference in the distribution of fat.

Adaptation to training in different sport disciplines can markedly influence body composition characteristics. The deposition of body fat is commonly significantly decreased in adolescent athletes of both sexes and there may also be differences in the distribution of subcutaneous fat, depending on the specific training emphases and muscle usage in various sport disciplines.[12,13]

The assessment of body size and shape of adolescent athletes has a number of important applications. These include the identification of talented athletes, the assessment and monitoring of the growing athlete, the monitoring of training and performance, and the determination of optimal adiposity and muscularity for events classified according to weight.[2]

IX. Assessment Challenges: Validity, Reliability and Efficacy

The assessment of growth in adolescents also presents numerous challenges, including the determination of appropriate choice between various methodologies or techniques. Due reference must be made to the validity, reliability and efficacy of an instrument and this should inform the decision-making process. Validity refers to the extent to which the measurement or method is a true indication of the variable being assessed.[14] Reliability (or repeatability, reproducibility) refers to the extent to which a method produces similar values on two or more occasions and may be expressed in terms of intra- or intertester reliability. The terms "precision" and "accuracy" are often used to reference the ability of a measurement technique to produce a constant or stable value.[15]

X. Anthropometry

A. Measurement of Body Size and Shape

Anthropometric measurements can be used to assess body size and proportions as well as total body and regional body composition of athletic populations. Measures include stature and body mass, proportions of body segments, circumferences, skinfold thickness, skeletal diameters, and segment lengths.[16] Anthropometry is the only method that has been validated against cadaveric material[17] and has numerous advantages over other assessment techniques. Anthropometry, which is noninvasive, does not impinge on performance, the equipment used is portable and therefore able to be used in a range of settings, and is also relatively inexpensive. An anthropometric profile of each athlete may be composed of either a small number of physical measurements or a more comprehensive grouping.[2]

B. Stature and Body Mass

The two most commonly employed anthropometric measurements are stature and body mass. The significance of each measure can be determined accurately only with due consideration of the other parameter. A range of factors, including diurnal variation, influences the measurement of stature. Therefore, a standardized procedure should take into account the time of the day when measurements are taken, recent participation in vigorous physical activity and a consistent postural position.

It is preferable to measure stretch stature using the following procedure. The measurement is the maximum distance from the floor to the vertex of the head (highest point on the skull when the head is held in the Frankfort plane). The barefoot subject is instructed to stand upright with heels together and arms hanging naturally at the sides. The subject's heels, buttocks and back should be in contact with the vertical surface and he or she is instructed to "look straight ahead" and "take a deep breath." A gentle stretch is applied by cupping the subject's head; firm traction is applied under the mastoid processes to ensure that the heels do not rise and a horizontal headpiece is depressed against the vertex. The vertical measure is taken to the nearest 0.1 cm.

The measurement of body mass is often considered simple and straightforward but there are numerous potential sources of error and measurement is subject to considerable variation. Every attempt should be made to standardize the measurement protocol. As for stature, a possible variation in the measurement of body mass is not surprising. Accuracy of measurement is largely dependent on the degree of hydration of body tissues, the time of last ingestion of food and drink and the recency of urination and bowel movement. An increase in body mass during adolescence may be attributable to any one of the various components of body composition, namely, skeletal weight, total body water, muscle tissue or adipose tissue. Measurement scales, preferably beam-type, should be regularly calibrated and mounted on a firm surface. Body weight should be recorded to the nearest 0.1 kg. Measurement of nude weight is optimal, however, if this is not possible, the athlete should wear a consistent amount of clothing of a known weight (for example, a bathing suit). Repeat measures may be useful to ensure reproducibility.

C. Proportions of Body Segments

Different parts of the developing human body do not grow at the same pace. Consequently, the relationships between body segments vary during different periods of growth. This results in varying proportionality of the individual. The variability among individuals also changes during various periods of growth, especially before and during puberty. The synchrony or asynchrony of growth can also vary among individuals as a result of level of trainability and the standard of athletic performance. Individual variability also changes during various periods of growth, especially before and during puberty.

Individual size and shape, including proportionality, predisposes individuals to certain sports. For example, a shorter stature with relatively short lower extremities can be advantageous for gymnasts. In contrast, a longer lower limb is suited to jumping, running and team sports such as basketball and volleyball. Adult proportions are usually established during puberty, and the evaluation of these morphological characteristics is an important tool for the selection of body types physically predisposed to a particular type of sport performance. In some cases, not only body stature, but also the proportionality of the figures of the parents has been considered in the selection of young athletes for specific tasks and training in certain sport disciplines.

Various indices relating the length of the trunk (usually assessed as sitting height) to the length of lower extremities, or to various breadth measures (biacromial, chest, bicristal or bitrochanteric breadth) have been used to characterize athletes for various sport disciplines. For example, relatively narrow shoulders characterize most runners but commonly they have long legs. In contrast, athletes in throwing and lifting disciplines have relatively broad shoulders and shorter legs. In some sports, such characteristics can be greatly advantageous to an athlete and also be related to particular positions in team sports, such as in football. For other team sports, a wide range of size and shape is catered for. It must be remembered that physical characteristics are but one of many groups of interacting factors influencing performance outcomes.

D. Circumferences

A range of circumference measures can be used to assess the adolescent athlete, but most involve the trunk and upper and lower extremities. Chest circumference at rest, during inspiration and expiration and the difference between the two latter measures give an important estimation of the respiratory capacity, which correlates significantly with vital capacity. Abdominal circumference at the level of the navel and maximal gluteal circumference reveal not only the absolute values at these sites but also characterize the distribution of fat. For example, the waist circumference and waist:hip ratio have been widely accepted as important for the evaluation of relative overweight and obesity, athletes included. The difference or relationship between chest and abdominal circumference characterizes the fitness status of the individual and is also used in adolescents.[18]

E. Skinfold Thickness

Various skinfold thicknesses are used to predict the amount of subcutaneous fat and also to define fat distribution. If it is possible to measure only a single site, the recommended location is under the chin, over the hyoid bone. More commonly, two (triceps and subscapular) or five skinfolds (triceps and sub-scapular plus biceps, suprailiac and calf) are assessed.[19] Other researchers commonly measure 10 or 11 skinfolds (with the addition of the submandib-ular skinfold, two sites on the thorax, abdomen and thigh).[7,20] The commonly cited maximum number of measured skinfolds is 93.[7,21]

A wide range of calipers has been used for the assessment of skinfold thickness, and most often the Harpenden or Lange caliper. The Harpenden caliper was originally designed to measure the thickness of leather and there was no extensive adaptation of the instrument for use in anthropometry. An assumption is that the pressure on the measured skinfold is always the same, irrespective of skinfold thickness or age of the individual being measured. However, there is considerable evidence to suggest that tissue compressibil-ity can vary. The modified Best caliper is arranged so that regular calibration is possible. By pressing the jaws of the caliper to a special hallmark, pressure can be checked and reset if necessary. This possibility is very important when measuring small children or infants, aged subjects, or subjects with different degrees of obesity.[7] In the measurement of predominantly lean young chil-dren or adolescent athletes, the measurement error due to nonhallmarked and noncalibrated calipers may be negligible.

F. Skeletal Diameters

Breadth measures characterize the robustness of the skeleton. As mentioned above, trunk breadths (biacromial, chest width and depth), and hip breadths (bicristal and bitrochanteric) are commonly measured. On the extremities, the humeral and wrist breadth on the arm, and the femoral and ankle breadth on the leg are also common measurements. These measures can vary mark-edly among athletes involved in various sport disciplines.

G. Segment Lengths

For a more detailed characterization of skeletal development and proportion-ality, individual segments on the arm (acromiale-humerale and humerale-ulnare) and leg (iliospinale-tibiale and tibiale-sphyrion) are ascertained.

These measurements are most often reserved for a more detailed charac-terization of the somatic development of a young athlete. The measurements addressed in this chapter are a relatively small number of the anthropometric measurements that may be taken depending on the research focus. The reader is urged to source more detail from standard textbooks in the area, e.g., *Anthropometrica* by Norton and Olds.[22]

H. Prediction of Adult Stature

Adult stature of a young person is best correlated with calculations of mid-parent stature (the difference in the mean adult statures of the parents.[1] However, there is greater variation in the size of young people born to parents of disparate heights than in young people of parents who are both of medium stature.[23] Numerous other methods can be employed to predict adult stature of a young person and rely on calculations that include growth history.

XI. Body Composition

The assessment of body composition in adolescents can be challenging because of differential maturation at a given chronological age. The reader is encouraged to source the extensive overviews, provided by a number of recent publications, of the assessment of body composition in pediatric populations.[16,24,25] An overview of the recognized elements in body composition assessment is referenced here. Commonly, body composition analysis involves subdividing body mass (weight) into two or more compartments according to elemental, chemical, anatomical or fluid components.[26,27] Traditionally, body composition assessment has been based on the two-compartment model in which the body is divided into fat mass (FM) and fat-free mass (FFM).[28–30] More recently, there has been widespread use of multi-compartment models coincidental with advances in technology related to body composition assessment.[31,32] Generally, the following components have composed such models: total body water (TBW) incorporating extracellular (ECW) and intracellular (ICW) water, FM, bone mineral (BM) and protein (P).

Another bias is the derivation of various regression equations using body density as the basic data for the calculation of the ratio of depot fat and fat-free lean body mass. There are numerous equations, but most of them have not been validated by a direct method (either anatomical or biochemical). Results using such equations may not differ markedly, however, the measurement error may be much greater. As concluded by many authors, it may be preferable to use direct results, that is, total body density or the sum of skinfolds as an indicator of body composition status rather than to confuse the results by additional calculations.

One of the assumptions of the two-compartment model is that the FM and FFM have constant densities (0.0900 kg/l and 1.100 kg/l, respectively).[33] Another assumption is that the relative amounts of the three major components of the FFM (aqueous, mineral, and protein) are known additives, and constant in all individuals.[34] This model has serious limitations when used on individuals (such as children and adolescents) who differ from the reference population in bone mineralization or hydration of their FFM. Adult values for the chemical composition of the FFM are not achieved until approximately 17–20 years of age. Overestimation of FM is common in children and adolescents when using the two-compartment model.[35]

All body composition assessment methods other than cadaveric approaches are indirect. Many body composition techniques are referred to as doubly indirect, meaning that they rely on another indirect method and are subject to the estimation errors inherent in that and subsequent iterations of the data and, at best, provide estimations or predictions of actual composition.

Body composition assessment methods range from simple and inexpensive field methods to highly complex and expensive laboratory procedures. Durnin[36] suggests that one carefully appraise exactly what aspect of body composition one wishes to assess in order to choose the best method in the circumstances. Important considerations for all assessment methods are:

- The degree of skill needed by the tester
- The type of equipment required
- The degree of cooperation expected of the subject
- The validity and reliability of the method

The more popular field methods for the assessment of body composition are anthropometric measures (including skinfolds and circumferences), and bioelectrical impedance analysis (BIA). In contrast, the laboratory procedures of hydrodensitometry, dual energy x-ray absorptiometry (DXA), total body electrical conductivity (TOBEC), total body water (TBW), magnetic resonance imaging (MRI) and total body potassium (TBK) are generally not available for routine assessments of large numbers of adolescent athletes.

A. Anthropometric Indices

Anthropometric indices include the Body Mass Index (BMI) and the waist to hip ratio (WHR). Apart from skinfolds, most measures are relatively simple and inexpensive and do not require a high degree of technical skill. However, high subject cooperation is required, which may present challenges in the assessment of younger athletes.

Potential sources of error in the use of anthropometric methods are the equipment, the technical skill of the tester, subject factors, and the prediction equation selected to estimate body composition. Prediction equations have been published for use in children and adolescents and use combinations of circumferences and skeletal diameters to predict body density.

B. Body Mass Index (BMI)

BMI is the most commonly employed anthropometric index to predict relative overweight. However, the value of the index in children and adolescents is regularly questioned. In children younger than 15 years of age, BMI is not totally independent of height and thus should be used with caution. The calculation of BMI may add little value in the assessment of adolescent athletes beyond the measurement of stature and body mass.[36] Individuals with the same BMI may have quite different body fat percentages because of variable proportions of skeleton and muscle in the same body mass. Prediction of body composition from BMI is also biased in subjects with either high[37] or low body fat content and gives more reliable results only in subjects with a normal range of body weight and BMI.

C. Skinfold Thickness

Measurement of skinfold thickness can be used to estimate regional fat distribution by determining the ratio of subcutaneous fat on the trunk and extremities. Skinfold calipers measure the double fold of skin and the underlying subcutaneous fat.[16] A popular and routinely used technique is to manipulate skinfold measures to derive body fat percentages. This is unnecessary, as satisfactory intra- and interindividual comparisons can be made using the sum of skinfolds from representative anatomical locations.[36]

Advantages of the skinfold measurement technique as a field measure include the portability of equipment and its relative affordability. However, the assessment of skinfold thickness requires a high degree of technical skill, including use of the same calipers to assess change in skinfolds. The same side of the body should also be used for consistency and the practitioner should accurately measure the same skinfold sites used in the chosen prediction equation.[16] Individuals should not be measured immediately after exercise and the menstrual cycle of young female athletes should be accounted for in repeated measurements. Durnin[36] has suggested that the equations developed by Durnin and Womersley[19] and Jackson et al. [37,38] are sufficiently valid for people as young as 10 years of age.

The equations for the calculation of total body fat from skinfolds depend on the changing relationship between subcutaneous fat (skinfolds) and total body fat assessed, for example, by densitometry during puberty and adolescence. At younger ages, such as 11 and 12 years, the same skinfolds correspond to lower total fat content than in 13- and 14-year-old boys.[7,10] Therefore, it is recommended that special regression equations be derived — at least for the individuals before and after the beginning of puberty, when the amount and distribution of fat undergoes relatively greatest change.[7] An ideal, however unlikely scenario, is equations for individual age categories and stages of sexual development. Moreover, there is also evidence that regression equations derived for untrained individuals do not give reliable results for highly trained individuals. This is because, when measuring five or ten common skinfolds, even when results are comparable, in the highly trained, the amount of fat over the buttocks or upper parts of thighs (sites not measured with calipers) is negligible, but in the untrained can be considerably higher. Therefore, we can gain a relatively higher percentage of fat that does not correspond to the real status in gymnasts when using equations for the general population.[39]

D. Densitometry

The hydrostatic weighing technique has often been referenced as the gold standard in body composition assessment. However, Durnin[36] maintains that the method is associated with composite errors in the calculated FFM. The method is based on the principle that the weight of the submerged human being is directly related to body density.[16] Body density represents a combination of the density of body fat and FFM. As is the case for all body composition measures, underwater weighing has a number of limitations, particularly for use with young people. The technique requires the subject to be submerged, to exhale air from the lungs and then hold the breath for at least 10 seconds underwater. The primary shortcomings of the technique relate to the assumptions of the hydrostatic method. These include the constancy of the density of FFM, which is affected by hydration status, and contribution of BM to FFM.[40] These components are variable throughout growth and development and depend also on the diet and level of physical fitness as a result of sport training. Moreover, more accurate results could be obtained only when simultaneously weighing the subjects under the water and measuring the air in respiratory passages[7,20,21] rather than later in the normal atmosphere, as is commonly the case. However, simultaneous measurements are particularly difficult, especially in younger children and those who have a fear of being totally submerged. Nevertheless, the approach has generally been relatively easy for most athletes of all ages.[7] An interesting new methodology involving air-displacement (BOD POD body composition system) has overcome many of the problems associated with underwater weighing. However, the technique requires a much more extensive evaluation.[41]

E. Total Body Water (TBW)

Measurements of TBW and extracellular water (ECW) are useful as body composition assessment techniques, however, one needs to be aware of the assumptions commonly made with respect to the water fraction of the FFM.[7,42] For adults, the water fraction of 73.2% is commonly used, but this value is not constant in adults. Some of the estimates include a range from 80% in neonates to adult values of 71–75% attained at the end of the adolescent period.[45] Higher levels of water content (that is, above the assumed values such as 73.2%) will result in an underestimation of percent body fat. Further, protocols need to ensure that no dehydration or superhydration situation exists due to increased exercise or increased fluid intake. Children are renowned for their predisposition to voluntary dehydration.[16] TBW measurements have not been used recently for the evaluation of body composition and the effect of exercise in adolescents. The hydration of lean fat-free body mass can vary before and after puberty and, compared with adults, can also undergo more marked changes before, during and after workload.

F. Absorptiometry (Dual Energy X-Ray Absorptiometry — DXA)

The analysis of total and regional body composition using the DXA procedure is based on the principle that when a beam of x-rays passes through the body, the beam is attenuated (or reduced in intensity) in proportion to the size and composition of the tissue components. Ogle et al.[44] compared DXA with anthropometric measures of body fat using the equations of Slaughter et al.[45] that account for the chemical immaturity of children. The findings from this work indicated a similar result for percentage BF in males but in contrast, an overestimation of percentage BF in females. The common recommendation is that further studies need to be undertaken to validate the accuracy of DXA measurements in children.

As advantages of the DXA technique, Heyward and Stolarczyk[46] identified high reliability, rapidity of measurement and minimal subject cooperation. The technique also accounts for differences in bone mineral density of subjects, an important consideration in the assessment of children and adolescents. Some of the disadvantages include further validation of the technique for children as opposed to adolescents and also the ethical issues associated with exposure to radiation, albeit minimal. Heyward[47] has indicated that estimates of FM depend on the manufacturer, the mode of data collection and the software used.

G. Bioelectrical Impedance Analysis (BIA)

Bioelectrical impedance is an indirect method of measuring total body water (TBW). The BIA method involves passing a low-level electrical current through the body and measuring the impedance or opposition to the flow of current. The electrolytes in the body water are excellent conductors of electricity. Using an equation (different for each instrument), TBW and therefore FFM are calculated and FM (and usually percent body fat) derived. Because adipose tissue is a relatively poor conductor of electricity due to its small water content, the resistance in an individual with large amounts of body fat will be higher than that of an individual with a greater percentage of FFM. More recent research has considered measurement across multiple frequencies (MFBIA) instead of the customary single frequency and also segmental versus whole-body bioimpedance. The limbs primarily influence electrical resistance, which suggests that the BIA technique may be relatively insensitive to differences in tissue composition of the trunk.[48]

Schaefer et al.[49] found higher intra- and interobserver reliability with BIA than with skinfold measures in youngsters with a mean age of 11.8 years; however, FFM estimates were similar for both BIA and anthropometry. Okasora et al.[50] compared BIA and DXA as methods of body composition assessment in children and found close correlation between percentage BF, FFM and body fat content. The limitation of this study was that equations used by the researchers were those of Brozek et al.[29] These equations are widely recognized as inappropriate for use in youths, as they do not account for the variability of the composition of the FFM in young individuals. Bland and Altman[51] plots or an analysis of the size of the prediction error should be utilized to determine if there is agreement between the two measures.

The BIA technique is recognized as a useful body composition assessment technique in children and adolescents because measurement is fast and non-invasive. It is also inexpensive, painless, requires little subject cooperation, and does not require a high level of technical skill.[49] However, the derived values using the BIA technique are as good as the prediction equation utilized in the software. That is, if the group of individuals being assessed is representative of the population from whom the algorithm was derived, the greater the potential value of the approach.[16] The equations of Houtkeeper et al.[52] are recommended for boys and girls 10–19 years of age. Further, the reliability of a method is dependent on the protocol used in the measurement. A number of factors influencing BIA measurements can also be influenced by the following factors:

- The level of hydration of the subject
- Posture
- Environmental or skin temperature
- Age
- Gender
- Athletic status
- Body composition status
- Ethnic origin

Ideally, if the BIA technique is used to assess changes in an individual over time, biological and environmental variables such as hydration status, timing and content of last ingested meal, skin temperature and menstrual cycle must be controlled for.[18]

XII. Summary

BIA, skinfolds and anthropometry are the most appropriate for use in the field. These techniques are most commonly used at present as they have satisfactory validity providing that appropriate equations are used for the specific population (gender, age category, level of adaptation to exercise and so on). The current best prediction equations have been noted in this paper. BIA may hold the advantage over skinfolds as the technique is less invasive, requires less technical skill, has both higher inter- and intra-tester reliability, is quicker and may be easier to administer to a wider range of individuals. When experimental assessment is required, densitometry or DXA measurement procedures are preferred. This is especially the case when longitudinal observations are made (especially during puberty) when the individual is engaged in sport training. Further development of methods for the evaluation of body composition and morphological characteristics essential for athletic performance are necessary, especially for adolescent athletes at the beginning of their sporting careers.

References

1. Rogol, A.D., Clark, P.A. and Roemmich, J.N., Growth and pubertal development in children and adolescents: effects of diet and physical activity, *Am. J. Clin. Nutr.*, 72, 5215, 2000.
2. Kerr, D.A., Ackland, T.R. and Schreiner, A.B., The elite athlete — assessing body shape size, proportion and composition, *Asia Pac. J. Clin. Nutr.*, 4, 25, 1995.
3. Ross, W.D. and Marfell-Jones, M.J., Kinanthoropometry, in *Physiological Assessment of High Performance Athletes*, Human Kinetics, Champaign, IL, 1992, 223.
4. Cooper H.E. and Nakashima I., Adolescence, in *Current Pediatric Diagnosis and Treatment*, 7th ed., Kempe, C.H., Silver H.K. and O'Brien D., Eds., Lange Medical Publications, Los Altos, CA, 1982, 164.
5. Rolland-Cachera, M-F., Prediction of adult body composition from infant and childhood measurement, in *Body Composition Techniques in Health and Disease*, Davies, P.S.W. and Cole, T.J., Eds., Cambridge University Press, Cambridge, 1995, 100.
6 Pařízková, J., and Hills, A.P., *Childhood Obesity*, CRC, Boca Raton, FL, 2001.
7. Pařízková, J., *Body Fat and Physical Fitness*. Martinus Nijhoff, B.V./Medical Division, The Hague, 1977.
8. Marshall, W.A., *Human Growth and its Disorders*. Academic, New York, 1977.
9. Tanner, J.M., Whitehouse, R.H., Marshall, W.A.and Carter, B.S., Prediction of adult height, bone age and occurrence of menarche, at age 4 to 16 with allowance for midparental height height, *Arch. Dis. Child.*, 50, 14, 1975.
10. Pařízková, J., Adaptation of functional capacity and exercise, in *Nutritional Adaptation in Man*. Blaxter, K. and Waterlow, J., Eds., John Libbey, London, 1985, 127.
11. Hills, A.P. and Byrne, N.M., Body composition, body satisfaction, eating and exercise behaviors of Australian adolescents, in *Physical Fitness and Nutrition during Growth*, Parizková J. and Hills, A.P., Eds., Karger, Basel, 1998, 44-53.
12. Pařízková, J., Changes in approach to the measurements of body composition, in *Body Composition Techniques in Health and Disease,* Davies, P.S.W. and Cole, T.J., Eds., Cambridge University Press, Cambridge, 1995, 222.
13. Pařízková, J., Physical working capacity and physical fitness methodology, in *Nutritional Status Assessment, A Manual for Population Studies,* Fidanza, F., Ed., Chapman and Hall, London, 1991, 101.

14. Hills, A.P., Byrne, N.M. and Parízková J., Methodological considerations in the assessment of physical activity and nutritional status of children and youth, in *Physical Fitness and Nutrition during Growth*, Parízková, J. and Hills, A.P., Eds., Karger, Basel, 1998, 155.

15. Solomons, N.W. and Mazariogos, M., Low-cost appropriate technologies for body composition assessment: a field researcher's view, *Asia Pac. J. Clin. Nutr.*, 4, 19, 1995.

16. Hills, A.P., Lyell, L. and Byrne, N.M., An evaluation of the methodology for the assessment of body composition in children and adolescents, in *Body Composition Assessment in Children and Adolescents*, Jurimae, T. and Hills, A.P., Eds., Karger, Basel, 2001, 1.

17. Clarys, J.P., Martin, A.D. and Drinkwater, D.T., Gross tissue weights in the human body cadaver dissection, *Hum. Biol.* 56, 459, 1985.

18. Hills A.P. and Byrne, N.M., Bioelectrical impedance: use and abuse, in *Proc. Int. Coun. Phys. Act. Fit. Res.*, Coetsee, M.F. and Van Heerden, H.J., Eds., Itala, South Africa, 1997, 23.

19. Durnin, J.V.G.A. and Womersley, J., Body fat assessed from total body density and its estimation from skinfold thickness: measurements on 481 men and women aged from 16–72 years, *Br. J. Nutr.*, 32, 77, 1974.

20. Parízková, J., Age trends in fatness in normal and obese children, *J. Appl. Physiol.*, 16, 173, 1961.

21. Keys, A. and Brozek, J., Body fat in adult man, *Physiol. Rev.*, 33, 245, 1953.

22. Norton, K. and Olds, T., *Anthropometrica*, University of New South Wales Press, Sydney, 1996.

23. Smith, D.W., *Growth and its Disorders*, W. B. Saunders, Philadelphia, 1977.

24. Claessens, A.L., Beunen, G. and Malina, R.M., Anthropometry, physical and body composition and maturity, in *Paediatric, Exercise Science and Medicine*, in Armstrong, N. and van Mechelen, W., Eds., Oxford University Press, Oxford, 2000, 11.

25. Zemel, B.S., Riley, E.M. and Stallings, V.A., Evaluation of methodology for nutritional assessment in children: anthropometry, body composition and energy expenditure, *Ann. Rev. Nutr.*, 17, 211, 1997.

26. Heymsfield, S.B. and Masako, W., Body composition in humans: advances in the development of multicompartment chemical models, *Nutr. Rev.*, 49, 97, 1991.

27. Wang, Z., Ma, R., Pierson, R.N., Heymsfield S.B., Five-level model: reconstruction of body weight at atomic, molecular, cellular and tissue-system levels from neutron activation analysis, *Basic Life Sci.*, 60, 125, 1993.

28. Behnke, A.R. and Wilmore, J.H., *Evaluation and Regulation of Body Build and Composition*, Prentice Hall, Englewood Cliffs, NJ, 1974.

29. Brozek, J. et al., Densitometric analysis of body composition: revision of some quantitative assumptions, *Ann. N.Y. Acad. Sc.*, 110, 113, 1963.

30. Siri, W.E., The gross composition of the body, in *Advances in Biological and Medical Physics*, Tobias, C.A. and Lawrence, J.H., Eds., Academic, New York, 1956, vol 4, 239.

31. Wells, J.C.K., Fuller, N.J., Dewit, O., Fewtrell, M.S., Elia, M.and Cole, T.J., Four-compartment model of body composition in children: density and hydration of fat-free mass and comparison with simpler models, *Am. J. Clin. Nutr.*, 69, 904, 1999.

32. Roemmich, J.N., Clark, P.A., Weltman, A.and Rogol, A.D., Alterations in growth and body composition during puberty. I. Comparing multicompartment body composition models, *J. Appl. Physiol.,* 83, 927, 1997.

33. Visser, M., Gallagher, D., Deurenberg, P., Wang, J., Pierson, R.N. and Heymsfield, S.B., Density and fat-free body mass: relationship with race, age and level of fatness. *Am. J. Physiol.,* 272, E781, 1997.

34. Classey, J.L., Kanaley, J.A., Wideman, L., Heymsfield, S.B., Teates, C.D., Gutgesell, M.E., Thorner, M.O., Hartman, M.L. and Weltman, A., Validity of methods of body composition assessment in young and older men and women, *J. Appl. Physiol.,* 86, 1728, 1999.

35. Reilly, J.J., Assessment of body composition in infants and children, *Nutr.,* 14, 821, 1998.

36. Durnin, J.V.G.A., Appropriate technology in body composition: a brief review, *Asia Pac. J. Clin. Nutr.,* 4, 1, 1995.

37. Jackson, A.S. and Pollock, M.L., Generalised questions for predicting body density in men, *Br. J. Nutr.,* 40, 497, 1978.

38. Jackson, A.S., Pollock, M.L. and Ward, A., Generalised equations for predicting body density of women, *Med. Sci. Sports Ex.,* 12, 175, 1980.

39. Pařízková, J. , Total body fat and skinfold thickness in children, *Metabolism,* 10, 794.

40. Lukaski, H.C., Methods for the assessment of human body composition: traditional and new, *Am. J. Clin. Nutr.,* 46, 537, 1997.

41. Elia, M. and Ward, L.C., New techniques in nutritional assessment: body composition methods, *Proc. Nutr. Soc.,* 58, 33, 1999.

42. Jensen, M.D., Research techniques for body composition assessment, *J. Am. Diet. Assoc.,* 92, 454, 1992.

43. Haschke, F., Body composition of adolescent males. Part II. Body composition of male reference adolescents, *Acta. Paed. Scand.,* 307, 13, 1983.

44. Ogle, G.D., Allen, J.R., Humphries, I.R.J., Lu, P.W., Briody, J.N., Morely, K., Howman-Giles, R. and Cowell, C.T., Body composition assessment by dual energy x-ray absorptiometry in subjects aged 4–26 years, *Am. J. Clin. Nutr.,* 61, 746, 1995.

45. Slaughter, M.H., Lohman, T.G., Boileau, R.A., Horswill, C.A., Stillman, R.J., Van Loan, M.D. and Bemben, D.A., Skinfold equations for estimation of body fatness in children and youth, *Hum. Biol.,* 60, 709, 1998.

46. Heyward, V.H. and Stolarczyk, L.M., *Applied Body Composition Assessment,* Human Kinetics, Champaign, IL., 1996.

47. Heyward, V.H., Practical body composition assessment for children, adults and older adults, *Int. J. Sp. Nutr.,* 8, 285, 1998.

48. Zhu, F., Schneditz, D., Wang, E. and Levin, N.W., Dynamics of segmental extracellular volumes during changes in body position by bioelectrical impedance, *J. Appl. Physiol.,* 85, 497, 1997.

49. Schaefer, F., Georgi, M., Zieger, A. and Scharer, K., Usefulness of bioelectric impedance and skinfold measurements in predicting fat-free mass derived from total body potassium in children, *Ped. Res.,* 35, 617, 1994.

50. Okasora, K., Takaya, R., Tokuda, M., Fukunaga, Y., Oguni, T., Tanaka, H., Konishi, K. and Tamai, H., Comparison of bioelectrical impedance analysis and dual energy x-ray absorptiometry for assessment of body composition in children, *Ped. Int.,* 41, 121, 1999.

51. Bland, J.M. and Altman, D.G., Statistical methods for assessing agreement between two methods of clinical measurement, *Lancet*, 1, 307, 1986.
52. Houtkeeper, L.B., Going, S.B., Lohman, T.G., Roche, A.F. and Van Loan, M., Bioelectrical impedance estimation of fat-free body mass in children and youth: a cross-validation study, *J. Appl. Physiol.*, 72, 366, 1992.

7

Anthropometry of Adult Athletes: Concepts, Methods and Applications

Robert M. Malina, Rebecca A. Battista and Shannon R. Siegel

CONTENTS

I.   Introduction

Anthropometry has a long tradition in physical anthropology and physical education. In physical anthropology, more appropriately human biology in the present context, anthropometry is used primarily to describe the external dimensions of populations and to assess growth and nutritional status. Anthropometry is also central to the study of constitution, a field that involves the interrelationships and interdependency among structural, functional and behavioral characteristics of the individual.[1,2] The study of physique is an aspect of an area of study sometimes labeled human constitution, which considers associations between physique, or body build and a variety of behavioral, occupational, disease and performance variables, primarily in adults. At present, anthropometric procedures are used to estimate physique.

In physical education, particularly the sport sciences, anthropometry is used to assess physical status, specifically in the context of health-related fitness and performance. Anthropometry was a primary tool in the development of the field of measurement (tests and measurements), along with measures of strength and other functional characteristics.[3] The assessment of physique is also an important tool in the sport sciences.

This chapter focuses on the application of anthropometry to adult athletes. It has four specific objectives. First, anthropometric studies of athletes are briefly reviewed in a historical context. Second, anthropometric concepts and methods are summarized. Third, the anthropometric characteristics of female athletes in seven sports are described and compared. And fourth, anthropometric data for athletes are applied in the context of secular change, seasonal variation and disordered eating.

II.   Anthropometric Studies of Athletes: Historical Overview

Historically, the study of elite athletes has had a central position in the sport sciences. The unique physical characteristics of elite athletes and their relationship to performance were basic questions and anthropometry was central to these studies. The first systematic studies of world class athletes took place in 1928 at the second Olympic Winter Games in St. Moritz[4] and at the ninth Olympic Summer Games in Amsterdam.[5] The studies at the Winter Games included primarily physiological measurements, although the body dimensions of male skiers and ice hockey players were reported.[6] The Amsterdam Summer Games included two primarily anthropometric investigations of male athletes among the 16 reported papers.[7,8] Extensive data for male swimmers and track-and-field athletes, many of whom represented the United States at the 1948 Olympic Games in London, included anthropometry, body composition and physiological variables.[9] Subsequently, anthropometric observations of elite athletes have been presented on a more or less regular basis. These included two independent studies of male participants at the 1960 Summer Olympic Games in Rome.[10,11] The focus was primarily on track-and-field athletes in both studies, although several swimmers,[11] weight lifters and wrestlers from the British Empire Commonwealth Games[10] were also included.

Surveys at the Summer Olympics in 1968 (Mexico City),[12] 1972 (Munich)[13] and 1976 (Montreal)[14] were more detailed. They included both male and female athletes, a broader array of sports and additional information to complement anthropometry and physiology. The Mexico City survey also included familial and genetic information,[12] while the Munich survey included detailed study of body composition in a limited number of male and female athletes in several sports.[15-17] The Montreal survey included a concerted effort to study Olympic athletes ≤18 years of age — 47 females and 17 males.[18]

The studies of Olympic athletes provide information about the body size and other dimensions, body proportions, physique (somatotype) and body composition of athletes in a variety of sports, more so for males than for females. These data have been summarized in the volume edited by Carter.[19]

Detailed anthropometric studies of elite athletes at specific competitions and in several countries have also been reported. For example, the anthropometric dimensions of 125 female track-and-field athletes at the eighth European Athletic Championships in 1966 were surveyed.[20] Others are the comprehensive anthropometric analysis of the best athletes, both adolescent and adult, in the former German Democratic Republic,[21] and anthropometric and somatotype studies of Dutch,[22] Indian,[23] Bulgarian,[24] Venezuelan[25] and Mexican[26] athletes. Two comprehensive studies of the anthropometric and somatotype characteristics of athletes in specific sports have been recently reported. These include male and female participants in aquatic sports (swimming, synchronized swimming, diving, water polo) at the sixth Federation Internationale de Natation Amateur (FINA) championships in 1991,[27] and male soccer players at the 1995 American Cup (la Copa América).[28] Much of the data on the body size and somatotypes of athletes of both sexes are summarized in Carter and Heath.[29]

Anthropometric studies of elite athletes thus have a relatively long history in the 20th century, spanning about 75 years. Earlier studies focused largely on male athletes in a limited number of sports, whereas more recent studies include athletes of both sexes in a greater number of sports. Given the time frame of the studies, the issue of secular changes in body size is of interest. Male track-and-field athletes at the 1972 Olympic Games, for example, were taller (2–3 cm) than those at the 1960 Olympic Games.[30] On the other hand, there were no secular differences in the body size of Olympic athletes ≤18 years of age at the Mexico City, Munich and Montreal Games.[31] Sampling variation associated with generally small numbers and changing ethnic composition are confounding factors in secular comparisons of Olympic athletes.

Secular comparisons of athletes within specific sports indicate both positive and negative trends. For example, American football players (all white) at the University of Texas in the 1960s were, on average, 6.6 cm taller and 16.1 kg heavier than those early in the 20th century (1899–1910).[32] The size of American professional football players is a topic of regular discussion in the sports media.[33] In a more restricted time period, basketball players at the University of Kentucky in 1968 were 5.1 cm taller and 9.4 kg heavier than those in 1948.[34] On the other hand, recent samples of elite artistic gymnasts are younger, shorter and lighter than those in the 1970s.[35,36]

Secular trends in the body size of athletes need to be interpreted in the context of recruiting and changing style of play in some sports (American football, basketball) and selection practices and changing technical demands in other sports (gymnastics, figure skating). Changes in methods of training and diet are also important. Dietary restriction has been implicated in the low body weights of artistic gymnasts and figure skaters. The well-documented use of anabolic steroids and other chemical substances in several Eastern European countries[37,38] is an additional factor that needs to be considered in evaluating earlier anthropometric data from these countries.

A related factor in secular comparisons of athletes is the enhanced opportunities in sport for girls and women. This is best exemplified in the United States in the effects of Title IX of the Education Amendments Act of 1972. The relevant section states as follows: "No person in the United States shall, on the basis of sex, be excluded from participation in, be denied the benefits of, or be subjected to discrimination under any educational program or activity receiving Federal financial assistance...."[39] The regulations implementing Title IX were put into effect in 1975 and specifically included high school and collegiate athletic programs. As a result, opportunities for girls to participate in sport at the high school level and to continue participation at the collegiate level were expanded. Implementation was incomplete and there were many gender equity lawsuits in an attempt to accommodate women athletes.[39] An item of interest is the comparison of athletes before and after the legislation went into effect. With Title IX, scholarship support was more available for women athletes at many colleges and universities and the better athletes were more highly recruited.

III.   Concepts and Methods

Anthropometry is a set of standardized techniques for systematically taking measurements of the body and parts of the body, i.e., for quantifying dimensions of the body. It involves the use of carefully defined body landmarks for measurements, specific subject positioning for the measurements and the use of appropriate instruments. Measurement, of course, is objective and nonjudgmental. Evaluation of measurements requires interpretation and is judgmental.

An important issue is the selection of measurements because the number of dimensions that can be taken on an individual is almost limitless.

Measurement selection depends on the purpose of a study and the specific question(s) under consideration. Each measurement should provide a specific bit of information that contributes to the question(s) under study. Measurement for the sake of measurement (i.e., just to have the data available) is not appropriate.

Several more commonly used anthropometric dimensions are subsequently described. Each provides a specific bit of information on the external physical characteristics, more appropriately, dimensions of the individual. Techniques of measurement are described in the Anthropometric Standardization Reference Manual.[40] Other dimensions can be measured, but the choice of measurements depends on the information desired in the context of a study.[41,42]

A. Overall Body Size

Weight and stature (height) are the two most often used measurements of growth. The terms stature and height are used interchangeably. Body weight is a measure of body mass; it is more appropriately called body mass, but the term "weight" is entrenched in the literature. Body weight is a composite of independently varying tissues. Although weight should be measured with the individual nude, this is often impractical; it is thus taken with the individual attired in ordinary indoor clothing without shoes (e.g., gym shorts and a T-shirt).

Stature, or standing height, is a linear measurement of the distance from the floor or standing surface to the top (vertex) of the skull. It is measured with the subject in a standard erect posture, without shoes. Stature is a composite of linear dimensions contributed by the lower extremities, the trunk, the neck and the head.

Stature and weight show diurnal variation — variation during the course of a day. This can be a problem in short-term longitudinal studies in which apparent changes might simply reflect variation in the time of the day at which the measurement was taken. Stature is greatest in the morning upon arising from bed and decreases as the individual assumes upright posture and walks about. The "shrinking" of stature occurs as a result of compression of the fibrous intervertebral discs. With the force of gravity imposed by standing and walking, the discs are gradually compressed. As a result, stature diminishes by a centimeter or more. The loss of stature is limited to the vertebral column and thus to sitting height (see below). Compressive forces associated with vigorous physical activity also contribute to the diurnal reduction in height.

For body weight, the individual is lightest in the morning, specifically after voiding the bladder upon arising. Body weight then increases gradually during the course of the day and is affected by diet and physical activity. Phase of the menstrual cycle also affects diurnal variation in body weight.

B. Components of Stature

Sitting height, as the name implies, is height while sitting and includes the head, neck and trunk. This measurement is especially of value when used with stature. Stature minus sitting height provides an estimate of length of the lower extremities (subischial length or leg length). By definition, lower extremity length is the distance between the hip joint and the floor, with the individual standing erect. Precise location of the hip joint landmark is difficult in the living individual. Hence, lower extremity length is most often defined as the difference between stature and sitting height.

C. Skeletal Breadths

Breadth or width measurements are ordinarily taken across specific bone landmarks and therefore provide an indication of the robustness, or sturdiness, of the skeleton. Four skeletal breadths are commonly used to provide information about the robustness of the extremity and trunk skeleton. Biacromial breadth measures the distance across the right and left acromial processes of the scapulae and provides an indication of shoulder breadth. Bicristal breadth measures the distance across the most lateral parts of the iliac crests and provides an indication of hip breadth. Breadths across the bony condyles of the femur (bicondylar breadth) and the humerus (biepicondylar breadth) provide information on the robustness of the extremity skeleton.

D. Limb Circumferences

Limb circumferences are used as indicators of relative muscularity. Note, however, that a circumference includes bone surrounded by a mass of muscle tissue that is ringed by a layer of subcutaneous adipose tissue. Thus, a circumference does not provide a measure of muscle tissue per se; however, because muscle is the major tissue composing a circumference (except perhaps in obese individuals), limb circumferences are used to indicate relative muscular development. The two more commonly used limb measurements are the arm and calf circumferences. The former is measured with the arm hanging loosely at the side and the measurement is taken at the point midway between the acromial process of the scapula and olecranon process of the ulna (tip of the elbow). The latter is measured as the maximum circumference of the calf, most often with the subject in a standing position and the weight evenly distributed between both legs. Arm circumference is also measured in the tensed or flexed state (see below).

E. Skinfold Thicknesses

Skinfold thicknesses are indicators of subcutaneous adipose tissue. They are measured in the form of a double fold of skin and underlying subcutaneous tissue with special calipers. Skinfolds can be measured at any number of body sites. Most often, to provide information on the relative distribution of subcutaneous fat in different areas of the body, they are measured on the extremities and on the trunk. More commonly used skinfold sites on the extremities include the following:

- Triceps — on the back of the arm over the triceps muscle at the same level as arm circumference
- Biceps – over the biceps muscle at the same level as arm circumference
- Mid-thigh – over the anterior thigh at the level midway between the inguinal crease and the proximal border of the patella
- Medial calf — on the inside of the calf at the level of calf circumference.

The forearm and lateral calf skinfolds are occasionally used. The lateral and medial calf skinfolds are used for estimating calf muscle circumference. More commonly used skinfold sites on the trunk include the following:

- Subscapular — on the back just beneath the inferior angle of the scapula
- Suprailiac — over the iliac crest in the midaxillary line
- Abdominal — a horizontal fold lateral and inferior to the umbilicus

The Heath-Carter anthropometric somatotype protocol[29] (see below) utilizes a suprailiac skinfold, but it is measured over the anterior superior iliac spine (supraspinale).

F.   Quality Control

Implicit in studies using anthropometry is the assumption that every effort is made to ensure the accuracy and reliability of measurement and standardization of technique. Also implicit is the assumption that the measurements are taken by trained individuals. This is essential to obtain accurate and reliable data and to enhance the utility of the data from a comparative perspective. Reliable and accurate data are especially critical in serial studies where the same individual is followed longitudinally over time, either short- or long term, in which the definition of rather small changes may be necessary and technical errors associated with measurement can mask true changes.

Error is the discrepancy between the measured value and its true quantity. Measurement error can be random or systematic. Random measurement error is a normal aspect of anthropometry and results from variation within and between individuals in technique of measurement, problems with instruments (e.g., calibration or random variation in manufacture) and errors in recording (e.g., transposition of numbers). Random error is non-directional — it is above or below the true dimension. In large-scale surveys, random errors tend to cancel each other and ordinarily are not a major concern. Systematic error, on the other hand, results from the tendency of a technician or a measuring instrument (e.g., an improperly calibrated skinfold caliper or weighing scale) to consistently under- or over-measure a particular dimension. Such error is directional and introduces bias into the data.

Replicate measurements of the same subject are used to estimate variability or error in measurement. Replicate measurements on the same individual are taken independently by the same technician after a period of time has lapsed, or are taken independently on the same individual by two different technicians. They provide an estimate of imprecision. Replicates by the same individual provide an estimate of within-technician measurement variability, whereas corresponding measurements taken on the same subject by two different individuals provide an estimate of between-technician measurement variability.

The technical error of measurement is a widely used measure of replicability.[43] It is defined as the square root of the squared differences of replicates divided by twice the number of pairs (i.e., the within-subject variance):

$$\sigma_e = \sqrt{\Sigma d^2 / 2N}$$

The statistic assumes that the distribution of replicate differences is normal and that errors of all pairs can be pooled. It indicates that, about two thirds of the time, the measurement in question should fall within the technical error measurement.

Technical errors are reported in the units of the specific measurement. Within technician (intra-observer) and between technician (inter-observer) technical errors of measurement for a variety of anthropometric dimensions in national surveys and several more local studies are summarized in Malina.[42]

Accuracy is another component of the measurement process. It refers to how closely measurements taken by one or several technicians approximate the "true" measurement. Accuracy is ordinarily assessed by comparing measurements taken by the technician(s) with those obtained by a well trained or "criterion" anthropometrist (i.e., the standard of reference). However, even well trained expert anthropometrists do in fact make errors!

G. Ratios and Indices

In addition to providing specific information in their own right, measurements can be related to each other as indices or ratios to express proportional relationships. Ratios are influenced by the relationship between the two dimensions and it is assumed that the two dimensions change in a linear manner. Ratios may yield spurious results when they are based on different types of dimensions, such as weight and stature, or arm circumference and stature or when the standard deviations of the dimensions differ considerably.[44] Body dimensions may also be expressed in the form of an index in which one of the measurements is expressed as a power function. Ratios and indices provide information on proportional relationships between the dimensions and thus on body proportions.

The body mass index (BMI) expresses the relationship between weight and stature: BMI = weight/stature² where weight is in kilograms (kg) and stature is in meters (m) squared (kg/m²). It relates reasonably well to total body fatness in the general adult population, but also to the lean tissue mass of the body. The BMI is widely used at present in surveys to screen for overweight and obesity. Its usefulness stems from the fact that it is independent of stature, i.e., the correlation between the BMI and stature approaches zero. The utility of the BMI with athletes is questionable; it is more appropriately an index of heaviness and not fatness.

The sitting height:stature ratio provides an estimate of relative trunk length and, conversely, relative leg length. It is calculated as:

$$\frac{\text{sitting height}}{\text{height}} \times 100.$$

The relationship of dimensions of the shoulders and hips is of interest in comparisons of sexual dimorphism. The degree of masculinity in the female physique, or the degree of femininity in the male physique, can be estimated with the androgyny index suggested by Tanner:[45]

Androgyny index = (3 × biacromial breadth) − bicristal breadth.

H. Corrected Limb Circumferences

Adjusting arm and calf circumferences for the thicknesses of skinfolds provides an estimate of limb musculature. Assuming the limb is a cylinder, the circumference is corrected for the outer perimeter of subcutaneous adipose tissue. The corrected circumference provides an estimate of lean tissue (muscle plus bone). Because muscle is the dominant tissue, the resulting estimates are generally referred to as estimated mid-arm muscle and calf muscle circumferences or areas.

Relaxed arm circumference is corrected for the thicknesses of the triceps and biceps skinfolds and calf circumference is corrected for the thicknesses of the medial and lateral calf skinfolds. Using skinfolds on the anterior and posterior aspects of the arm and the medial and lateral aspects of the calf provides a better estimate of relative muscularity because subcutaneous adipose tissue is unevenly distributed on the extremities. It should be noted that, in surveys of nutritional status, arm circumference is ordinarily corrected only for the thickness of the triceps skinfold.

Calculations for correcting arm and calf circumferences are as follows:[42]

1. Estimated mid-arm muscle circumference (cm) = $C_a - \pi/2 \, (S_t + S_b)$
2. Estimated mid-arm muscle area (cm²) = $1/4\pi \, [C_a - \pi/2 \, (S_t + S_b)]$, where C_a is relaxed arm circumference (cm) and S_t and S_b are the triceps and biceps skinfolds (cm), respectively.
3. Estimated calf muscle circumference (cm) = $C_a - \pi/2 \, (S_m + S_l)$
4. Estimated calf muscle area (cm²) = $1/4\pi \, [C_a - \pi/2 \, (S_m + S_l)]$, where C_a is calf circumference (cm) and S_m and S_l are the medial and lateral calf skinfolds (cm), respectively.

I. Heath-Carter Anthropometric Somatotype

The Heath-Carter method for estimating somatotype combines both photoscopic and anthropometric procedures.[29] In practice, however, the Heath-Carter method is used primarily in its anthropometric form. Anthropometry is more objective and obtaining standardized somatotype photographs is difficult and costly. Somatotype components and the dimensions used in the Heath-Carter anthropometric protocol to derive each component are as follows:

- Endomorphy — described as relative fatness or leanness, is derived from the sum of three skinfolds — the triceps, subscapular and supraspinale. It has a continuum from lowest (relative leanness) to highest (relative fatness) values.
- Mesomorphy — refers to relative musculoskeletal development adjusted for stature. It is described as expressing fat-free mass relative to stature. Mesomorphy is derived from biepicondylar and bicondylar breadths, flexed arm circumference (in contrast to relaxed arm circumference) corrected for the thickness of the triceps skinfold and calf circumference corrected for the thickness of the medial calf skinfold. Correcting the circumferences is simply a matter of subtracting the skinfold thickness from the circumference. The four measurements of the upper and lower extremities are then adjusted for stature.
- Ectomorphy — the relative linearity of build. It is based on the reciprocal ponderal index (height divided by the cube root of body weight).

Although the components are described separately, the three together are components of a single entity, the individual's somatotype. Each component contributes variably to a somatotype. Hence, it is relative fatness, relative musculoskeletal development, or relative linearity in reference to the physique as a whole, which is a composite of the three components.

The algorithms for estimating a somatotype with the Heath-Carter anthropometric protocol are as follows:[29]

- Endomorphy = $-0.7182 + 0.1451(X) - 0.00068(X^2) + 0.0000014(X^3)$, where X is the sum of the triceps, subscapular and supraspinale skinfolds; to adjust for stature, X is multiplied by 170.18/height (cm);

- Mesomorphy = $(0.858$ biepicondylar + 0.601 bicondylar + 0.188 corrected arm circumference + 0.161 corrected calf circumference) $-$ (stature x 0.131) + 4.50, where corrected arm and calf circumferences are the respective limb circumferences minus the triceps and medial calf skinfolds, respectively;

- Ectomorphy = HWR $\times 0.732 - 28.58$, where HWR = stature/$\sqrt[3]{}$ weight. If HWR < 40.75 but > 38.25, ectomorphy = HWR $\times 0.463 - 17.63$. If HWR < 38.25, a rating of 0.1 is assigned.

If the calculation for any component is zero or negative, a value of 0.1 is assigned, because by definition a rating cannot be zero or negative.

The principles of quality control in anthropometry described in the preceding chapter also apply to the estimate of somatotype. Intra- and interobserver measurement variability can influence the reproducibility of somatotype components in the Heath-Carter anthropometric protocol. Errors are less than 0.5 somatotype units when the body dimensions are measured by experienced technicians.[46]

IV. Anthropometric Characteristics of Female Athletes

Consideration of the anthropometric characteristics of female athletes is important for several reasons. First, data for recent samples of female athletes in a variety of sports are relatively limited. Second, there has been a major change in the population of female athletes since Title IX legislation in the United States and wider social acceptance of women in the role of athlete. It is of interest, therefore, to compare the characteristics of female athletes over time. Third, anthropometry provides a relatively simple means of monitoring soft tissue and body composition changes associated with training and competition. This assumes, of course, that the data are collected by experienced anthropometrists with due attention to quality control. And fourth, many of the women athletes were followed during the course of a season or several seasons. This permits examination of the use of anthropometry to monitor changes in soft tissues and body composition during the season and variation with year in school.

Selected anthropometric characteristics of female athletes in seven sports are subsequently described. Anthropometric dimensions of 387 intercollegiate women athletes at the University of Texas at Austin, 295 whites

(European American ancestry and including several of Hispanic American ancestry) and 92 blacks (African-American ancestry), were measured from fall 1985 through fall 1995. They represented all of the athletes participating in the respective sports, which included swimming, diving, tennis, golf, basketball, volleyball and track and field. Sample sizes by sport and by race and position or event within three sports are indicated later. Over the interval of the survey, the teams in each of the sports were nationally competitive and were quite successful at the national intercollegiate level, including 19 national championships. The sample included several Olympians, world record holders, national champions and All-Americans. Most of the sample was on scholarship support for their athletic abilities (at the time of the surveys, the Department of Intercollegiate Athletics for Women at the University of Texas served the needs of about 100 scholarship athletes per year).[47] Hence, the athletes as a group can be regarded as reasonably elite.

In addition to weight, height and sitting height, four skeletal breadths (biacromial, bicristal, biepicondylar, bicondylar), three limb circumferences (arm relaxed, arm flexed, calf) and nine skinfolds (triceps, biceps, forearm, subscapular, suprailiac, supraspinale, anterior thigh, medial calf, lateral calf) were measured on all athletes. All measurements were made by the same individual (RMM). The sitting height:height ratio and the androgyny index were calculated. Relaxed arm and calf circumferences were corrected for the triceps and biceps and medial and lateral calf skinfolds, respectively, to estimate limb muscularity. The sum of eight skinfolds (excluding supraspinale) was used as an indicator of overall subcutaneous adipose tissue. Percentage body fat was estimated from four skinfolds (triceps, subscapular, suprailiac, medial calf) using an equation developed for female swimmers.[48] Finally, somatotypes were estimated with the Heath-Carter anthropometric protocol.[29]

A sample of 123 students enrolled at the same university as the athletes was also measured in 1987.[49] The battery included weight, height, sitting height, four skeletal breadths, three limb circumferences and four skinfolds (triceps, subscapular, supraspinale, medial calf). The sitting height:height ratio androgyny index and Heath-Carter somatotypes were calculated for the nonathletes.

A. Athletes, Nonathletes and Variation among Sports

Means and standard deviations for age and the selected anthropometric characteristics of the athletes in seven sports and the nonathletes are indicated in Table 7.1. With the exception of divers, who are similar to the nonathletes, athletes in the other sports are, on average, taller and heavier than nonathletes. Swimmers, basketball players and volleyball players have better developed arm musculature than athletes in the other sports. On the other hand, basketball and volleyball players and track-and-field athletes have better developed calf musculature than athletes in the other sports. The

TABLE 7.1

Age and Selected Anthropometric Characteristics of Female Athletes in Seven Sports and a Sample of Nonathletes

Variable	Swimming (n = 87)		Diving (n = 19)		Tennis (n = 29)		Golf (n = 32)		Basketball (n = 57)		Volleyball (N = 47)		Track & Field (n = 116)		Nonathletes (n = 1 23)	
	Mean	SD	Mean	SD	Mean	SD	Mean	SD	Mean	SD	Mean	SD	Mean	SD	Mean	SD
Age, yrs	18.8	0.9	19.5	1.6	19.0	0.9	19.0	0.9	19.5	1.2	19.1	0.9	19.4	1.2	18.7	0.6
Height, cm	171.8	5.7	163.4	5.3	167.9	5.7	166.6	6.7	176.7	9.2	177.9	5.6	167.0	5.5	163.3	5.9
Weight, kg	63.0	5.1	57.8	6.5	60.1	6.8	60.0	5.8	70.0	8.8	70.3	7.5	60.2	12.2	56.9	8.2
Sit Ht/Ht, %	52.7	1.0	53.7	1.2	52.8	1.1	52.9	1.2	51.4	1.2	51.6	1.2	51.8	1.4	52.7	1.0
Biacromial, cm	39.5	1.5	37.7	1.1	37.1	1.8	36.9	1.8	39.4	1.8	39.3	1.5	37.8	1.9	36.1	1.6
Bicristal, cm	28.2	1.3	27.3	1.4	28.0	1.4	28.1	1.3	28.3	2.1	28.2	1.6	26.9	1.9	27.5	1.8
Androgyny Index	90.3	4.0	85.7	3.1	83.1	4.9	82.6	5.0	89.8	4.7	89.8	4.0	86.6	5.1	80.9	4.3
Arm Muscle, cm	25.1	1.5	23.6	1.4	22.6	1.7	22.3	0.9	24.6	1.4	24.4	1.4	23.1	2.6		
Calf Muscle, cm	30.4	1.4	30.3	1.9	30.2	1.6	29.7	1.5	32.4	2.1	32.5	1.9	31.7	2.3		
Sum 8 Skf, mm	91.2	16.7	97.4	23.6	100.3	21.5	113.7	23.1	87.1	20.9	91.3	23.4	74.7	32.2		
Fat, %	16.5	1.6	17.4	2.6	17.7	2.4	19.1	2.2	16.4	2.2	16.9	2.7	15.4	3.8		
Endomorphy	3.0	0.6	3.5	0.9	3.6	0.9	4.2	0.8	3.0	0.8	3.1	0.9	2.8	1.2	4.6	1.4
Mesomorphy	3.8	0.7	4.2	0.7	3.6	0.9	3.7	0.8	3.5	1.1	3.4	1.0	3.7	1.3	3.3	1.1
Ectomorphy	3.0	0.7	2.4	1.0	2.9	0.9	2.6	0.8	2.9	1.0	3.0	0.9	2.9	1.2	2.7	1.3

trends in estimated limb muscle circumferences probably reflects sport-specific body size variation and the specific demands of the respective sports.

Swimmers, tennis players, golfers and nonathletes are similar in the proportions of trunk length to height, or conversely, relative leg length, whereas divers have, on average, relatively shorter lower extremities (higher sitting height:height ratio). Ratios for basketball players, volleyball players and track-and-field athletes are, on average, lower, indicating proportionally longer legs. This reflects, to some extent, the racial composition of the sample. Black athletes are represented in these three sports, and blacks have, on average, lower sitting height:height ratios, i.e., relatively longer lower extremities. Shoulder–hip relationships indicate higher androgyny indices in the athletes in all sports than in the nonathletes. Swimmers, volleyball players and basketball players are most androgynous in build, followed by track-and-field athletes as a group, divers, tennis players and golfers.

Among athletes, golfers have, on average, the largest sum of eight skinfolds and estimated relative fatness, whereas track-and-field athletes have the lowest sum and estimated relative fatness. Standard deviations are reasonably large, indicating overlap among athletes in the seven sports.

Golfers are slightly more mesomorphic and less endomorphic than nonathletes. Athletes in other sports tend to be less endomorphic and more mesomorphic than the nonathletes, but only slightly more ectomorphic.

The heights and weights (mean ± one standard deviation) for the athletes in each sport are plotted relative to the new Centers for Disease Control and Prevention[50] reference values for the American population in Figure 7.1. The reference values are for females 19.5 years of age. Mean heights and weights of divers are similar to the reference median. Mean heights of tennis players, golfers and track-and-field athletes as a group approximate the 75th percentile, while their mean weights are slightly above the medians. Mean height of swimmers exceeds the 90th percentile and mean weight is slightly below the 75th percentile. Mean heights of basketball players and volleyball players exceed the 97th percentile and are between the 75th and 90th percentiles for body weight. Thus, the athletes as a group tend to carry less weight for height than young adult American women, with the exception of divers. The position of the heights and weights of child and adolescent female athletes in these sports compared to United States reference values is similar to that of adult athletes.[51,52] The same is true for other characteristics of young athletes. In other words, the size, proportions, body composition and somatotype characteristics of elite young athletes are generally consistent with those reported in adult athletes participating in the same sport or position or event within a sport.[29,31,51,53] This emphasizes an important role for constitutional factors in the selection or exclusion process for sport.

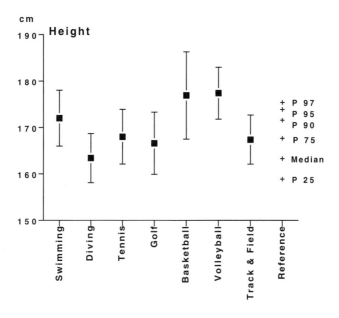

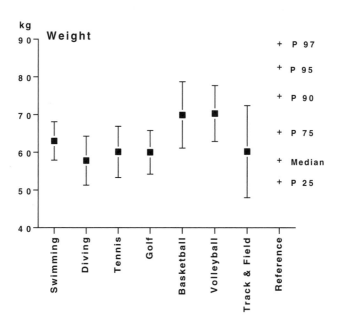

FIGURE 7.1
Heights (top) and weights (bottom) of athletes in seven sports (means±standard deviations) compared with reference data for young adult American women 19.5 years of age. Reference values are from the new Centers for Disease Control and Prevention growth charts.[50]

B. Variation within Specific Sports

Athletes in some sports show variation in anthropometric characteristics associated with specific events or positions within a sport. This variation probably reflects the performance demands of the specific events or positions. This is readily evident by stroke among swimmers, by event in track-and-field athletes and by position among volleyball and basketball players. An additional potential source of variation is the ethnic or racial distribution of athletes in some sports, specifically basketball and track and field.

1. Swimming

Characteristics of swimmers by stroke are summarized in Table 7.2. All swimmers in the sample were white. Allowing for small sample sizes in the butterfly and individual medley, freestyle and backstroke swimmers tend to be slightly taller and heavier than specialists in the breaststroke, butterfly and individual medley. Estimated arm and calf muscle circumferences do not differ among swimmers specializing in different strokes, except for somewhat smaller estimated values in the small sample of medley swimmers. Swimmers specializing in different strokes are, on average, generally similar in the sitting height:height ratio, the androgyny index, subcutaneous adipose tissue and relative fatness and somatotype.

Mean heights and weights (± one standard deviation) of swimmers by stroke are compared with United States reference values in Figure 7.2. Freestyle and backstroke swimmers approximate the 90th percentile for height and the 75th percentile for weight. Heights of breaststroke, butterfly and

TABLE 7.2

Age and Selected Anthropometric Characteristics of Female Swimmers by Stroke

Variable	Freestyle (n = 37) Mean	SD	Backstroke (n = 18) Mean	SD	Breaststroke (n = 17) Mean	SD	Butterfly (n = 9) Mean	SD	Medley (n = 6) Mean	SD
Age, yrs	18.8	0.8	18.9	1.0	18.7	0.7	19.1	1.0	18.9	1.4
Height, cm	173.4	6.0	172.7	4.2	169.4	4.8	169.8	6.7	169.3	6.2
Weight, kg	63.5	5.4	64.5	5.3	61.5	5.2	62.2	4.4	60.5	3.0
Sit Ht/Ht, %	52.7	0.9	52.6	1.0	52.5	1.3	53.2	0.8	52.7	0.8
Biacromial, cm	39.7	1.4	39.8	1.5	39.3	1.5	38.5	1.4	39.3	1.6
Bicristal, cm	28.4	1.3	28.3	1.2	28.0	1.4	28.0	1.2	26.8	1.4
Androgyny Index	90.8	3.7	91.0	4.0	89.9	4.1	87.4	3.3	91.0	5.8
Arm Muscle, cm	25.2	1.6	25.1	1.1	25.0	1.6	25.5	1.9	24.3	0.3
Calf Muscle, cm	30.4	1.4	30.7	1.4	30.4	1.5	30.6	1.5	29.9	1.6
Sum 8 Skf, mm	88.8	15.1	93.9	20.5	88.1	14.1	91.4	20.0	105.9	9.3
Fat, %	16.3	1.6	16.8	1.9	16.4	1.3	16.4	1.9	17.5	0.8
Endomorphy	2.9	0.7	3.2	0.7	3.1	0.5	3.0	0.8	3.4	0.3
Mesomorphy	3.7	0.6	3.8	0.6	3.9	0.5	4.0	1.0	3.9	0.6
Ectomorphy	3.2	0.8	3.0	0.5	2.9	0.6	2.8	1.0	3.0	0.7

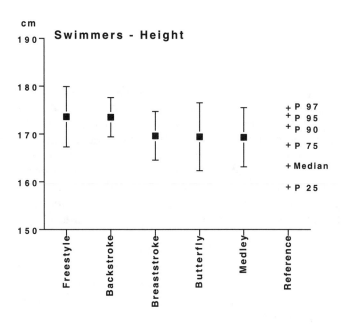

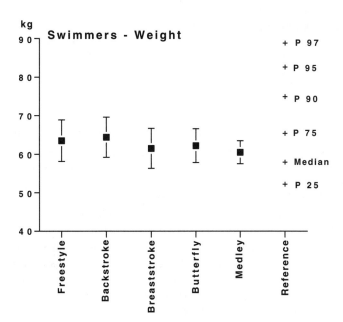

FIGURE 7.2
Heights (top) and weights (bottom) of swimmers by stroke (means ± standard deviations) compared with reference data for young adult American women 19.5 years of age. Reference values are from the new Centers for Disease Control and Prevention growth charts.[50]

individual medley specialists fall between the 75th and 90th percentiles, whereas weights fall between the median and 75th percentiles.

2. Basketball

The total sample of basketball players (n = 57) included 30 whites and 27 blacks. The players were classified into three positions: guards, wings or forwards and post players or centers. Sample sizes by race within position are thus small. Nevertheless, characteristics of basketball players by position and race are summarized in Table 7.3. As expected, there is variation in anthropometric characteristics by position. Height and weight increase, on average, from guards to wings to post players. Within each position, black basketball players have proportionally longer lower extremities (lower sitting height:height ratio). Black and white players at the wing position are most similar in body size, estimated muscle circumferences, the androgyny index, fatness and somatotype. There is some ethnic variation among players at the other two positions. Among guards, blacks are somewhat taller, more androgynous and less endomorphic and have less fatness. Among post players, whites are taller and more ectomorphic, whereas blacks are more androgynous and mesomorphic.

Relative to reference data for young adult American women, guards have heights that fall, on average, between the median and 75th percentile and weights that approximate the 75th percentile (Figure 7.3). Mean heights of wings are at the 95th percentile, but weights are between the 75th and 90th percentiles. Mean heights of post players exceed the 97th percentile, but mean weights are between the 90th and 95th percentiles.

3. Volleyball

The number of black volleyball players is small (n = 9), so that ethnic comparisons by position are not possible. The black players are represented among three of the four positions. Anthropometric characteristics by position are summarized in Table 7.4. Middle blockers are, on average, tallest and heaviest, followed in order by outside hitters, setters and back row specialists. Although middle blockers are taller and heavier, estimated arm muscle does not differ from setters and back row specialists. Outside hitters have, on average, the largest estimated arm muscle circumference. There is little difference in calf muscle among volleyball players by position, except for somewhat smaller estimates in setters. The androgyny index and fatness show the same trend. Proportional differences in the legs and trunk are small. Outside hitters and back row specialists are most mesomorphic, whereas middle blockers and setters have balanced somatotypes.

Relative to reference values for young adult American women, outside hitters and middle blockers have heights that exceed the 97th percentile and weights that are just below the 90th percentile (Figure 7.4). Setters and back

TABLE 7.3

Age and Selected Anthropometric Characteristics of Female Basketball Players by Position and Race

	Guard				Wing/Forward				Post			
	White (n = 13)		Black (n = 7)		White (n = 6)		Black (n = 11)		White (n = 11)		Black (n = 9)	
Variable	Mean	SD	Mean	SD	Mean	SD	Mean	SD	Mean	SD	Mean	SD
Age, yrs	19.4	0.9	19.6	1.2	19.3	0.9	19.8	1.5	19.6	1.4	19.6	1.6
Height, cm	166.9	3.9	169.4	2.6	176.6	3.5	175.7	3.8	188.6	7.5	183.3	4.9
Weight, kg	61.4	6.6	62.0	3.4	71.1	5.5	69.5	4.2	77.6	4.9	79.1	6.8
Sit Ht/Ht, %	52.7	0.7	51.2	0.9	52.3	0.7	50.3	0.8	51.1	1.0	50.6	1.1
Biacromial, cm	37.5	1.3	38.0	1.0	40.1	1.5	39.6	0.9	40.7	1.6	40.9	1.0
Bicristal, cm	27.4	1.5	26.0	1.4	28.8	1.3	27.6	1.5	31.0	1.3	28.6	1.9
Androgyny Index	85.1	3.7	88.1	3.3	91.3	3.9	91.1	2.9	91.0	5.3	94.0	3.1
Arm Muscle, cm	23.6	1.6	24.9	0.7	25.0	0.9	24.8	1.2	24.7	1.7	25.2	0.7
Calf Muscle, cm	30.7	2.0	32.2	2.1	32.7	1.2	32.3	1.5	32.8	1.5	34.5	2.2
Sum 8 Skf, mm	95.4	20.1	70.7	11.9	80.7	8.1	77.6	16.8	97.1	24.1	91.7	23.9
Fat, %	16.9	2.1	14.9	1.2	16.1	1.4	15.5	1.7	17.4	2.6	17.1	2.5
Endomorphy	3.3	0.9	2.7	0.4	2.9	0.6	2.9	0.7	3.0	0.9	2.9	0.8
Mesomorphy	3.8	0.9	4.0	0.7	3.9	0.7	3.7	0.6	2.5	1.4	3.6	1.0
Ectomorphy	2.5	1.0	2.8	0.6	2.6	0.8	2.7	0.6	3.8	1.3	2.7	0.9

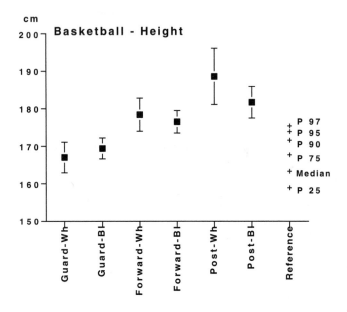

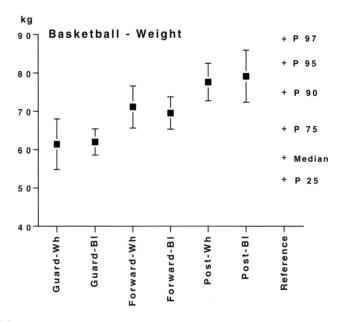

FIGURE 7.3

Heights (top) and weights (bottom) of basketball players by race (Wh = White, Bl = Black) within position (means ± standard deviations) compared with reference data for young adult American women 19.5 years of age. Reference values are from the new Centers for Disease Control and Prevention growth charts.[50]

TABLE 7.4

Age and Selected Anthropometric Characteristics of Female Volleyball Players by Position

Variable	Outsider Hitter (n = 24)		Middle Blocker (n = 12)		Setter (n = 6)		Back Row (n = 5)	
	Mean	SD	Mean	SD	Mean	SD	Mean	SD
Age, yrs	19.2	1.0	18.7	0.7	19.2	0.8	19.2	0.5
Height, cm	178.5	5.3	181.8	2.0	173.7	5.0	170.8	3.5
Weight, kg	71.1	8.2	73.3	4.0	66.1	7.6	64.0	5.5
Sit Ht/Ht, %	51.5	1.3	51.2	1.2	52.3	0.8	52.3	1.1
Biacromial, cm	39.5	1.5	40.0	1.3	38.9	1.4	37.8	1.4
Bicristal, cm	28.2	1.5	29.2	1.6	27.7	1.0	26.7	1.7
Androgyny Index	90.1	4.1	90.7	3.7	89.0	3.7	86.6	4.1
Arm Muscle, cm	24.8	1.2	24.0	0.9	23.9	2.0	24.0	1.9
Calf Muscle, cm	32.8	1.9	32.3	1.2	31.7	2.9	32.5	2.6
Sum 8 Skf, mm	90.5	26.4	99.6	22.2	91.4	13.0	75.1	13.3
Fat, %	16.9	3.0	17.8	2.6	17.0	1.9	14.9	1.3
Endomorphy	3.1	1.0	3.3	0.9	3.2	0.5	2.4	0.5
Mesomorphy	3.5	1.0	3.1	0.8	3.4	1.5	3.6	1.0
Ectomorphy	3.0	0.9	3.2	0.7	2.9	1.4	2.7	0.9

row specialists have heights that approximate the 95th and 90th percentiles, respectively and weights that approximate the 75th percentile for nonathletic women.

4. Track and Field

Although many track-and-field athletes participated in more than one event, their primary event was used for classification. Sprints include 100 and 200 meters (100 and 220 yards) and hurdlers at these distances. Middle distance runs include 800 and 1500 meters (half mile and mile). Some sprinters and middle distance runners also ran in the 400 meters (440 yards). Distance runs include cross-country and 3,000, 5,000 and 10,000 meters. Cross-country is a fall sport, whereas other distance runs are included in the indoor and out-door seasons. Almost all athletes in field events participated in more than one event. They were simply classified as jumpers (long jump, high jump, heptathletes) and throwers (discus, shotput, javelin). There are five white sprinters and only one black distance runner.

Anthropometric characteristics of track-and-field athletes by event and race are summarized in Table 7.5 (running events) and Table7. 6 (field events). Middle-distance and distance runners do not differ in height and weight; sprinters are slightly taller and heavier. Among runners, sprinters have the best developed arm musculature and, to a lesser extent, calf musculature. Ethnic variation in height among runners is negligible. Among sprinters and middle distance runners, black athletes have proportionally longer legs, are somewhat more androgynous and have less fatness. Somatotypes of black and white middle-distance runners do not differ, while distance runners are

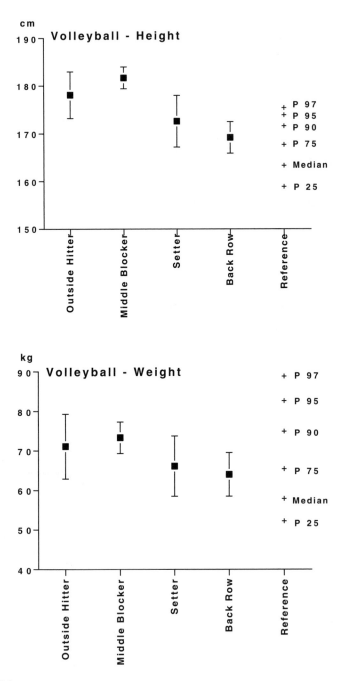

FIGURE 7.4
Heights (top) and weights (bottom) of volleyball players by position (means ± standard deviations) compared with reference data for young adult American women 19.5 years of age. Reference values are from the new Centers for Disease Control and Prevention growth charts.[50]

TABLE 7.5

Age and Selected Anthropometric Characteristics of Female Track and Field Athletes by Running Event and Race

	Sprint				Middle Distance				Distance	
	White (n = 5)		Black (n = 38)		White (n = 6)		Black (n = 5)		White (n = 29)	
	Mean	SD	Mean	SD	Mean	SD	Mean	SD	Mean	SD
Age, yrs	21.1	1.4	19.3	1.4	18.9	0.6	18.6	0.8	19.3	1.2
Height, cm	168.1	3.5	166.0	4.9	165.1	4.0	164.7	7.2	164.7	4.7
Weight, kg	57.3	4.1	59.2	6.1	53.0	2.6	54.7	8.2	52.2	3.8
Sit Ht/Ht, %	52.3	1.7	51.3	0.9	51.8	1.2	50.8	0.9	52.6	1.1
Biacromial, cm	37.1	1.4	37.9	1.7	37.2	1.1	37.3	1.3	36.5	1.2
Bicristal, cm	26.9	1.4	26.0	1.4	26.6	1.1	26.2	1.4	26.8	1.3
Androgyny Index	84.3	5.0	87.8	4.5	84.9	3.1	85.6	4.1	82.7	3.2
Arm Muscle, cm	23.5	1.3	23.4	1.7	21.5	1.1	21.5	1.1	20.7	1.1
Calf Muscle, cm	31.9	1.1	31.9	1.9	30.6	1.8	31.6	1.8	30.4	1.4
Sum 8 Skf, mm	64.6	8.3	61.6	11.0	62.4	17.2	57.8	5.0	66.6	16.2
Fat, %	14.1	0.3	14.1	1.4	13.8	1.6	13.6	0.7	14.2	1.6
Endomorphy	2.4	0.2	2.4	0.5	2.3	0.9	2.2	0.2	2.4	0.7
Mesomorphy	3.3	0.2	3.8	0.7	3.3	0.4	3.2	0.9	2.8	0.8
Ectomorphy	3.3	0.2	2.6	0.6	3.6	0.5	3.3	1.6	3.7	1.0

TABLE 7.6

Age and Selected Anthropometric Characteristics of Female Track and Field Athletes by Field Event and Race

	Jumps				Throws			
	White (n = 9)		Black (n = 7)		White (n = 11)		Black (n = 5)	
	Mean	SD	Mean	SD	Mean	SD	Mean	SD
Age, yrs	19.3	0.9	20.0	1.3	19.5	1.1	18.7	0.5
Height, cm	172.4	4.1	167.0	4.9	170.8	6.7	174.2	2.2
Weight, kg	60.9	5.7	60.9	5.6	77.1	9.8	94.0	24.5
Sit Ht/Ht, %	52.1	1.4	50.3	1.4	53.3	1.1	51.6	1.2
Biacromial, cm	39.0	1.2	37.6	1.7	39.5	1.4	42.2	2.5
Bicristal, cm	27.4	1.2	26.1	1.2	29.3	1.7	30.3	2.8
Androgyny Index	89.6	3.9	86.7	4.4	89.1	3.7	96.4	5.4
Arm Muscle, cm	23.6	1.6	23.0	1.7	26.6	1.4	29.1	3.2
Calf Muscle, cm	31.8	2.4	32.7	2.1	32.8	2.2	36.4	3.4
Sum 8 Skf, mm	73.0	14.1	65.4	11.3	138.6	34.8	141.3	53.6
Fat, %	15.1	1.8	14.6	1.4	22.4	4.1	23.9	7.8
Endomorphy	2.4	0.7	2.7	0.7	4.8	1.4	5.4	2.2
Mesomorphy	3.2	0.9	3.8	0.6	5.5	1.3	7.1	2.4
Ectomorphy	3.5	1.1	2.5	0.6	1.1	0.8	0.8	1.0

somewhat less mesomorphic and more ectomorphic than middle-distance runners. Among sprinters, blacks are more mesomorphic and less ectomorphic.

Comparisons of field athletes must be tempered by the small sample sizes (Table 7.6). Black throwers are tallest, followed by white jumpers, white throwers and black jumpers. Estimated arm muscle is larger in throwers than in jumpers, but estimated calf muscle does not differ except for larger mean in the small sample of black throwers, which reflects their larger body size. The same trend is apparent for the androgyny index. Black and white jumpers do not differ in body weight, but black jumpers have less fatness. Black throwers are heavier than white throwers, but differences in fatness between black and white throwers are negligible. Black jumpers are more mesomorphic and white jumpers are somewhat more ectomorphic. Black throwers are more mesomorphic and endomorphic than white throwers.

Mean heights and weights (± one standard deviation) of track-and-field athletes by event and race are compared to United States reference values in Figure 7.5. Sprinters, middle-distance runners, distance runners and black jumpers have heights that fall, on average, between the median and 75th percentile of the reference. White jumpers and throwers have heights at the 90th percentile, while black throwers have a mean height at the 95th percentile. In contrast, body weights of track-and-field athletes are more variable. Middle-distance and distance runners have mean weights that fall between the median and 25th percentile. Sprinters have mean weights that approximate the median, while jumpers have mean weights slightly above the median. White and black throwers, as expected, have mean weights above the 90th and 97th percentiles, respectively. The wide range of variation in the small sample of black throwers should be noted.

V.   Secular Comparisons of Athletes

Data for two comparative samples of female athletes are considered in secular comparisons. The first includes 67 athletes (66 white, 1 black) who were participants in the First National Intercollegiate Track and Field Championships in San Marcos, Texas, in 1969.[54,55] The athletes represented seven colleges and universities in the southern part of the United States and about two-thirds of the athletes at the competition. At the time of the competition, the 880-yard and 1-mile runs (800 and 1500 meters, respectively) were classified as "distance" runs. At present, they are classified as middle distance.

The second sample includes 108 intercollegiate athletes at the University of Texas at Austin who were measured in 1973–1974 and 1978–1979. This sample included athletes in swimming, diving, tennis, basketball, volleyball and track and field. The track and field sample included seven black athletes. With the exception of six cross-country (distance) runners and one thrower,

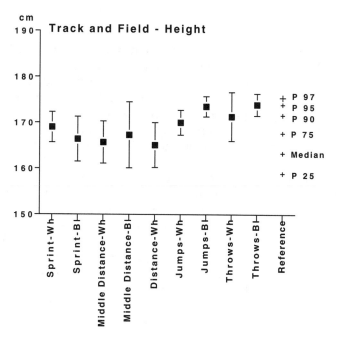

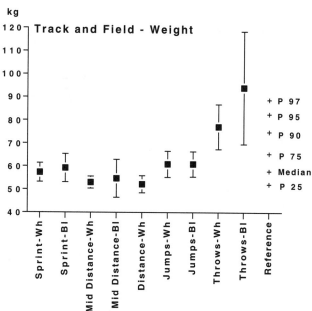

FIGURE 7.5

Heights (top) and weights (bottom) of track and field athletes by race (Wh = White, Bl = Black) within event (means ± standard deviations) compared with reference data for young adult American women 19.5 years of age. Reference values are from the new Centers for Disease Control and Prevention growth charts.[50]

the events of the other track-and-field athletes were not specified. Some of the data have been published previously.[56,57]

The athletes at the 1969 championships and at the University of Texas from 1986 through 1995 were measured by the same individual (RMM). The sample of athletes in the 1970s was measured by two individuals. Intra- and interobserver technical errors of measurement for the common core of dimensions (weight, height, sitting height, skeletal breadths, limb circumferences and four skinfolds) derived from several independent studies are generally smaller than estimates in the United States Health Examination Survey.[42,43]

The athletes studied in 1969 and the 1970s represent the pre-Title IX era. Although some athletes were measured in 1978 and 1979, the impact of Title IX legislation was just starting. Thus, the data summarized in Tables 7.7 through 7.9 can be viewed as comparisons of pre- and post-Title IX athletes. The more recent sample of university athletes (1986–1995) is different from those of earlier studies in terms of opportunity, selection and recruitment, scholarship support and greater social acceptability of females in the role of athlete. Note there has been, on average, no significant secular increase in the heights of adolescents and young adults in the United States since the 1960s.[50]

TABLE 7.7

Age and Selected Anthropometric Characteristics of Female Athletes in Three Sports at the Same University*

Sport/Variable	Mean	SD	Mean	SD
Swimming	1970s (n = 24)		1990 (n = 87)	
Age, yrs	19.3	1.2	18.8	0.9
Height, cm	170.3	4.5	171.8	5.7
Weight, kg	57.8	4.8	63.0	5.1
Sit Ht/Ht, %	52.2	1.3	52.7	1.0
Androgyny Index	85.8	3.8	90.3	4.0
Diving	1970s (n = 6)		1990 (n = 19)	
Age, yrs	20.2	1.0	19.5	1.6
Height, cm	162.5	3.9	163.4	5.3
Weight, kg	55.3	3.8	57.8	6.5
Tennis	1970s (n = 10)		1990 (n = 29)	
Age, yrs	19.5	1.5	19.0	0.9
Height, cm	168.1	5.4	167.9	5.7
Weight, kg	62.4	8.5	60.2	6.8
Sit Ht/Ht, %	52.4	1.0	52.8	1.1
Androgyny Index	80.2	2.2	83.1	4.9

* Measured between 1973 and 1978 (mid-1970s) and between 1986 and 1995 (1990). All athletes were white.

The more recent sample of swimmers is only slightly taller (1.5 cm) but considerably heavier (5.2 kg) and has a higher androgyny index than the sample from the mid-1970s. In contrast, the two samples of tennis players do not differ in body size and relative sitting height, but the more recent sample is somewhat more androgynous. The six divers in the mid-1970s do not differ in mean height and weight from the more recent sample (Table 7.7). Biacromial and bicristal breadths are not available for the earlier sample of divers. Diving and tennis have a tradition of social acceptability for women, whereas many elite young swimmers in the 1960s often "retired" in their teens due to the lack of opportunities at the collegiate level. Hence, small differences in body size over time might be expected in divers and tennis players.

Athletes in the two team sports in the post-Title IX sample are taller and heavier and have especially higher androgyny indices than athletes in the corresponding sports in the mid-1970s (Table 7.8). Relative sitting height differs only slightly, but suggests that the more recent samples have proportionally longer lower extremities.

Comparisons of track-and-field athletes are summarized in Table 7.9. Differences in body size and proportions over time vary by event and are confounded in part by ethnic variation. Except for the greater height of the small sample of distance runners in 1978, current samples of white athletes in the other events tend to be, on average, taller, but body weights do not appreciably differ. Sitting height:height ratios in the current samples of white sprinters, middle-distance runners and jumpers suggest proportionally longer lower extremities. In contrast, the two samples of throwers do not differ in relative sitting height and the earlier sample of distance runners has proportionally longer lower extremities than the current sample. The androgyny index is larger in the current sample of track-and-field athletes

TABLE 7.8

Age and Selected Anthropometric Characteristics of Female Basketball and Volleyball Players at the Same University*

Sport/Variable	Mean	SD	Mean	SD	Mean	SD
Basketball	**1970s (n = 18)**		**1990 (n = 30, Wh)**		**1990 (n = 27, Bl)**	
Age, yrs	19.9	0.9	19.5	1.1	19.7	1.4
Height, cm	172.2	7.6	176.8	11.2	176.6	6.7
Weight, kg	64.2	9.1	69.3	9.3	70.7	8.3
Sit Ht/Ht, %	52.3	1.3	52.0	1.1	50.7	1.0
Androgyny Index	80.4	4.7	88.5	5.2	91.3	3.7
Volleyball	**1970s (n = 29)**		**1990 (n = 38, Wh)**		**1990 (n = 9, Bl)**	
Age, yrs	19.9	1.2	19.1	0.9	18.9	0.6
Height, cm	168.9	8.5	178.2	5.9	176.8	4.2
Weight, kg	61.8	5.6	69.7	7.1	72.9	8.8
Sit Ht/Ht, %	52.2	1.4	51.9	1.1	50.5	1.4
Androgyny Index	83.2	3.9	89.4	4.1	91.2	3.5

* Measured between 1973 and 1979 (mid-1970s) and between 1986 and 1995 (1990). All players in the mid-1970s were white.

TABLE 7.9

Age and Selected Anthropometric Characteristics of Intercollegiate Female Track-and-Field Athletes*

Event/Variable	Mean	SD	Mean	SD	Mean	SD
Sprint	**1969 (n = 24)**		**1990 (n = 5, Wh)**		**1990 (n = 43, Bl)**	
Age, yrs	20.1	1.3	21.1	1.4	19.3	1.4
Height, cm	165.0	4.1	168.1	3.5	166.0	4.9
Weight, kg	56.7	5.5	57.3	4.1	59.2	6.1
Sit Ht/Ht, %	53.2	1.0	52.3	1.7	51.3	0.9
Androgyny Index	82.0	4.2	84.3	5.0	87.8	4.5
Middle Distance	**1969 (n = 12)**		**1990 (n = 6, Wh)**		**1990 (n = 5, Bl)**	
Age, yrs	20.9	3.5	18.9	0.6	18.6	0.8
Height, cm	161.7	4.4	165.1	4.0	164.7	7.2
Weight, kg	52.5	4.7	53.0	2.6	54.7	8.2
Sit Ht/Ht, %	52.8	1.2	51.8	1.2	50.8	0.9
Androgyny Index	80.0	3.4	84.9	3.1	85.6	4.1
Distance	**1978 (n = 6, Wh)**		**1990 (n = 29, Wh)**			
Age, yrs	18.2	0.8	19.3	1.2		
Height, cm	168.3	6.5	164.7	4.7		
Weight, kg	52.8	6.2	52.2	3.8		
Sit Ht/Ht, %	51.7	0.8	52.6	1.1		
Jumps	**1969 (n = 12)**		**1990 (n = 9, Wh)**		**1990 (n = 7, Bl)**	
Age, yrs	20.2	1.1	19.3	0.9	20.0	1.3
Height, cm	166.0	4.7	172.4	4.1	167.0	4.9
Weight, kg	58.4	3.4	60.9	5.7	60.9	5.6
Sit Ht/Ht, %	52.5	1.0	52.1	1.4	50.3	1.4
Androgyny Index	85.5	4.4	89.6	3.9	86.7	4.4
Throws	**1969 (n = 19)**		**1990 (n = 11, Wh)**		**1990 (n = 5, Bl)**	
Age, yrs	21.3	1.4	19.5	1.1	18.7	0.5
Height, cm	168.1	5.3	170.8	6.7	174.2	2.2
Weight, kg	74.0	11.3	77.1	9.8	94.0	24.5
Sit Ht/Ht, %	53.3	0.9	53.3	1.1	51.6	1.2
Androgyny Index	87.6	3.2	89.1	3.7	96.4	5.4
Total Samples	**1969 (n = 67)**		**1978 (n = 14, Wh)**		**1978 (n = 7, Bl)**	
Age, yrs	20.7	1.9	19.1	1.2	19.6	0.9
Height, cm	165.5	5.0	171.5	6.7	166.2	4.0
Weight, kg	61.2	11.0	60.1	10.4	53.0	3.7
Sit Ht/Ht, %	53.0	1.0	51.9	1.0	50.8	0.9
Androgyny Index	83.7	4.6				
Total Samples			**1990 (n = 60, Wh)**		**1990 (n = 56, Bl)**	
Age, yrs			19.4	1.2	19.3	1.3
Height, cm			167.3	5.7	166.7	5.4
Weight, kg			58.6	10.8	61.9	13.5
Sit Ht/Ht, %			52.6	1.3	51.1	1.1
Androgyny Index			85.3	4.6	88.1	5.2

* Measured in 1969 and 1978 and between 1986 and 1995 (1990). The 1969 sample included only one black athlete (see text for details).

in each event than in athletes measured in 1969 (measurements needed to derive the index are not available for the 1978 sample).

With the exceptions of tennis players and divers, post-Title IX athletes tend to be taller than pre-Title IX athletes and are especially more androgynous. The secular change in the androgyny index is apparently real because mean androgyny scores for nonathlete females in 1969 (80.7 ± 2.7), 1975 (79.3 ± 4.3) and 1987 (80.9 ± 4.3) do not differ,[57] and are similar to those for other samples, e.g., Oxford University students (78.9 ± 4.6)[45] and Edinburgh women 20–24 years of age (81.8 ± 4.0).[58] It is thus reasonable to assume that there been no secular change in the androgyny index of nonathletic women from about 1950 to 1990.

VI. Seasonal Changes

Changes in body composition in response to specific training programs or during a season are important in studies of athletes. For example, among university swimmers (several of whom are included in the preceding anthropometric comparisons), body composition was estimated with densitometry at three points during the season. Decreases in weight (–1.3 ± 1.8 kg), fat mass (–2.4 ± 1.2 kg) and relative fatness (–3.8 ± 1.9%) and an increase in fat-free mass (1.1 ± 1.8 kg) occurred during the early part of the season (October–December). Weight training with emphasis on high repetition and low resistance typically preceded swim training early in the season. The changes in body composition that occurred during the first part of the season, when training was more intense, were generally maintained during the second part as the swimmers tapered for the national championships (December to March). Changes in weight (0.8 ± 1.2 kg), fat mass (0.8 ± 1.5 kg) and relative fatness (1.2 ± 2.0 kg) were small and fat-free mass, on average, did not change (0.0 ± 1.1 kg), although there was considerable variation among individuals.[59]

The changes in body composition of female swimmers during a swim season were generally consistent with those observed in college age female and male athletes and nonathletes and indicated similar responses in males and females. Much of the comparative literature on changes in body composition with training reports only differences between means, so that it is difficult to evaluate individual variation in changes. Using data reported by Wilmore,[60] differences between pre- and posttraining mean values in nine studies of males 18-23 years ranged from –0.2 kg to +1.4 kg for fat-free mass (overall mean of +0.8 kg) and –0.4% to –3.0% for relative fatness (overall mean of –1.7%). Corresponding differences for 10 studies of females 18–22 years ranged from –1.7 kg to +1.5 kg for fat-free mass (overall mean of +0.3 kg) and –2.1% to +3.1% for relative fatness (overall mean of –0.4%). Note, however, training protocols varied among studies, as did the quality and level of training among athletes.

Given the time commitment required of athletes, it is often not practical to estimate body composition with commonly used laboratory methods (densitometry, total body water, DEXA) on a regular basis during the course of a season. Hence, it may be necessary to monitor changes in body composition indirectly with anthropometry. Results based on several indirect procedures for female distance runners and basketball players followed through the season are summarized subsequently. The procedures include body weight, the sum of eight skinfolds (triceps, biceps, forearm, subscapular, suprailiac, anterior mid-thigh, medial calf and lateral calf), relative fatness predicted from an equation developed on female swimmers,[48] estimated midarm muscle circumference (relaxed arm circumference corrected for the thicknesses of the triceps and biceps skinfolds) and estimated calf muscle circumference (calf circumference corrected for the thicknesses of the medial and lateral calf skinfolds).

A. Distance Runners

Changes (means and standard deviations) in indirect estimates of body composition of female distance runners during the season are shown in Table 7.10. The runners are grouped by year in school. On average, runners declined in body weight, subcutaneous fat and relative fatness from the beginning of the school year through the latter part of the cross-country season (mid-August–late October). Subsequently, weight and fatness increased, on average, from the cross-country to the outdoor season (late October–April) and from the outdoor season to the next school year (April–August). It appears that freshman distance runners experienced somewhat greater changes in weight and fatness during their first season of competition. The change in body weight of freshman runners was accompanied by gains in estimated arm muscle, which was somewhat greater than those of sophomore and junior distance runners. The gains probably reflected the effects of more intensive training (compared with the high school level), weight training and late adolescent growth in muscle mass. Changes in arm muscle of sophomore and junior runners during the season were, on average, relatively small. Corresponding changes in estimated calf muscle were less than those in the arm. Calf musculature appeared to increase, on average, from the cross-country to the outdoor season and the gains were greater in the older runners.

The preceding summarizes average changes in the distance runners. There was, however, considerable variation among individuals. Changes in individual athletes during the season are illustrated in Figure 7.6. The athletes are grouped by year in school and are ordered based on weight change during the cross-country season (mid-August to late October) in all panels of the figure. About one half of the runners lost weight during the competitive season with the largest losses approaching 3 kg. Almost all of the runners lost subcutaneous adipose tissue and showed a reduction in relative

TABLE 7.10

Changes (Means and Standard Deviations) in Body Weight and Anthropometric Indicators of Body Composition in Distance Runners during the Course of a Season

Variable	August-October		October-April		April-August	
	Mean	SD	Mean	SD	Mean	SD
Body Weight, kg						
F*	-0.5	1.4	1.5	1.3	0.0	0.9
S	-0.1	0.8	0.4	0.9	0.4	1.0
J	-0.5	1.4	0.7	0.5	0.2	1.3
Sum of 8 Skinfolds, mm						
F	-4.8	6.4	3.7	6.1	4.9	7.2
S	-4.2	3.4	0.8	7.3	6.0	6.1
J	-8.1	7.0	2.4	5.7	3.0	8.3
Fat, %						
F	-0.6	0.6	0.4	0.6	0.6	0.8
S	-0.4	0.2	0.1	0.7	0.5	0.7
J	-0.6	0.5	0.1	0.6	0.4	0.7
Arm Muscle, cm						
F	0.5	0.5	0.6	0.5	0.2	0.4
S	0.1	0.7	0.0	0.4	0.0	0.3
J	-0.1	0.3	0.3	0.5	0.1	0.6
Calf Muscle, cm						
F	0.2	0.2	0.2	0.4	-0.1	0.5
S	-0.0	0.4	0.3	0.5	-0.1	0.5
J	0.0	0.5	0.5	0.5	-0.1	0.3

* Runners are grouped by school year: freshman (F, n = 6), sophomore (S, n = 5), junior (J, n = 6).

fatness and 11 showed an increase in estimated calf muscle (top row of Figure 7.6). Changes from the end of the cross-country season (late October) to the outdoor season (April) are shown in the middle row of Figure 7.6. In contrast to the cross-country season, 11 runners gained weight and nine gained in subcutaneous adipose tissue and relative fatness. Changes in estimated calf muscle were small and nine runners showed a slight decline. From the outdoor season (April) to the next school year (mid-August), most of the runners gained in weight and fatness (bottom row of Figure 7.6). Changes in estimated calf muscle during this interval were small.

B. Basketball Players

Corresponding changes during the season in basketball players are summarized in Table 7.11. As in the description of distance runners, the basketball players are grouped by year in school. Body weight increased from early in the school year (September, beginning of systematic conditioning prior to formal basketball practice) to the middle of the season (February), especially in the freshmen and sophomores, while the sum of skinfolds and relative fatness, on average, declined. The decrease in fatness during the first half of

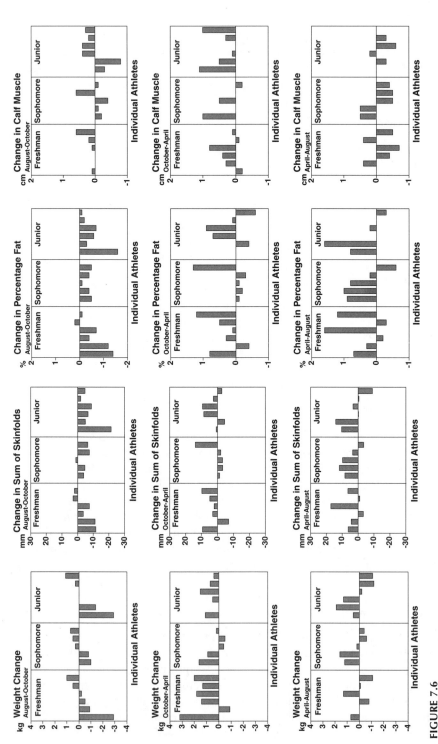

FIGURE 7.6

Changes in anthropometric indicators of body composition in individual distance runners during a season. Runners are grouped by year in school and are ordered based on weight change during the cross-country season (mid-August to late October) in all panels of the figure. Thus, individuals have the same position in all panels.

TABLE 7.11

Changes (Means and Standard Deviations) in Body Weight and
Anthropometric Indicators of Body Composition in Basketball
Players during the Course of a Season

Variable	September-February Mean	September-February SD	February-September Mean	February-September SD
Body Weight, kg				
F*	1.4	2.6	−1.3	2.3
S	1.8	2.3	0.1	2.8
J	0.1	2.0	0.3	2.6
Sum of 8 Skinfolds, mm				
F	-2.3	10.2	−0.5	10.9
S	−4.1	7.0	8.7	11.4
J	−10.3	8.2	7.3	12.2
Fat, %				
F	−0.3	1.1	0.0	1.1
S	−0.5	0.7	0.9	1.4
J	−1.0	1.0	0.8	1.2
Arm Muscle, cm				
F	0.7	0.6	−0.3	0.7
S	0.3	0.8	0.2	0.6
J	0.1	0.5	0.0	0.6
Calf Muscle, cm				
F	0.7	0.8	−0.4	0.3
S	0.6	0.7	−0.3	0.8
J	0.5	0.7	−0.4	0.5

* Players are grouped by school year: freshman (F, n = 14), sophomore
(S, n = 13), junior (J, n = 12).

the season was greatest in the juniors and progressively less in sophomores
and freshmen. From mid-season to the next school year (February to September), body weight declined in the freshman, but was stable in the sophomores and juniors. In contrast, the freshmen showed, on average, virtually
no change in fatness over this span, while the sophomores and juniors
increased. Estimated arm and calf muscle increased, on average, from the
beginning of the school year to mid-season and freshmen showed greater
gains than sophomores and juniors. Estimated calf muscle tended to increase
more than arm muscle in the sophomores and juniors, while both muscle
circumferences increased to the same extent in freshmen. Changes in estimated muscle circumferences reflect the effects of weight training prior to
the start of the basketball season. From mid-season until the next school year,
estimated calf muscle declined slightly in the three groups, while arm muscle
was more variable.

As in distance runners, there was considerable variation among individuals in changes in the anthropometric indicators during the season. This is
illustrated in Figure 7.7. The athletes are grouped by year in school and are
ordered based on weight change from September to February in all panels
of the figure. The majority of basketball players gained weight during the

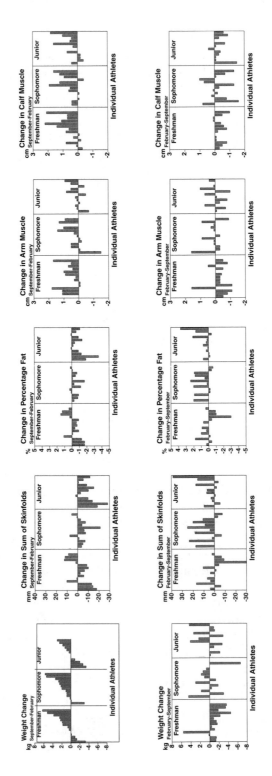

FIGURE 7.7

Changes in anthropometric indicators of body composition in individual basketball players during a season. Players are grouped by year in school and are ordered based on weight change during the cross-country season (mid-August to late October) in all panels of the figure. Thus, individuals have the same position in all panels.

first part of the year, which included preseason training prior to formal practices and the early part of the competitive season. Weight change was accompanied by a loss in absolute and relative fatness and a gain in estimated arm and calf muscle in about three fourths of the players (top row of Figure 7.7). During the interval from February to September, which included the final month and one half of the season and then the off season, individual responses were more variable. Most of the freshman continued to lose weight, which was accompanied by decreases in estimated arm and calf muscle circumferences and variable changes in estimated fatness (about one half of the freshman declined and the other half gained in fatness). In contrast to the freshmen, about one half of sophomore and junior basketball players gained weight while the other half lost weight during the interval from February to September. The changes in weight were accompanied by decreases in estimated calf muscle and gains in subcutaneous adipose tissue and relative fatness in most of the older players. Changes in estimated arm muscle were variable (lower row of Figure 7.7).

Although distance runners and basketball players differ considerably in size, physique and body composition and there is considerable individuality in responses during the season, changes in indirect estimates of body composition over the year show some similarities. Freshmen athletes tend to experience significant changes in body composition, specifically gains in estimated arm and calf muscle, which can be viewed as indirect indicators of fat-free mass. These gains most likely reflect the effects of more intensive and specialized training (in contrast to training at the high school level) and especially regular weight training, although late adolescent growth in muscle mass is a possible contributory factor. Reductions in fatness are concentrated largely in the early part of the respective seasons for each sport.

VII.   Disordered Eating

Many female athletes have concerns about body weight, some of which is self generated. Coaches, the media, others in the sports system and society are additional sources of stress associated with weight, especially social preferences for thinness. This may lead to the initiation of weight controlling behaviors associated with eating disorders among athletes, who are a population that is identified at risk.[61]

Changes in anthropometric indicators and somatotype over the course of almost 2 years in a distance runner who developed disordered eating are summarized in Table 7.12. Although there was recovery after the outdoor season (II to III), the disordered eating resumed during the next season (IV to V). Over the interval for which data were available (I to V), weight decreased by 9% and subcutaneous fatness decreased by 47%. Changes in estimated arm and calf muscle were relatively small, which probably reflects

TABLE 7.12

Changes in Anthropometric Indicators of Body Composition
and Somatotype in a Distance Runner Who Developed
Disordered Eating

	Aug I	Apr II	Aug III	Oct IV	Apr V
Weight, kg	55.6	51.4	56.2	53.3	50.8
Sum 8 Skinfolds, mm	67.2	39.9	59.5	44.5	35.5
Arm Muscle, cm	19.5	18.5	20.7	18.6	18.5
Calf Muscle, cm	30.3	30.6	32.0	30.5	30.6
Endomorphy	2.0	1.4	1.8	1.2	1.1
Mesomorphy	2.1	1.9	2.7	2.1	1.9
Ectomorphy	4.9	5.7	4.7	5.3	5.9

nutritional recovery (III) and the effects of regular activity and training in maintaining muscle mass, more so in the calf than in the arm.

Changes in somatotype reflected soft tissue, specifically subcutaneous fatness. Endomorphy and mesomorphy declined by 45% and 10%, respectively, whereas ectomorphy increased by about 20% over the observation period (I–V). Somatotype changes are in the same direction as those reported in the Minnesota Experiment in which adult males (25.5 ± 3.5 years) underwent 6 months of semistarvation — average daily energy intake during the experiment was 1530 kcal, including about 50 g protein and 30 g fat.[62] Of course, the subjects were not intensively training during the experiment. After 6 months of semistarvation, endomorphy and mesomorphy declined by about 48% and 29%, respectively, while ectomorphy increased by about 67%. These changes suggest that endomorphy and ectomorphy are strongly influenced by the amount of subcutaneous tissue.

VIII. Summary

Anthropometry is basically a standardized set of techniques for taking dimensions of the body and its parts. Measurements are objective and non-judgmental, whereas evaluation of the measurements requires interpretation and judgment. Anthropometric studies of adult athletes have a long tradition in the sport sciences. Initial studies largely documented the body dimensions of athletes in a variety of sports, males more than females. The study of somatotype (physique) has expanded considerably with the development of the Heath-Carter anthropometric protocol.

Selected anthropometric characteristics of female athletes in seven sports show variation between and within sports and between ethnic groups (blacks and whites) within sports by position and event. There is also secular variation in female athletes in several sports, particularly swimming, basketball and volleyball. The secular changes probably reflect more opportunities for women in sport, especially after Title IX legislation in the mid-1970s, selection and recruitment, scholarship support and greater social acceptability of females in the role of athlete. As a result, more females are likely to persist in sport beyond the high school years. In contrast, there has been no secular increase in the heights of United States adolescents and young adults.

Anthropometirc indicators of body composition are valuable for monitoring changes during the course of a season or from year to year. Seasonal changes show similarity in distance runners and basketball players. Freshman athletes tend to experience significant changes in estimated arm and calf muscle circumferences, which probably reflect the effects of more intensive and specialized training (in contrast to training at the high school level) and especially regular weight training. Late adolescent growth in muscle mass is also a contributory factor. Reductions in fatness are concentrated largely in the early part of the respective seasons for each sport when training is more intense. The anthropometric indicators also provide potentially useful information in monitoring individuals who might be at risk for disordered eating.

Acknowledgments

The assistance of Christine M. Bonci and Randa C. Ryan of the Department of Intercollegiate Athletes for Women at the University of Texas at Austin is greatly appreciated. The data for the athletes surveyed between 1985 and 1995 are categorized as standard of care data, which are not generated for research purposes but as a result of general health and safety procedures taken for an athletic population training and competing in a collegiate environment. The athletes signed a standard release of information waiver as part of their participation. The Human Subjects Committee of the University of Texas at Austin has designated standard of care data exempt from committee review.

Albert B. Harper, Bruce W. Meleski, Richard F. Shoup and Anthony N. Zavaleta participated in the collection of the data in 1969 and the 1970s. Diane Merrett assisted in preliminary analyses. Their contributions are gratefully acknowledged. Thanks and appreciation are also extended to Rita Wellens for use of her dissertation data.

References

1. Tanner, J.M., Growth and constitution, in: *Anthropology Today,* Kroeber, A.L., Ed. University of Chicago Press, Chicago, 1953, pp. 750-770.

2. Damon, A. (1970) Constitutional medicine, in *Anthropology and the Behavioral and Health Sciences*, Von Mering, O. and Kasdan, L., Eds. University of Pittsburgh Press, Pittsburgh, 1970, pp. 179-205.

3. Malina, R.M., Anthropometry in physical education and sport sciences, in *History of Physical Anthropology: An Encyclopedia, Volume One*, Spencer, F., Ed. Garland Publishing, New York, 1997, pp. 90-94.

4. Knoll, W., Ed., Die sportärztlichen Ergebnisse der II. Olympischen Winterspiele in St. Moritz 1928, Haupt, Bern, 1928.

5. Buytendijk, F.J.J., Ed., *Ergebnisse der sportärztlichen Untersuchungen bei den IX Olympischen Spielen in Amsterdam 1928*, Julius Springer, Berlin, 1929.

6. Mülly, K., Die Form des Körpers, als Ausdruck seiner Funktion, in: *Die sportärztlichen Ergebnisse der II. Olympischen Winterspiele in St. Moritz 1928*, Knoll, W., Ed. Haupt, Bern, 1928, as cited in Carter (19).

7. Dybowska, J. and Dybowski, W., Anthropolodische Untersuchungen an Teilnehmern der Wettkämpfe der IX. Olympiade in Amsterdam 1928, in *Ergebnisse der sportärztlichen Untersuchungen bei den IX Olympischen Spielen in Amsterdam 1928*, Buytendijk, F.J.J., Ed. Julius Springer, Berlin, 1929, pp. 1-29.

8. Kohlrausch, W., Zusammenhange von Körperform und Leistung. Ergebnisse der anthropometrischen Messungen an den Athleten der Amsterdamer Olympiade, in *Ergebnisse der sportärztlichen Untersuchungen bei den IX Olympischen Spielen in Amsterdam 1928*, Buytendijk, F.J.J.,, Ed. Julius Springer, Berlin, 1929, pp. 30-47.

9. Cureton, T.K., *Physical Fitness of Champion Athletes*, University of Illinois Press, Urbana, 1951.

10. Tanner, J.M., *The Physique of the Olympic Athlete*, George Allen and Unwin, London, 1964.

11. Correnti, V. and Zauli, B., *Olimpionici 1960: Ricerche di Antropologia Morfologica sull'Atletica Leggera*, Tipolitografia Marves, Rome, 1964.

12. de Garay, A.L., Levine, L. and Carter, J.E.L. *Genetic and Anthropological Studies of Olympic Athletes*, Academic Press, New York, 1974.

13. Jungmann, H., Ed., *Sportwissenschaftliche Untersuchungen während der XX. Olympischen Spiele, München, 1972*, Karl Demeter, Hamburg, 1976.

14. Carter, J.E.L., Ed., *Physical Structure of Olympic Athletes. Part I. The Montreal Olympic Games Anthropological Project*, Karger, Basel, 1982.

15. Novak, L.P., Bestit, C., Mellerowicz, H. and Woodward, W.A., Maximal oxygen consumption, body composition and anthropometry of selected Olympic male athletes, in: *Sportwissenschaftliche Untersuchungen während der XX. Olympischen Spiele, München, 1972*, Jungmann, H., Ed., Karl Demeter, Hamburg, 1976, pp. 57-68.

16. Novak, L.P., Bestit, C., Mellerowicz, H. and Woodward, W.A., Working capacity (WC170), body composition and anthropometry of Olympic female athletes, in: *Sportwissenschaftliche Untersuchungen während der XX. Olympischen Spiele, München, 1972*, Jungmann, H., Ed., Karl Demeter, Hamburg, 1976, pp. 69-78.

17. Novak, L.P., Bestit, C., Mellerowicz, H. and Woodward, W.A., Maximal aerobic power, body composition and anthropometry of Olympic runners and road cyclists, in: *Sportwissenschaftliche Untersuchungen während der XX. Olympischen Spiele, München, 1972*, Jungmann, H., Ed., Karl Demeter, Hamburg, 1976, pp. 79-90.

18. Malina, R.M., Bouchard, C., Shoup, R.F., Demirjian, A. and Larivière, G., Growth and maturity status of Montreal Olympic athletes less than 18 years of age, in *Physical Structure of Olympic Athletes. Part I. The Montreal Olympic Games Anthropological Project,* Carter, J.E.L., Ed. Karger, Basel, 1982, pp. 117-127.

19. Carter, J.E.L., Ed., *Physical Structure of Olympic Athletes. Part II. Kinanthropometry of Olympic Athletes,* Karger, Basel, 1984.

20. Eiben, O., *The Physique of Woman Athletes.* Hungarian Scientific Council for Physical Education, Budapest, 1972.

21. Tittel, K. and Wutscherk, H., *Sportanthropometrie: Aufgaben, Bedeutung, Methodik und Ergebnisse biotypologischer Erhebungen,* Johann Ambrosius Barth, Leipzig, 1972.

22. Maas, G.D., *The Physique of Athletes: An Anthropometric Study of 285 Top Sportsmen from 14 Sports in a Total of 774 Athletes,* Leiden University Press, Leiden, 1974.

23. Sodhi, H.S. and Sidhu, L.S., *Physique and Selection of Sportsmen,* Punjab Publishing House, Patiala, 1984.

24. Toteva, M., *Somatotypology in Sports,* National Sports Academy, Sofia, 1982.

25. Perez, B.M., *Los Atletas Venezolanos Su Tipo Fisico: Un Estudio Biotipologico de las Especialidades de Natacion, Baloncesto, Volibol, Atletismo, Levantamiento de Pesas y Gimnasia.,* Universidad Central de Venezuela, Caracas, 1981.

26. Calzada, J.L. del O., *Los Deportistas de Alto Rendimiento: Un Enfoque Antropologico,* Instituto Nacional de Antropologia e Historia, Mexico, D.F., 1990.

27. Carter, J.E.L. and Ackland, T.R., Eds., *Kinanthropometry in Aquatic Sports: A Study of World Class Athletes,* Human Kinetics, Champaign, Ill., 1994.

28. Rienzi, E. and Mazza, J.C., Eds., *Futbolista Sudamericano de Elite: Morfologia, Analisis del Juego y Performance,* Biosystem Servicio Educativo, Rosario, Argentina, 1998.

29. Carter, J.E.L. and Heath, B.H., *Somatotyping: Development and Applications,* Cambridge University Press, Cambridge, 1990.

30. Kunze, D., Hughes, P.C.R. and Tanner, J.M., Anthropometrische untersuchungen an sportlern der XX. Olympischen 1972 in München, in: *Sportwissenschaftliche Untersuchungen während der XX. Olympischen Spiele, München, 1972,* Jungmann, H., Ed., Karl Demeter, Hamburg, 1976, pp. 33-56.

31. Malina, R.M et al., Growth status of Olympic athletes less than 18 years of age: young athletes at the Mexico City, Munich and Montreal Olympic Games, in: *Physical Structure of Olympic Athletes. Part II. Kinanthropometry of Olympic Athletes,* Carter, J.E.L., Ed. Karger, Basel, 1984, pp. 183-201.

32. Malina, R.M., Comparison of the increase in body size between 1899 and 1970 in a specially selected group with that in the general population. *Am. J. Phys. Anthropol.,* 37, 135, 1972.

33. Noonan, D., Really big football players, *The New York Times* Magazine, December 14, 64, 1997.

34. Jokl, E., Rupp, A., Lancaster, H., Johnson, H., Adams, K. and Mooney, S., Basketball 20 years ago and today: a comparative analysis of physiques and performances of University of Kentucky basketball teams, 1948 and 1968, *J. Health Phys. Educ. Rec.,* 40, 65, 1969 (April).

35. Malina, R.M., Growth and maturation of female gymnasts, *Spotlight on Youth Sports,* Michigan State University, 19 (3), 1, 1996.

36. Claessens, A.L., Elite female gymnasts: a kinanthropometric overview, in: *Human Growth in Context*, Johnston, F.E., Zemel, B. and Eveleth, P.B., Eds. Smith-Gordon, London, 1999, pp. 273-280.

37. Franke, W.W. and Berendonk, B., Hormonal doping and androgenization of athletes: A secret program of the German Democratic Republic government, *Clin. Chem.*, 43, 1262, 1997.

38. Kalinski, M.I., Dunbar, C.C. and Szygula, Z., Research on anabolic steroids in the former Soviet Union. *Med. Sci. Sports Exerc.*, 33 (suppl.), S338, 2001 (abstract).

39. Pieronek, C., A clash of titans: college football v. Title IX. *J. Coll. Univ. Law*, 3, 351, 1994.

40. Lohman, T.G., Roche, A.F. and Martorell, R., Eds., *Anthropometric Standardization Reference Manual*, Human Kinetics, Champaign, Ill., 1988.

41. Malina, R.M., Physical anthropology, in: *Anthropometric Standardization Reference Manual*, Lohman, T.G., Roche, A.F. and Martorell, R., Eds. Human Kinetics, Champaign, Ill., 1988, pp. 99-102.

42. Malina, R.M., Anthropometry, in: *Physiological Assessment of Human Fitness*, Maud, P.J. and Foster, C., Eds. Human Kinetics, Champaign, Ill., 1995, pp. 205-219.

43. Malina, R.M., Hamill, P.V.V. and Lemeshow, S., Selected body measurements of children 6–11 years, Vital and Health Statistics, Series 11, No. 123, Department of Health, Education and Welfare, Washington, D.C., 1973.

44. Malina, R.M., Ratios and derived indicators in the assessment of nutritional status, in: *Anthropometric Assessment of Nutritional Status*, Himes, J.H., Ed. Wiley-Liss, New York, 1991, pp. 151-171.

45. Tanner, J.M., Current advances in the study of physique: Photogrammetric anthropometry and an androgyny scale, *Lancet*, 1, 574, 1951.

46. Bouchard, C., Reproducibility of body composition and adipose tissue measurements in humans, in *Body Composition Assessments in Youth and Adults*, Roche, A.F., Ed. Ross Laboratories, Columbus, Ohio, 1985, pp. 9-13.

47. Ryan, R.C., Menstrual status in elite female athletes: An evaluation of multiple sports, unpublished doctoral dissertation, University of Texas at Austin, 1996.

48. Meleski, B.W., Shoup, R.F. and Malina, R.M., Size, physique and body composition of competitive female swimmers 11 through 20 years of age, *Hum. Biol.*, 54, 609, 1982.

49. Wellens, R.E., Activity as a temperamental trait: Relationship to physique, energy expenditure and physical activity habits in young adults, unpublished doctoral dissertation, University of Texas at Austin.

50. Centers for Disease Control and Prevention, National Center for Health Statistics CDC growth charts: United States, 2000. http://www.cdc.gov/growthcharts.htm.

51. Malina, R.M., Physical growth and biological maturation of young athletes, *Exerc. Sports Sci. Rev.*, 22, 389, 1994.

52. Malina, R.M., Growth and maturation of young athletes — is training for sport a factor?, in: *Sports and Children*, Chan, K-M. and Micheli, L.J., Eds. Williams and Wilkins Asia-Pacific, Hong Kong, 1998, pp. 133-161.

53. Carter, J.E.L., Somatotypes of children in sports, in: *Young Athletes: Biological, Psychological and Educational Perspectives*, Malina, R.M., Ed. Human Kinetics, Champaign, IL., 1988, pp. 153-165.

54. Malina, R.M., Harper, A.B., Avent, H.H. and Campbell, D.E., Physique of female track-and-field athletes, *Med. Sci. Sports*, 3, 32, 1971.

55. Malina, R.M. and Zavaleta, A.N. androgyny of physique in female track-and-field athletes, *Ann. Hum. Biol.*, 3, 441, 1976.

56. Malina, R.M. and Shoup, R.F., Anthropometric and physique characteristics of female volleyball players at three competitive levels, *Humanbiologia Budapestinensis*, 16, 105, 1985.

57. Malina, R.M. and Merrett, D.M.S. Androgyny of physique of women athletes: comparisons by sport and over time, in: *Essays on Auxology*, Hauspie, R., Lindgren, G. and Falkner, F., Eds. Castlemead Publications, Hertfordshire, U.K., 1995, pp. 355-363.

58. Milne, J.S., Age differences in the androgyny score, *Br. J. Prevent. Med.*, 26, 231, 1972.

59. Meleski, B.W. and Malina, R.M., Changes in body composition and physique of elite university level swimmers during a competitive season, *J. Sports Sci.*, 3, 33, 1985.

60. Wilmore, J.H., Appetite and body composition consequent to physical activity, *Res. Q.*, 54, 415, 1983.

61. Sundgot-Borgen, J., Risk and trigger factors for the development of eating disorders in female elite athletes, *Med. Sci. Sports Exerc*, 26, 414, 1994.

62. Keys, A., Brozek, J., Henschel, A., Mickelsen, O. and Taylor, H.L., *The Biology of Human Starvation*, University of Minnesota Press, Minneapolis, 1950.

8

Body Composition and Gender Differences in Performance

Samuel N. Cheuvront, Robert J. Moffatt and Keith C. DeRuisseau

CONTENTS

I.   Introduction

The comparison between men's and women's athletic performances has gained considerable attention over the past 30 years. The foundation for this interest is rooted in the extreme contrast between women's historical and present-day sports participation. The first Olympic Games of 1896 included no women athletes. One hundred years later, women represented 36% of more than 10,000 athletes competing from around the world in the Games of the XXVI Olympiad. Although the societal role of women in U.S. sports changed drastically in the mid-1970s as the result of legislation (Title IX) for equal opportunities in organized sports, recent history shows us that women are still competing for true sport equality. The marathon is one example of an Olympic event historically thought to be too difficult for women. It was not added as an Olympic sport for women until 1984. Other sports requiring strength and power, such as the hammer throw, weightlifting and pole vault were likewise added for women only in the most recent 2000 Olympic Summer Games.

The progression of world record performances in many athletic events for women has improved at a faster rate than for men over the same duration. Comparative analyses of these performances inspired many to conclude that women would soon perform as well as or better than men in athletic contests. However, the reality of disproportionate improvements in women's sports is best explained by a historical social sports bias.[1-4] The accelerated improvements in women's performances have now reached a plateau similar to that of men. The consistent performance edge that men still retain over women in almost all sports can be explained primarily by considerable differences in body composition and developmental physiology.

II.   Gender and Strength

Skeletal muscle accounts for approximately 50% and 40% of body mass in males and females, respectively.[5] Because muscle mass is proportional to strength,[6] men are generally stronger than women. However, numerous reports demonstrate the adaptability of skeletal muscle to various exercise regimens in both genders. To better understand quantitative gender differences in strength, knowledge of qualitative differences in muscle morphology, histochemistry and hormonal influences on muscle development is essential.

A. Factors Influencing Strength Development

1. Muscle Fiber Type

Differences in fiber characteristics of one muscle group between genders may not be reflected in another muscle.[7] Therefore, an important consideration is the muscle group sampled when comparing males and females. Several studies have reported similar[7-12] and different[10,13] fiber type distributions of selected muscle groups between males and females. Table 8.1 includes fiber type distributions and areas of male and female athletes along

TABLE 8.1

Mean Skeletal Muscle Characteristics of Athletic, Active and Sedentary Males and Females

Sport	Gender	Age	n	Muscle	%Type I	Type I F_a	Type II F_a	Total F_a	Reference
Bodybuilding	F	36.6	5	BB	49.9	4,760	5,010		8
Bodybuilding	M	33.1	8	BB	40.1	7,526	11,398		
Bodybuilding	M	24.8	11	BB	41.9	7,500	11,650	9,899	7
Bodybuilding	M	28.0	5	VL	52.0	6,830	10,400	8,400	12,14
Weight lifting	M	25.0	4	DEL	52.6				15
				VL	46.1				
Weight lifting	M	20.3	8	VL	44.0	4,550	7,430		16
Weight/Power lifting	M	26.8	8	VL	59.0			9,300	17
Power lifting	M		3	VL	45.0	4,430	7,290†		18
Field Hockey	F	22.8	5	VL	48.2	4,305	4,679†		11
Running/Cycling	M	21.8	8	VL	40.0			6,500	17
Cycling	M	24.0	4	DEL	50.7				15
				VL	61.4				
Sprinting	F	19.5	2	GAST	27.4	3,752	3,930		9
Sprinting	F	18.0–26.0	3	VL	39.0	3,200*	3,500*		19
Sprinting	M	19.5	2	GAST	24.0	5,878	6,034		9
Pentathlon	F	18.0–26.0	6	VL	54.0	3,700*	3,000*		19
Mid distance running	F	18.0–26.0	9	VL	63.0	3,300*	2,600*		19
Mid distance running	F	19.9	7	GAST	60.6	6,069	5,642		9
Mid distance running	M	22.9	7	GAST	51.9	6,099	7,117		9
Distance running	F	18.0–26.0	4	VL	73.0	3,500*	2,200*		19
Distance running	M	24.2	5	GAST	69.4	6,613	7,627		9
Distance running	F	23.0	5	VL	62.0	3,900*	3,200*†		20
				DEL	54.0	3,100*	3,500*†		
Distance running	M		3	VL	44.3	4,609	5,224†		18
Running	M	23.0	8	VL	58.9				15
Swimming	M	21.0	5	DEL	74.3				15
				VL	57.7				

TABLE 8.1 (CONTINUED)
Mean Skeletal Muscle Characteristics of Athletic, Active and Sedentary Males and Females

Sport	Gender	Age	n	Muscle	%Type I	Type I F_a	Type II F_a	Total F_a	Reference
Swimming	F	17.0	4	VL	49.0	4,500*	4,200*†		9
				DEL	62.0	3,300*	3,800*†		9
Long-high jump	F	22.3	3	GAST	48.7	4,163	5,113		9
Long-high jump	M	29.0	2	GAST	46.7	4,718	6,523		9
Javelin	F	20.7	3	GAST	41.6	4,864	4,569		9
Javelin	M	25.3	3	GAST	50.4	5,585	5,771		9
Shotput, discus	F	23.5	2	GAST	51.2	5,192	5,851		9
Shotput, discus	M	26.8	4	GAST	37.7	7,702	9,483		9
Elite canoeists	M		9	DEL	53.0				21
Canoeists	M	26.0	4	DEL	58.4				15
				VL	61.4				
Kayak/Canoe paddlers	M & F	24.6	9	VL	43.3				22
				BB	43.9				
Orienteers	M	52.0	11	DEL	63.1				15
				VL	68.8				
Orienteers	M	24.0	8	VL	68.1	4,040	4,220		23
			7	GAST	67.1	3,500	4,290		
			4	DEL	68.3	4,600	6,010		
PE students	M	25.0	31	VL	50.0				24
PE students	F	29.0	7	VL	52.0				14
PE students	F	26.0	10	VL	52.0	4,400	4,480	4,400	12
PE students	M	27.0	11	VL	52.0	5,680	7,240	6,200	12,14
PE students	F	25.0	20	VL	52.0	5,200*	4,700*		20
	F		16	DEL	56.0	4,000*	4,800*†		
Untrained	F	21.0	8	BB	38.7	3,750*	4,375*	4,112	7
Untrained	F	21.5	4	VL	36.4	2,784	3,392		11
Untrained	F	22.2	10	GAST	51.0	3,875	4,193		9

Untrained	F	19.4	22	VL	49.1				13
Untrained	M	17.8	40	VL	55.9				
Untrained	M	26.4	8	VL	48.0	4,560	5,070		16
Untrained	M	22.5	13	BB	38.5	5,000*	7,500*	6,248	7
Untrained	M	27.3	11	GAST	52.6	5,699	4,965		9
Untrained	M	26.0	8	VL	39.0			5,400	17
Untrained	M		10	VL	42.1				25
Untrained	M	27.0	12	DEL	46.0	5,000	4,800		15
				VL	36.1				
Untrained	M		5	VL	35.5	3,303	4,105†		18
Untrained	M & F	19.0-30.0	10	VL	47.0	4,474	4,497		26
Untrained	F	26.0	25	VL	52.0*	4,000*	3,600*†		20
Untrained	F		8	DEL	52.0	4,000*	4,600*†		
Untrained	M	16-18	69	VL	53.9	4,840	5,270		23
Untrained	M		4	VL	35.5				

VL = Vastus Lateralis; BB = Biceps Brachii; DEL = Deltoid; GAST = Gastrocnemius

F$_a$ = Fiber Area

* = Values estimated from figures

† = Type IIa fibers

with less active and sedentary individuals. Komi and Karlsson,[13] in a study investigating mono- and dizygotic twins, showed a greater distribution of Type I fibers from the vastus lateralis of males compared with females. The males also demonstrated greater individual variations in fiber type distributions compared with the females.[13] Miller et al.[10] observed similar fiber distributions in the biceps brachii muscle in males and females, but a higher proportion of Type II fibers in the vastus lateralis of the males.

A common technique for fiber type analysis involves a tissue sample from muscle biopsy followed by staining for the enzyme myfibrillar ATPase.[15] Skeletal muscle consists of two main groups of fibers when stained for this enzyme. Using this technique, an assumption must be made that the biopsied muscle sample is representative of the entire muscle. Reports indicating similar fiber type distributions between males and females have involved bodybuilders,[7,8,12] field hockey players,[11] track athletes,[9] and physical education students.[12] Untrained individuals often possess a similar distribution of Type I and Type II fibers.[16] Costill et al.[9] did report a greater distribution of Type I fibers in female middle-distance runners than in males, but no differences among other groups of athletes.

In comparing different groups of athletes, those individuals participating in endurance events typically possess a greater percentage of oxidative fibers.[15,18-20] As would be expected, there is an effect of exercise specificity with regard to skeletal muscle adaptation to exercise.[20] However, the notion that a particular fiber type distribution is not a predictor for athletic success has been indicated.[9,22] One example of this point involved a group of elite paddlers in which the fiber distribution between the deltoid and vastus lateralis muscles was similar.[22]

2. Muscle Fiber Number

It is generally acknowledged that the number of muscle fibers does not become altered after birth.[8] The mechanism for an increase in muscle size is therefore believed to result from hypertrophy of existing muscle fibers rather than hyperplasia. A study comparing male and female bodybuilders did find evidence of an increased estimated fiber number when comparisons were made with untrained individuals.[8] The observed increase in fiber number was similar between the males and females. However, differences in fiber number between certain muscle groups of males and females have been reported. Sale et al.[7] found males (untrained and body builders) to possess a greater fiber number in the biceps brachii muscle than untrained females. In the anterior tibialis muscle, fewer numbers of fibers have also been observed in females than in males.[29] Females possess a greater amount of noncontractile tissue within the muscle tissue, which must be taken into account when estimating fiber number.[7] Schantz et al.[14] did not find differences in fiber number between males and females. However, these authors did not correct for noncontractile tissue within the muscle sample.[7] The increased amount of noncontractile tissue in female muscle was not shown to exert a large impact on force generation.[10]

3. Muscle Fiber Area

Many studies report smaller mean muscle fiber areas in females than in males. Thus, this is a primary factor responsible for increased muscle cross-sectional area in males.[7–10] It must be noted that high individual variability in fiber cross-sectional areas have been reported, which are not always reflected in the mean values.[18] Type II fibers (particularly oxidative fibers) are larger than Type I fibers, [11] an observation particularly apparent among weight lifters.[15,16,18] Type I fibers have been shown to be of similar size in male weightlifters, endurance athletes, and untrained individuals.[16] However, female athletes have been shown to possess greater Type I fiber areas than their untrained counterparts.[11] Type I fibers have been reported to be larger than Type II fibers in the vastus lateralis muscle of athletic[19,20] and untrained[30] females. It has been suggested that the greater mean fiber area in males compared with females may be the result of differences in activity patterns.[7]

4. Training

It is generally accepted that exercise training does not increase the number of muscle fibers. Fiber type distribution has[26] and has not[31–35] been shown to be affected by exercise training. In a group of males and females who underwent 15 weeks of cycling training, an increase and decrease in the percent of Type I and Type II fibers, respectively, was observed.[26] The majority of studies have not demonstrated conversions between Type I and Type II muscle fibers. Studies using electrical stimulation or cross-innervation of muscle fibers have demonstrated the ability to convert fibers between Type I and Type II. Training studies involving humans have typically not shown this effect; in general, there are no fiber type conversions when fibers are classified as two main groups.[27] As a result of exercise training, the fiber distribution of subgroups within the Type II group may undergo conversions. The Type II muscle fiber population possesses the greater ability to adapt in size and oxidative capacity than the Type I fibers.[18] Type II fiber conversions have been demonstrated in both genders. For example, the conversion of Type IIb to Type IIa fibers was observed following cycling training in males[27] and in females undergoing 24 weeks of cross-country running[28] and following 20 weeks of strength training.[30]

There is, however, limited evidence in humans suggesting a Type I to Type II fiber conversion.[23] Following a period of aerobic training, male runners decreased the percentage of Type I fibers and increased the percentage of Type II fibers. Following anaerobic training, the opposite change in fiber distribution occurred. It was suggested that conversions between Type I and

Type II fibers may occur, with the formation of Type IIc fibers serving as intermediary transition fibers between the types.[23]

Fiber areas of the vastus lateralis have been shown to be influenced by:

- 5 months of cycling exercise in a group of male subjects[34]
- 15 weeks of cycling exercise in a group of males and females[26]
- 20 weeks of resistance exercise in females[30]
- Following 24 weeks of cross-country running in a group of females[28]

In other studies, the mean fiber areas of the vastus lateralis have not been shown to be affected by strength[31,33] or sprint[35] training. Thorstensson et al.[35] observed an increase in mean areas of Type I and Type II fibers in three out of four subjects undergoing 8 weeks of spring training. However, the average of the four subjects did not indicate significant differences. Seven[31] and 8[33] weeks of strength training influenced the fiber area ratios of the vastus lateralis, but had no effect on fiber area or distribution.

5. The Role of Testosterone

Men and women experience similar improvements in relative strength gains from resistance training,[36,37] although men are still 25–60% stronger than women in absolute weight lifted.[10,37] Strength differences between the sexes are often attributed to androgen hormones. In a cross-sectional study of male and female adolescents 11–18 years of age, Ramos et al.[38] report an increase in testosterone and growth hormone levels with maturation in males, but not females. Testosterone levels and absolute strength were, however, positively correlated for both sexes. Females participating in strength training programs have demonstrated significant gains in strength despite only small increases in muscle hypertrophy.[39,40] Brown and Wilmore[39] observed average lean body mass increases of less than 1 kg following 6 months of strength training, despite increases in strength of 15–45%. In women performing 3 weeks of intensive heavy resistance training, significant strength improvements were observed posttraining without significant changes in circulating testosterone. More importantly, strength was improved with minimal changes in muscle hypertrophy.[41] It was concluded that strength gains were the result of increased voluntary activation of the trained muscles.

Why are men stronger than women? Although many structural characteristics of muscle can potentially contribute to force production and growth (fiber type, fiber length, pennation angle), only muscle fiber cross-sectional area (CSA) differs between men and women.[8,10,12,42] In general, men have muscle CSAs that are 25–45% greater than women, depending on the muscle examined.[8,10] Voluntary strength has been shown to correlate positively with muscle CSA.[24] Expressed relative to lean body mass, males still possess greater strength, however, strength is similar between genders when expressed relative to muscle CSA.[10,13] Therefore, gender differences in strength are directly attributable to differences in skeletal muscle architecture — specifically muscle fiber CSA.[10,36,42] Because skeletal muscle possesses androgen receptors,[43] the higher concentration of circulating testosterone in men than in women and the well known effects of androgen-stimulated protein synthesis probably explain this physiological difference in CSA. It probably also explains the absolute performance differences in strength between men and women.

B. Gender Differences in Strength Performance

The amount of body mass as contractile tissue determines muscle strength, which varies almost exactly with muscle mass to the two-thirds power.[6] The 25–45% greater absolute muscle mass and CSA of skeletal muscle in men is also remarkably similar to the absolute differences in strength between men and women. Ford et al.[6] compared male and female world champion weight-lifters (1993–1997) on various body dimensions and performance in the combined snatch and clean and jerk lifts. They reported that strength per "cross-sectional area" (defined as body weight divided by height) was reduced in proportion to the amount of body mass carried as noncontractile tissue. For example, unlimited-class champions (no weight limit) lifted only 6% more weight than the heaviest limited-class competitors despite being 61% heavier. This was explained by a larger fraction of their mass carried as noncontractile tissue.[6] Ford et al.[6] also concluded that the women weight-lifters had 30% less contractile tissue than the men, which is consistent with general observations between men and women (25%),[5] and approximates the differences in world record weightlifting performances for men and women matched for body mass in Table 8.2. Therefore, the absolute strength differences between men and women are the collective result of differences in body composition. Women carry less mass as contractile tissue (more body fat) and have smaller muscle CSAs due to genetic differences in circulating androgens.

III. Gender and Endurance

Physical differences between the sexes contributed for decades to the mistaken belief that women were too fragile to compete in endurance sports.[1,45] Although societal influences (training and participation in sports) may have made the biggest impact historically,[1-4] large gender differences in aerobic performance diminished when classic analyses like that of Sparling et al.[46] clearly showed the importance of expressing oxygen uptake relative to body weight when comparing men and women on aerobic power parameters. But when the contribution of body fat to gender differences in aerobic capacity

TABLE 8.2

World Record Performances in Olympic-Style Weightlifting*

Weight Class (kg)	Combined Totals (kg)[a]		Difference (%)[b]
	Men	Women	
56–58	302.5	235.0	– 29
62–63	325.0	240.0	– 35
69	357.5	255.0	– 40
75–77	372.5	285.0	– 31

[a] = Combined clean and jerk and snatch lifts
[b] = [(women's total–men's total) / women's total]; (-) indicates women lift less
* All data from reference 44

is controlled, men still retain an endurance performance advantage of biological origin.

A three-tiered model that includes aerobic power (VO_{2max}), lactate threshold, and economy of movement[47] explains the physiological determinants of endurance performance. Taken together, these three variables determine how long an athlete can sustain any given exercise power output.

A. Factors Influencing Endurance Development

1. VO2max

Oxygen consumption increases directly as a function of exercise intensity. It is therefore intuitive that athletes wishing to run, cycle, or swim faster in prolonged exercise events must obtain and use larger quantities of oxygen to fuel their added energy (ATP) requirement. Maximal oxygen consumption (VO_{2max}) is defined as the point at which oxygen consumption reaches a plateau despite an increase in exercise intensity.[48] VO_{2max} results when both the rate of oxygen transport (cardiac output) and oxygen utilization (arteriovenous oxygen difference) are maximal. Defined properly, VO_{2max} is equal to the product of maximum cardiac output (Qmax) and maximum arteriovenous oxygen difference ($A-VO_{2diff}$). Q_{max} is itself the product of maximum heart rate (HR_{max}) and maximum stroke volume (SV_{max}) expressed in L/min^{-1} and $A-VO_{2diffmax}$ is the difference between the oxygen content of arterial and venous blood in ml O_2 /100 ml^{-1} blood (oxygen extraction and utilization).

Among the general population, absolute (L/min^{-1}) VO_{2max} values for men are 30–60% greater than those for women.[1,46,49] However, this difference is drastically reduced to roughly 20% and 10% when expressed relatively as ml • kg^{-1}/min^{-1} and $ml/kgLBM^{-1}/min^{-1}$, respectively.[1,46,49] Values in all categories contrast somewhat less when trained[46] or elite[50] men and women are compared. To illustrate the importance of body composition on VO_{2max}, Table 8.3 was constructed using data collected on accomplished male and female

TABLE 8.3

Physiological Comparisons between Elite Men and Women Marathon Runners for Indices of VO_{2max}.[a]

	TBM (kg)	BF (%)	LBM* (kg)	HR$_{max}$ (b/min)	SV$_{max}$* (ml/b)	Q$_{max}$* (L/min)	A-VO$_2$diff$_{max}$[b] (ml/100 ml)	Hb[c] (g/dL)	VO$_{2max}$* (L/min)	VO$_{2max}$ (ml/kg/min)	VO$_{2max}$* (ml/kgLBM/min)
Men	61.7	6	58.0	185	157	29.1	15	15.0	4.36	70.7	75.2
Women	54.6	13	47.5	186	115	21.4	15	13.5	3.22	59.0	67.8
Diff.	7.1	7	10.5	1	42	7.7	0	1.5	1.14	11.7	7.4

[a] = all data from references 51, 52, 53, 54 except where indicated

[b] = male value from reference 52; female value assumed equal (reference 59)

[c] = male value from reference 51; female value estimated as 10% lower (reference 55)

* = calculated value

All abbreviations defined in chapter text

marathon runners.[51–54] VO_{2max} is 26% (L/min^{-1}), 17% (ml/kg^{-1}/min^{-1}) and 10% (ml/kgLBM^{-1}/min^{-1}) greater for men than women in this example. Therefore, accounting for the smaller total body mass (TBM), lean body mass (LBM) and the larger body fat (BF) in the female runners reduces the difference in VO_{2max} between the sexes by at least two thirds. Gender differences in components of the oxygen transport and utilization system also play a large role.

Women have a smaller heart, lower hemoglobin concentration, and a smaller blood volume than men.[55–58] The smaller left ventricular mass of women, coupled with a smaller blood volume, reduces preload and compromises the Frank-Starling mechanism, thus resulting in a smaller stroke volume and cardiac output. This is supported by the literature[56–58] and apparent from the stroke volume and cardiac output data in Table 8.3 calculated using the Fick equation. Men also carry more blood oxygen (20 ml O_2/100 ml^{-1} blood) than women (18 ml O_2/100 ml^{-1} blood) (calculated using a binding capacity of 1.34 ml O_2/g^{-1} Hb). Thus, the convective oxygen delivery potential is greater for men. Differences in cardiac muscle architecture and hemodynamics probably best explain remaining differences in VO_{2max} between men and women from Table 8.3. Of course, these numbers are not intended for definitive interpretation, as much of the data from Table 8.3 is 1) derived rather than measured, 2) undoubtedly varies within the population considered and 3) does not include other potential gender differences that may affect VO_{2max}, such as pulmonary capacity. What these data do support is a significant contribution by body composition to the differences in VO_{2max} observed between men and women.

Although a strong inverse correlation exists between VO_{2max} and finishing time for marathon runners,[60,61] a large aerobic capacity is only one factor that determines success in endurance exercise. Consider that, in 1969, Derek Clayton set a world record for the men's marathon that stood for 12 years, even though his measured VO_{2max} was less (69 ml/kg^{-1}/min^{-1}) than many elite women competitors today.[50,62] The present world's best time for women is still ~12 minutes slower than this 1969 men's mark. In addition, the predictive capacity of VO_{2max} on endurance performance wanes heavily when the distribution of aerobic capacities is more homogenous.[62,63] Other important factors must also contribute to endurance exercise success.

2. *Lactate Threshold*

The inability to sustain exercise at VO_{2max} intensities throughout prolonged exercise is a key limitation to endurance performance. Because higher exercise intensities require obligatory carbohydrate to rapidly provide ATP commensurate with activity needs, a mismatch between pyruvate production and utilization is reflected in an accumulation of blood lactate.[64] The inflection point where blood lactate concentrations increase continuously at a constant exercise power output is commonly referred to as the lactate threshold.[65] The closer individual athletes can exercise to their VO_{2max} without incurring a mismatch between lactate production and clearance, the higher their lactate threshold.

An inverse relationship exists between the duration of exercise and the %VO_{2max} that can be sustained.[66,67] For prolonged bouts of exercise (> 2 hrs), values between 68–88 %VO_{2max} have been reported, with more highly trained athletes representing the higher values.[61,66,67] There appears to be no gender difference in lactate threshold,[68,69] which is corroborated by women athletes competing at relative exercise intensities (%VO_{2max}) similar to men's in endurance events.[61,70] This is also logical because the mitochondrial density and enzymatic characteristics of endurance-trained muscle are highly correlated with endurance performance,[71] but are likewise not significantly different between men and women when controlling for training status.[72-75]

3. Exercise Economy

Exercise economy refers to the relationship between speed of movement and energy expenditure (VO_2).[76] Performance technique is one key to good exercise economy. This is especially important for prolonged intense exercise because the physiological demands of endurance and ultraendurance sports lead to deterioration in exercise economy, especially in the latter stages of competition.[77] Examples of "unwanted" energy-costing movements are a larger vertical component in running,[78] excessive drag in swimming[79] and the engagement of muscle groups that contribute negligibly to propulsion in cycling.[80] Because large interindividual differences exist for exercise economy,[76] two athletes with the same VO_{2max} may require very different steady-state oxygen needs for the same submaximal running, swimming or cycling speed. Reciprocal logic dictates that an economical athlete with a moderate VO_{2max} might perform as well as or better than a less economical athlete with a high VO_{2max} — especially during prolonged exercise requiring enormous, but limited, energy needs. Such a difference, in addition to lactate threshold, explains how athletes with "modest" VO_{2max} values (< 70 ml/kg^{-1}/min^{-1}) can compete and even set world records in endurance events usually dominated by those with very high VO_{2max} values.

Most[81-84] studies examining the oxygen cost of running at any relative intensity find no gender differences in running economy. We might assume that the same is true of other endurance sports, however, gender differences in body weight, surface area, and density (body fat) might potentially impact swimming economy and performance. Zamparo et al.[85] demonstrated that men experience greater "torque" than women when in water, which is the tendency for the upper body to rise due to the relational configuration of the center of mass to the center of volume (lungs). Because body density explained a large portion of the variability in torque, the higher body fat and gynoidal distribution of fat in women could equate to a reduced body drag when swimming, owing to less torque (more buoyant, horizontal position). The smaller differences in swimming performances between men and women (Table 8.4) when compared with running (Table 8.5) and the fact that

TABLE 8.4

World and American Record Performances in
Long Distance Swimming

Distance (km)	Time (hr:min:sec)		Difference (%)[c]
	Men	Women	
0.4[a]	0:03:40	0:04:03	+ 9.4
0.8[a]	0:07:46	0:08:16	+ 6.0
1.5[a]	0:14:41	0:15:52	+ 7.4
5.0[b]	1:05:07	1:04:27	− 1.0
10.0[b]	1:54:05	2:00:48	+ 5.6
15.0[b]	3:21:23	3:22:44	+ 0.7
20.0[b]	4:34:57	4:31:00	− 1.5
25.0[b]	5:50:05	5:40:21	− 2.9
30.0[b]	7:05:27	6:48:26	− 4.2

[a] = World records–data from reference 86
[b] = American records–data from reference 87
[c] = [(women's time–men's time) / women's time];
(+) indicates women swim slower, (-) indicates
women swim faster

TABLE 8.5

World Record Performances in Long
Distance Running

Distance (km)	Time (hr:min:sec)		Difference (%)[c]
	Men	Women	
1.5[a]	0:03:26	0:03:50	+ 10.4
3.0[a]	0:07:20	0:08:06	+ 9.5
5.0[a]	0:12:39	0:14:28	+ 12.6
10.0[a]	0:26:22	0:29:31	+ 10.7
42.0[a]	2:05:42	2:20:43	+ 10.7
100.0[b]	6:10:20	7:23:28	+ 26.5
500.0[b]	60:23:00	77:53:46	+ 22.5
1000.0[b]	136:17:00	192:27:06	+ 29.2

[a] = Data from reference 86
[b] = Data from reference 88
[c] = [(women's time–men's time)/women's
time]; (+) indicates women run slower

women actually outperform men when swimming distances beyond 20 km,
make this a plausible hypothesis. Additionally, although the economy of
swimming, cycling and running is each an important contributor to triathlon
success, improvement in swimming economy alone is believed to hold particular promise toward enhancing triathlon performance.[63]

4. Training

The qualitative physiological responses of women to aerobic training appear equal to those of men, provided that the exercise training stimulus (intensity, frequency, duration) is the same and initial fitness is similar. Relative improvements in VO_{2max},[57,82,89,90] maximal heart rate,[82,89,90] stroke volume,[57,91] A-VO_{2diff}[59] and mitochondrial adaptations[74,75] are similar between the sexes. Likewise, similar slow-twitch (oxidative) muscle fiber percentages between endurance-trained men and women are observed (Table 8.1). Because men and women adapt equally to exercise stress and have similar lactate thresholds and exercise economies, gender differences in endurance performance are the result of differences in VO_{2max} that are explained largely by underlying differences in body composition. It is therefore interesting and controversial that women are still believed by some to be better suited for endurance sports than men.

5. The Role of Estrogen

The augmentation of peripheral fat store mobilization and utilization during prolonged exercise is an attractive means by which to delay muscle glycogen depletion and enhance endurance performance.[92] This beneficial shift in energy partitioning between carbohydrate and lipid substrates has been observed in women relative to men and is the impetus for the belief that women may be better adapted for endurance and ultraendurance sports. Initial theories of differences in energy metabolism between men and women ironically included the greater availability of lipid afforded by the higher body fat percentages of women.[93] More favorable theories now implicate circulating estrogens as the link to this alteration in substrate metabolism.

In untrained men and women during low- (35% VO_{2max}) and high- (80% VO_{2max}) intensity exercise, Blatchford et al.[94] and Froberg et al.[95] reported higher circulating free fatty acids and glycerol and lower respiratory exchange ratios (RER) in women than in their male counterparts. This resulted in fat utilization estimates of 59% for men and 73% for women.[94] Horton et al.[96] observed similar (42% for men and 51% for women) differences in fat utilization between the sexes during 2 hours of cycling at 40% VO_{2max}, which was again estimated using indirect calorimetry. Froberg et al.[95] reported significantly longer times to exhaustion (~ 17 minutes) for "physically active," but untrained, women when compared with men at 80% VO_{2max}. However, these differences in performance disappeared when exercise intensity was increased to 90% VO_{2max}. In contrast, Friedman and colleagues[97] ran untrained men and women on a treadmill at 75% VO_{2max} over 10 km and observed no differences in circulating free fatty acids, glycerol, or RER.

Costill et al.[98] tested male and female distance runners matched for training mileage, VO_{2max}, and muscle fiber composition before comparing substrate utilization during 60 minutes of treadmill running at 70% VO_{2max}. No differences in free fatty acids, glycerol, or RER were observed. Another study comparing trained men and women matched for fitness also reported no gender differences in RER after 90 minutes of treadmill running at 65% VO_{2max}.[99] However, Tarnopolsky et al.[100] reported gender differences in substrate utilization between six men and women matched for VO_{2max} and on a 3-day controlled diet. After running ~15 km at 65%VO_{2max}, significant differences in mean RER (0.94 men vs. 0.87 women) indicated that men utilized more carbohydrate than women, which was corroborated with muscle biopsy data showing that males used 25% more glycogen than women. It was concluded that females relied more on lipid fuel reserves (intramuscular) than equally trained men under identical relative exercise intensities. This was also the only study to report menstrual cycle phase (midfollicular), although this was not quantified by hormone assay.

Nicklas et al.[101] compared untrained eumennorrheic women at 70% VO_{2max} during midfollicular and midluteal cycle phases, which were confirmed by resting estradiol and progesterone concentrations. Estradiol levels were >300% higher in the luteal than the follicular phase (larger area under the estrogen curve), and RER values were significantly lower (0.71 luteal vs. 0.86 follicular) at rest. Run time to exhaustion was not significantly different between phases, but the trend (P < 0.09) for greater endurance observed in the luteal phase has been significant in related studies of both humans[102] and animals.[103-105] The proposed mechanism behind this alteration in metabolism appears to involve estrogen only,[103] despite higher circulating progesterone levels, also in the luteal phase. Estrogen appears to upregulate lipoprotein lipase (LPL) activity, as evidenced when 24 healthy females showed 150% greater LPL activity in the luteal vs. follicular phase.[106] This is also consistent with reports of improved endurance in the luteal phase.[101,102]

The evidence of Tarnopolsky et al.[100] seems conflicting, as it was gathered during the midfollicular phase of the menstrual cycle. Because estrogen levels were not measured, it is impossible to know if the women were closer to ovulation and the luteal phase or still in the early stages of the follicular phase. The control and documentation of menstrual cycle phase is therefore imperative when comparing men and women on energy metabolism and endurance performance. Many of the discrepancies in the literature reviewed may therefore be the result of menstrual cycle phase differences. Any degree of oligomenorrhea or amenorrhea, which is not an uncommon response to intense endurance training,[107,108] would also negate the "estrogen advantage" and could account for the more consistent effects of estrogen on substrate metabolism observed in untrained women.[94,95,97] While considerable evidence of an estrogen influence on lipid metabolism, and possibly also endurance, is well established, the more practical question of whether this translates into real-life record performance differences between men and women is more controversial.

B. Gender Differences in Endurance Performance

In 1992, Whipp and Ward[109] published a brief but highly controversial analysis of the progression in distance-running world records between men and women. Accordingly, they proposed that women would eventually run as fast as men at all distances from 200 meters to the marathon. However, the predictive slopes between men and women intersected much sooner for running distances beyond 10 km — especially for the marathon.[109] Sparling et al.[3] reevaluated running performances for men and women from 1.5 km to 42.2 km, examining world best times and the 100th best world times as performance indices for men and women between 1980 and 1996. They concluded that the rate of improvement in distance running for women had reached a plateau since the mid 1980s and was equal to that of men.[3] When plotting the mean running velocities for the top 50 times in 1996 for 1.5 km, 10 km, and 42.2 km, a consistent difference of ~ 13% between men and women was reported. Figure 8.1 is a comparative plot of the world record progression in the marathon between men and women between 1908 and 2000. Consistent with the findings of Sparling et al.,[3] the steep slope of improvement in women's marathon performance between 1964 and 1984 (28.5%) leveled off between 1984 and 2000 (1.4%). The difference in world record performances between men and women from 1984 (10%) and 2000 (11%) is also nearly identical. Despite this evidence, the idea that women might perform better than men at distances beyond 42.2 km still persists.

Men and women matched closely for VO_{2max} and 42 km performance time were recently compared for performance over 90 km.[110] The fact that the women ran the 90 km distance significantly faster (171 min) than their male counterparts (192.6 min) could not be explained by gender differences in VO_{2max}, training, running economy, or fatty acid metabolism. Bam et al.[111] found similar results when comparing existing race data from a large sample of men and women matched for 56 km performance, age, and training. Furthermore, the ~20% smaller body mass of the women in both studies could not explain the advantage since, although energy expenditure is constant and proportional to body mass (1 kcal/kg^{-1}/km^{-1}),[78,112] the women exercised at a slightly higher fractional percentage of VO_{2max}, thus producing similar power outputs.[110,111] What remains, however, is the fact that when men and women are matched for aerobic fitness, the women inherently represent a relatively more fit athlete than the males, because body compositional and physiological differences between men and women ordinarily make for a 10–60% aerobic fitness advantage in men. These findings are intriguing and it can be argued that women matched for aerobic fitness and performance to men from 42–56 km will perform better at longer (90 km) distances. However, this does not represent the usual competitive condition.

From Table 8.5 it is apparent that the best individual running performances of men and women at distances from 1.5–42.2 km are consistently ~ 10%

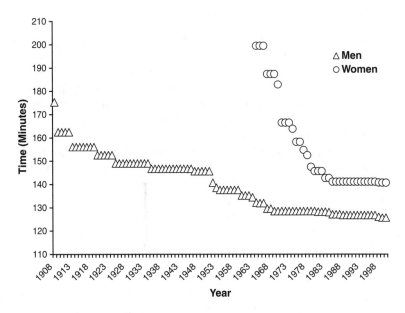

FIGURE 8.1
Progression in men's and women's world record performances for marathon running between 1908 and 2000. Data compiled from reference 86.

slower for women. At distances from 100–1000 km, the differences are actually even larger (20–30% slower for women). Table 8.4 suggests that women do have a genuine performance advantage over men in the water. Overall, differences in endurance swim records between the sexes are smaller than for running (< 10%), while women are 1–4% faster than men at distances from 20–30 km. In fact, a woman (Penny Dean) still holds the world record for the prestigious 20-plus-mile open water English Channel swim. Times in this race are quite variable, however, as differences in weather and tide can push swimmers from side to side and add additional horizontal swimming miles on any given attempt. Although comparisons of individual performances do not necessarily reflect population differences, Tables 8.4 and 8.5 and this literature review clearly illustrate that biological differences in VO_{2max} probably explain the superior performances of men in endurance running. This same difference in aerobic capacity may be, however, overshadowed by a more ideal female body composition (less torque[85]) for endurance swimming.

IV. Summary

The body compositional (body fat and muscle CSA) and physiological (hemoglobin concentration and cardiac muscle architecture) differences between men and women are fundamental gender differences of biological origin. Men are generally stronger than women and possess a larger aerobic capacity. Although the hormonal (estrogen) and morphological (body fat) characteristics of women may provide a qualitative advantage over men in endurance sports, only empirical evidence in ultraendurance swimming lends quantitative support to this idea when comparing the world's best men's and women's performances. The similar plateau in sports performance for men and women over the past 20 years suggests growing gender equality in sports participation. If this is so, then the remaining strength and endurance performance gaps between men and women are unlikely to narrow.

REFERENCES

1. Drinkwater, B.L. Women and exercise: physiological aspects. *Exerc. Sports Sci. Rev.,* 12, 21, 1984.
2. Kuscsik, N. The history of women's participation in the marathon. *Ann. NY Acad. Sci.,* 301, 862, 1977.
3. Sparling, P.B., O'Donnell, E.M. and Snow, T.K. The gender difference in distance running performance has plateaued: an analysis of world rankings from 1980–1996. *Med. Sci. Sports Exerc.,* 30, 1725, 1998.
4. Sparling, P.B., Nieman, D.C. and O'Connor, P.J. Selected scientific aspects of marathon racing: an update on fluid replacement, immune function, psychological factors and the gender difference. *Sports Med.,* 15, 116, 1993.
5. Wilmore, J. and Costill, D.L., Growth, development, and the young athlete, In: *Physiology of Sport and Exercise,* 2nd ed., Human Kinetics, Champaign, IL, 1999, p. 516-543.
6. Ford, L.E., Detterline, A.J., Ho, K.K. and Cao, W. Gender and height related limits of muscle strength in world weightlifting champions. *J. Appl. Physiol.,* 89, 1061, 2000.
7. Sale, D.G., MacDougall, J.D., Alway, S.E. and Sutton, J.R., Voluntary strength and muscle characteristics in untrained men and women and male bodybuilders, *J. Appl. Physiol.,* 62, 1786, 1987.
8. Alway, S.E., Grumbt, W.H., Gonyea, W.J. and Stray-Gundersen, J., Contrasts in muscle and myofibers of elite male and female bodybuilders, *J. Appl. Physiol.,* 67,24, 1989.
9. Costill, D.L., Daniels, J., Evans, W., Fink, W., Krahenbuhl, G. and Saltin, B., Skeletal muscle enzymes and fiber composition in male and female track athletes, *J. Appl. Physiol.,* 40, 149, 1976.
10. Miller, A.E.J., MacDougall, J.D., Tarnopolsky, M.A. and Sale, D.G., Gender differences in strength and muscle fiber characteristics, *Eur. J. Appl. Physiol.,* 66, 254, 1993.
11. Prince, F.P., Hikida, R.S. and Hagerman, F.C., Muscle fiber types in women athletes and nonathletes, *Pflügers Arch.,* 371, 161, 1977.
12. Schantz, P., Fox, E.R., Hutchinson, W., Tydén, A. and Åstrand, P.O., Muscle fibre type distribution, muscle cross-sectional area and maximal voluntary strength in humans, *Acta Physiol. Scand.,* 117, 219, 1983.

13. Komi, P.V. and Karlsson, J., Skeletal muscle fiber types, enzyme activities and physical performance in young males and females, *Acta Physiol. Scand.*, 103: 210, 1978.

14. Schantz, P., Fox, E.R., Norgren, P and Tydén, A., The relationship between the mean muscle fibre area and the musle cross-sectional area of the thigh in subjects with large differences in thigh girth, *Acta Physiol. Scand.*, 113, 537, 1981.

15. Gollnick, P.D., Armstrong, R.B., Saubert IV, C.W., Piehl, K and Saltin, B., Enzyme activity and fiber composition in skeletal muscle of untrained and trained men, *J. Appl. Physiol.*, 33, 312, 1972.

16. Edstrom, L. and Ekblom, B., Differences in sizes of red and white muscle fibres in vastus lateralis of musculus quadriceps femoris of normal individuals and athletes. Relation to physical performance, *Scand. J. Clin. Lab. Invest.*, 30, 175, 1972.

17. Tesch, P.A., Thorsson, A. and Kaiser, P., Muscle capillary supply and fiber type characteristics in weight and power lifters, *J. Appl. Physiol.*, 56, 35, 1984.

18. Prince, F.P., Hikida, R.S. and Hagerman, F.C., Human muscle fiber types in power lifters, distance runners and untrained subjects, *Pflügers Arch.*, 363, 19, 1976.

19. Gregor, R.J., Edgerton, V.R., Perrine, J.J., Campion, D.S and DeBus, C., Torque-velocity relationships and muscle fiber composition in elite female athletes, *J. Appl. Physiol.*, 47, 388, 1979.

20. Nygaard, E., Skeletal muscle fibre characteristics in young women, *Acta Physiol, Scand.*, 112, 299, 1981.

21. Tesch, P., Piehl, K., Wilson, G and Karlsson, J., Physiological investigations of Swedish elite canoe competitors, *Med. Sci. Sports*, 8, 214, 1976.

22. Clarkson, P.M., Kroll, W. and Melchionda, A.M., Isokinetic strength, endurance and fiber type composition in elite American paddlers, *Eur. J. Appl. Physiol.*, 48, 67, 1982.

23. Jansson, E., Sjödin, B. and Tesch, P., Changes in muscle fibre type distribution in man after physical training, *Acta Physiol. Scand.*, 104, 235, 1978.

24. Tesch, P. and Karlsson, J., Isometric strength performance and muscle fibre type distribution in man, *Acta Physiol. Scand.*, 103, 47, 1978.

25. Halkjaer-Kristensen, J. and Ingemann-Hansen, T., Variations in single fibre areas and fibre composition in needle biopsies from the human quadriceps muscle, *Scand. J. Clin. Lab. Invest.*, 41, 391, 1981.

26. Simoneau, J.A., Lortie, G., Boulay, M.R., Marcotte, M., Thibault, M.C and Bouchard, C., Human skeletal muscle fiber type alteration with high-intensity intermittent training, *Eur. J. Appl. Physiol.*, 54, 250, 1985.

27. Andersen, P. and Henriksson, J., Training-induced changes in the subgroups of human Type II skeletal muscle fibers, *Acta Physiol. Scand.*, 99, 123, 1977.

28. Ingjer, F., Effects of endurance training on muscle fiber ATP-ase activity, capillary supply and mitochondrial content in man, *J. Physiol.*, 294, 419, 1979.

29. Henriksson-Larsén, K., Distribution, number and size of different types of fibres in whole cross-sections of female m tibialis anterior. An enzyme histochemical study, *Acta Physiol, Scand.*, 123, 229, 1985.

30. Staron, R.S., Malicky, E.S., Leonardi, M.J., Falkel, J.E., Hagerman, F.C and Dudley, G.A., Muscle hypertrophy and fast fiber type conversions in heavy resistance-trained women, *Eur. J. Appl. Physiol.*, 60, 71, 1989.

31. Costill, D.L., Coyle, E.F., Fink, W.F., Lesmes, G.R and Witzmann, F.A., Adaptations in skeletal muscle following strength training, *J. Appl. Physiol.: Respirat. Environ. Exercise Physiol.*, 46, 96, 1979.

32. Dons, B., Bollerup, K., Bonde-Petersen, F and Hancke, S., The effect of weight-lifting exercise related to muscle fiber composition and muscle cross-sectional area in humans, *Eur. J. Appl. Physiol.*, 40, 95, 1979.

33. Thorstensson, A., Hultén, B., Von Döbelm, W and Karlsson, J., Effect of strength training on enzyme activities and fibre characteristics in human skeletal muscle, *Acta Physiol. Scand.*, 96, 392, 1976.

34. Gollnick, P.D., Armstrong, R.B., Saltin, B., Saubert IV, C.W., Sembrowich, W.L and Shepherd, R.E., Effect of training on enzyme activity and fiber composition of human skeletal muscle, *J. Appl. Physiol.*, 34, 107, 1973.

35. Thorstensson, A., Sjödin, B. and Karlsson, J., Enzyme activities and muscle strength after "spring training" in man, *Acta Physiol. Scand.*, 94, 313, 1975.

36. Cureton, K.J., Collins, M.A., Hill, D.W and Mcelhannon Jr., F.M., Muscle hypertrophy in men and women, *Med. Sci. Sports Exerc.*, 20, 338, 1988.

37. Lewis, D.A., Kamon, E. and Hodhson, J.L. Physiological differences between genders: implications for sports conditioning. *Sports Med.* 3: 357, 1986.

38. Ramos, E., Frontera, W.R., Llopart, A and Feliciano, D. Muscle strength and hormonal levels in adolescents: gender related differences. *Int. J. Sports Med.*, 19, 526, 1998.

39. Brown, C.H. and Wilmore, J.H. The effects of maximal resistance training on the strength and body composition of women athletes, *Med. Sci. Sports*, 6, 174, 1974.

40. Capen, E.K., Bright, J.A. and Line, P.A. The effects of weight training on strength, power, muscular endurance and anthropometric measurements on a select group of college women, *J. Assn. Phys. and Mental Rehab.*, 15, 169, 1961.

41. Hakkinen, K., Pakarinen, A. and Kallinen, M. Neuromuscular adaptations and serum hormones in women during short-term intensive strength training. *Eur. J. Appl. Physiol.*, 66, 553, 1993.

42. Abe, T., Brechue, W.F., Fujita, S and Brown, J.B. Gender differences in FFM accumulation and architectural characteristics of muscle. *Med. Sci. Sports Exerc.*, 30, 1066, 1998.

43. Dube, J.Y., Lesage, R. and Tremblay, R.R. Androgen and estrogen binding in rat skeletal and perineal muscles. *Can. J. Biochem.*, 54, 50, 1976.

44. *Guinness World Records, 2001.* Bantam Books, New York, 2001.

45. American College of Sports Medicine opinion statement on the participation of the female athlete in long-distance running. *Med. Sci. Sports*, 11, ix, 1979.

46. Sparling, P.B. A meta-analysis of studies comparing maximal oxygen uptake in men and women. *Res. Q.*, 51, 542, 1980.

47. Pate, R.R. and Branch, J.D. Training for endurance sport. *Med. Sci. Sports Exerc.*, 24, S340, 1992.

48. Howley, E.T., Bassett, D.R. and Welch, H.G. Criteria for maximal oxygen uptake: review and commentary. *Med. Sci. Sports Exerc.*, 27, 1292, 1995.

49. Saltin, B. and Astrand, P. Maximal oxygen uptake in athletes. *J. Appl. Physiol.*, 23, 353, 1967.

50. Joyner, M.J. Physiological limiting factors and distance running: influence of gender and age on record performances. *Exerc. Sport Sci. Rev.*, 103, 1993.

51. Costill, D.L. and Fox, E.L. Energetics of marathon running. *Med. Sci. Sports Exerc.*, 1, 81, 1969.

52. Fox, E.L. and Costill, D.L. Estimated cardiorespiratory response during marathon running. *Arch. Environ. Health*, 24, 316, 1972.
53. Wells, C.L., Hecht, L.H. and Krahenbuhl, G.S. Physical characteristics and oxygen utilization of male and female marathon runners. *Res. Q. Exerc. Sport*, 52, 281, 1981.
54. Wilmore, J.H. and Brown, C.H. Physiological profiles of women distance runners. *Med. Sci. Sports*, 6, 178, 1974.
55. Martin, R.P., Haskell, W.L. and Wood, P.D. Blood chemistry and lipid profiles of elite distance runners. *Ann. Amer. Acad. Sci.*, 301, 346, 1977.
56. Spirito, P., Pelliccia, A., Proschan, M.A., Granata, M., Spataro, A., Bellone, P., Caselli, G., Biffi, A., Vecchio, C and Maron, B.J. Morphology of the "athlete's heart" assessed by echocardiography in 947 elite athletes representing 27 sports. *Amer. J.Cardiol.*, 74, 802, 1994.
57. Mier, C.M., Domenick, M.A., Turner, N.S and Wilmore, J.H. Changes in stroke volume and maximal aerobic capacity with increased blood volume in men and women. *J. Appl. Physiol.*, 80, 1180, 1996.
58. Pavlik, G., Olexo, Z, Banhegyi, A., Sido, Z and Frenkl, R. Gender differences in the echocardiographic characteristics of the athletic heart. *Acta Physiol. Hung.*, 86, 273, 1999.
59. Cunningham, D.A., McCrimmon, D. and Vlach. L.F. Cardiovascular response to interval and continuous training in women. *Eur. J. Appl. Physiol.*, 41, 187, 1979.
60. Christensen, C.L. and Ruhling. R.O. Physical characteristics of novice and experienced women marathon runners. *Br. J. Sports Med.*, 17, 166, 1983.
61. Maughan, R.J. and Leiper, J.B. Aerobic capacity and fractional utilization of aerobic capacity in elite and non-elite male and female marathon runners. *Eur. J. Appl. Physiol.*, 52, 80, 1983.
62. Pollock, M.L. Submaximal and maximal working capacity of elite distance runners. Part I: cardiorespiratory aspects. *Ann. NY Acad. Sci.*, 301, 310, 1977.
63. Sleivert, G.G. and Rowlands, D.S. Physical and physiological factors associated with success in the triathlon. *Sports Med.*, 22, 8, 1996.
64. Holloszy, J.O. and Coyle, E.F. Adaptations of skeletal muscle to endurance exercise and their metabolic consequences. *J. Appl. Physiol.*, 56, 831, 1984.
65. Brooks, G.A. Current concepts in lactate exchange. *Med. Sci. Sports Exerc.*, 23, 895, 1991.
66 Costill, D.L. Metabolic responses during distance running. *J. Appl. Physiol.*, 28, 251, 1970.
67. Farrell, P.A., Wilmore, J.H., Coyle, E.F., Billing, J.E and Costill, D.L. Plasma lactate accumulation and distance running performance. *Med. Sci. Sports*, 11, 338, 1979.
68. Iawaoka, K., Hatta, H., Atomi, Y and Miyashita, M. Lactate, respiratory compensation thresholds and distance running performance in runners of both sexes. *Int. J. Sports Med.*, 9, 306, 1988.
69. Bhambhani, Y.N., Buckley, S.M. and Susaki, T. Detection of ventilatory threshold using near infrared spectroscopy in men and women. *Med. Sci. Sports Exerc.*, 29, 402, 1997.
70. Davies, C.T.M. Thermoregulation during exercise in relation to sex and age. *Eur. J. Appl. Physiol.*, 42, 71, 1979.
71. Davies, K.J.A., Packer, L. and Brooks, G.A. Biochemical adaptation of mitochondria, muscle and whole-animal respiration to endurance training. *Arch. Biochem. Biophys.*, 209, 539, 1981.

72. Berthon, P.M., Howlett, R.A., Heigenhauser, G.J and Spriet, L.L. Human skeletal muscle carnitine palmitoyltransferase I activity determined in isolated intact mitochondria. *J. Appl. Physiol.*, 85, 148, 1998.

73. Carter, S.L., Rennie, C.D., Hamilton, S.J and Tarnopolsky, M.A. Changes in skeletal muscle in males and females following endurance training. *Can. J. Physiol. Pharmacol.*, 79, 386, 2001.

74. Costill, D.L., Fink, W.J., Flynn, M. and Kirwan, J. Muscle fiber composition and enzyme activities in elite female distance runners. *Int. J. Sports Med.*, 8, 103, 1987.

75. Fink, W.J., Costill, D.L. and Pollock, M.L. Submaximal and maximal working capacity of elite distance runners: Part II. Muscle fiber composition and enzyme activities. *Ann. NY Acad. Sci.*, 301, 323, 1977.

76. Daniels, J.T. A physiologist's view of running economy. *Med. Sci. Sports Exerc.*, 17, 332, 1985.

77. Hausswirth, C., Bigard, A.X. and Guezennec, C.Y. Relationships between running mechanics and energy cost of running at the end of a triathlon and a marathon. *Int. J. Sports Med.*, 18, 330, 1997.

78. Margaria, R., Cerretelli, P., Aghemo, P and Sassi, G. Energy cost of running. *J. Appl. Physiol.*, 18, 367, 1963.

79. Holmer, I. Energy cost of the arm stroke, leg kick and whole stroke in competitive swimming style. *J. Appl. Physiol.*, 33, 105, 1974.

80. Faria, I.E. Applied physiology of cycling. *Sports Med.*, 1, 187, 1984.

81. Brandford, D.R. and Howley, E.T. Oxygen cost of running in trained and untrained men and women. *Med. Sci. Sports*, 9, 41, 1977.

82. Burke, E.J. Physiological effects of similar training programs in males and females. *Res. Q.*, 48, 510, 1977.

83. Daniels, J. and Daniels, N. Running economy of elite male and elite female runners. *Med. Sci. Sports Exerc.*, 24, 483, 1992.

84. Daniels, J., Krahenbuhl, G., Foster, C., Gilbert, J and Daniels, S. Aerobic responses of female distance runners to submaximal and maximal exercise. *Ann. NY Acad. Sci.*, 301, 726, 1977.

85. Zamparo, P., Antonutto, G., Capelli, C., Francescato, M.P., Girardis, M., Sangoi, R., Soule, R.G and Pendergast, D.R. Effects of body size, body density, gender and growth on underwater torque. *Scand. J. Med. Sci. Sports*, 6, 273, 1996.

86. *Sports Illustrated 2001 Sports Almanac*. Bishop Books: New York, NY, 2000.

87. USA Swimming–American long distance records. At http://www.usa-swimming. org/fast_times/2000longdistance.PDF (accessed August, 2001).

88. Runner's World all-time outdoor ultradistance best–track. At http://www. runnersworld.com /stats/ultra.html (accessed August, 2001).

89. Dolgener, F.A., Kolkhorst, F.W. and Whitsett, D.A. Long slow distance training in novice marathoners. *Res. Q. Exerc. Sport.*, 65, 339, 1994.

90. Eddy, D.O., Sparks, K.L. and Adelizi, D.A. The effects of continuous and interval training in women and men. *Eur. J. Appl. Physiol.*, 37, 83, 1977.

91. Kilbom, A. and Astrand, I. Physical training with submaximal intensities in women. II. Effect of cardiac output. *Scand. J. Clin. Lab Invest.*, 28, 163, 1971.

92. Lambert, E.V., Hawley, J.A., Goedecke, J., Noakes, T.D and Dennis, S.C. Nutritional strategies for promoting fat utilization and delaying the onset of fatigue during prolonged exercise. *J. Sports Sci.*, 15, 315, 1997.

93. Bjorntorp, P.A. Sex differences in the regulation of energy balance with exercise. *Am. J. Clin. Nutr.*, 49, 958, 1989.

94. Blatchford, F.K., Knowlton, R.G. and Schneider, D. Plasma FFA responses to prolonged walking in untrained men and women. *Eur. J. Appl. Physiol.*, 53, 343, 1985.

95. Froberg, K. and Pedersen, P.K. Sex differences in endurance capacity and metabolic response to prolonged, heavy exercise. *Eur. J. Appl. Physiol.*, 52, 446, 1984.

96. Horton, T.J., Pagliassotti, M.J., Hobbs, K and Hill, J.O. Fuel metabolism in men and women during and after long-duration exercise. *J. Appl. Physiol.*, 85, 1823, 1998.

97. Friedman, B. and Kindermann, W. Energy metabolism and regulatory hormones in women and men during endurance exercise. *Eur. J. Appl. Physiol.*, 59, 1, 1989.

98. Costill, D.L., Fink, W.J., Getchell, L.H., Ivy, J.L and Witzmann, F.A. Lipid metabolism in skeletal muscle of endurance-trained males and females. *J. Appl. Physiol.*, 47, 787, 1979.

99. Powers, S.K., Riley, W. and Howley, E.T. Comparison of fat metabolism between trained men and women during prolonged aerobic work. *Res. Q. Exerc. Sport*, 51, 427, 1980.

100. Tarnopolsky, L.J., MacDougall, J.D., Atkinson, S.A., Tarnopolsky, M.A and Sutton, J.R. Gender differences in substrate for endurance exercise. *J. Appl. Physiol.*, 72, 15, 1992.

101. Nicklas, B.J., Hackney, A.C. and Sharp, R.L. The menstrual cycle and exercise: performance, muscle glycogen and substrate responses. *Int. J. Sports Med.*, 10, 264, 1989.

102. Jurkowski, J.E., Jones, N.L., Toews, C.J and Sutton, J.R. Effects of menstrual cycle on blood lactate, O_2 delivery and performance during exercise. *J. Appl. Physiol.*, 51, 1493, 1981.

103. Hatta, H., Atomi, Y., Shinohara, S., Yamamoto, Y and Yamada, S. The effects of ovarian hormones on glucose and fatty acid oxidation during exercise in female ovariectomized rats. *Horm. Metab. Res.*, 20, 609, 1988.

104. Kendrick, Z.V. and Ellis, G.S. Effect of estradiol on tissue glycogen metabolism and lipid availability in exercised male rats. *J. Appl. Physiol.*, 71, 1694, 1991.

105. Kendrick, Z.V., Steffen, C.A., Rumsey, W.L and Goldberg, D.L. Effect of estradiol on tissue glycogen metabolism in exercised oophorectomized rats. *J. Appl. Physiol.*, 63, 492, 1987.

106. De Mendoza, S.G., Nucete, H., Salazar, E., Zerpa, A and Kashyap, M.L. Plasma lipids and lipoprotein lipase activator property during the menstrual cycle. *Horm. Metab. Rev.*, 11, 696, 1979.

107. Boyden, T.W., Pameter, R.W., Stanforth, P., Rotkis, T and Wilmore, J.H. Sex steroids and endurance running in women. *Fert. Steril.*, 39, 629, 1983.

108. Shangold, M., Freeman, R., Thysen, B and Gatz, M. The relationship between long distance running, plasma progesterone and luteal phase length. *Fert. Steril.*, 31, 130, 1979.

109. Whipp, B.J. and Ward, S.A. Will women soon outrun men? *Nature*, 355, 25, 1992.

110. Speechly, D.P., Taylor, S.R. and Rogers, G.G. Differences in ultra-endurance exercise in performance-matched male and female runners. *Med. Sci. Sports Exerc.*, 28, 359, 1996.

111. Bam, J., Noakes, T.D., Juritz, J and Dennis, S.C. Could women outrun men in ultramarathon races? *Med. Sci. Sports Exerc.*, 29, 244, 1997.

112. Kram, R. Muscular force or work: what determines the metabolic energy cost of running? *Exerc. Sports Sci. Rev.*, 28, 138, 2000.

Section Four

Physical Activity Needs
Assessment of Athletes

9

Laboratory Methods for Determining Energy Expenditure of Athletes

Robert G. McMurray

CONTENTS

I. Introduction

The central function of nutrition is to provide sufficient energy to sustain life. The energy is needed for muscle contraction, as well as to build tissues, digest food and to create enzymes and hormones. All of these processes will ultimately generate heat. Thus, metabolism and heat production can be viewed in the same perspective. For decades, the basic unit of energy in humans has been the *kilocalorie* (kcal). This is the amount of heat required to increase one kilogram of water 1° Celsius. However, the S.I. Unit (le Système International d'Unités) of the *kiloJoule* (kJ) is becoming more acceptable.[1] Conversion between systems is simple, as 1 kcal is equal to 4.184 kJ. Although these two units are used in the literature, other units of measure have been used. The kilogram-meter, or kgm, is a unit of energy used frequently on cycle ergometers. It is determined by multiplying the kilograms of resistance times the number of revolutions per minute, times the distance traveled per revolution. Thus, someone pedaling at 60 rpm on a standard cycle ergometer with a resistance of 2 kg would be working at 720 kgm.

Kgm can be converted to either kcal or kJ easily as there are 427 kgm per kcal or about 102 kgm per kJ. Using the example above, exercising at 720 kpm would equal 1.69 kcal or 7.06 kJ. Some researchers have also reported *watts* (w); however, the watt is a unit of power (Joules/second) and should not be used in energy production equations.

Energy derived from the complete combustion of each major nutrient is different. Fats produce the most energy per gram (9.4 kcal or 39.3 kJ/g), protein produces about 5.65 kcal or 23.7 kJ/g, while carbohydrates yield only 4.3 kcal/18 kJ/g.[2] These values are determined using a bomb calorimeter, which is a strong steel cylinder, resistant to high pressures, with a highly insulated water bath surrounding it.[3] The food substance is sealed in the cylinder containing high-pressure oxygen. The food is electronically ignited and the heat production is computed by measuring the increase in the water temperature in the water bath, taking into consideration the volume of water encircling the calorimeter. In contrast to the bomb calorimeter, human metabolism is not as efficient at assimilating and using these substrates. Thus, for practical purposes, the energy production of carbohydrates and proteins is about 4 kcal/g (17 kJ/g), while fats produce approximately 9 kcal/g (37 kJ/g).

II. Methods for the Measurement of Metabolic Rate

The energy output of humans can be measured by *direct* and *indirect* calorimetry.[4-6] The direct calorimetry method measures heat production. The method is accurate, but most organizations do not have the expensive, complicated facilities and equipment needed to use this method. Indirect methods, which rely on the measurement of oxygen uptake, are less expensive, smaller, and more portable. In addition, studies have shown good agreement between direct and indirect calorimetry. Because the advantages of indirect calorimetry are considerable, its use gained popularity in the early 1900s.[6-8]

A. Direct Calorimetry

Direct calorimetry, which directly assesses heat production, typically requires a small room with highly insulated walls.[4,6,8] These units are a larger version of the bomb calorimeter. The walls of the unit contain a series of finned pipes through which water is pumped at a constant rate. The heat generated by the subject is measured by the difference between the incoming and outgoing water temperatures measured to the 0.01°C, knowing the volume and rate of the water flow. Oxygen is continuously supplied and carbon dioxide is removed by chemical absorbent. Direct calorimeters come in several sizes and types ranging from suit calorimeters, like those used by astronauts, to small chambers and even larger rooms. Using direct calorimetry to measure metabolic rate takes considerable time, as it takes at least 30 minutes for the heat loss and heat production to equilibrate.[6] In addition, it appears that the methods work best for steady-state activities. The method is highly accurate, but is limited only to resting measures or those activities that have minimal range of movement. The methods will not work for most sports or activities, in varying environments, or in large-scale studies.

B. Indirect Calorimetry

The underlying principle of *indirect calorimetry* is that the production of energy requires oxygen.[4-6] Thus, if the oxygen uptake is measured, energy production can then be estimated and, through mathematical conversion, the results can be presented either in kcal or kJ. Indirect calorimetry appears to be the method of choice for measuring energy expenditure at rest or during activity.[5] This method is based on four assumptions:[4]

1. The individual is not in a starvation state.
2. Because the individual is not starving, protein makes up only a very small portion of the energy and can therefore be ignored.
3. The contribution of anaerobic metabolism to the energy production is quite small.
4. When using a combination of carbohydrates, fats, and proteins as a source of energy, approximately 4.82 kcal (20 kJ) of energy is liberated per liter of oxygen used.[8]

For convenience, the 4.82 kcal/L O_2 has been rounded to 5 kcal or 21 kJ per liter of oxygen. The equipment to obtain the oxygen uptake is much less expensive than that used for direct calorimetry and has been found to have an error as little as 1% compared with direct calorimetry.[7] There are actually two general indirect calorimetry methods. One employs a closed circuit system while the other uses an open-circuit system. Both appear to be equally valid; however, the open-circuit system has proven to be more beneficial for activities involving movement.

1. Closed-Circuit Spirometry

The closed circuit system, or closed-circuit spirometry, uses a spirometer, an airtight cylinder, filled with 100% oxygen and an absorbent that is used to remove the CO_2 exhaled in each breath.[2] The person simply breathes through the spirometer. Because O_2 is absorbed by the body, and any CO_2 produced is removed from the spirometer, the volume of gas in the spirometer is reduced. The difference between the initial and the final volumes of oxygen in the spirometer is the oxygen uptake. That oxygen uptake is multiplied by 5 kcal/L to obtain the energy use. Some problems are inherent with this system.[9] Temperature of the gas will affect the volume in the spirometer. A

1°C rise in temperature will cause a 10,000 ml volume to increase to 10,034 ml.[9] Because expired air is at a higher temperature than inspired, this could be a critical factor in underestimating metabolic rate. The system must be airtight so volumes will not change inappropriately. The CO_2 absorbent must be adequate or the CO_2 production will simply replace the oxygen uptake and reduce the measured oxygen uptake. Inadequate CO_2 absorbent will also increase respiration and reduce any exercise performance. Similarly, at high metabolic rates, the CO_2 absorbent may not be able to keep pace with the respiratory CO_2 output, once again reducing exercise performance. Because the equipment is a closed circuit, the apparatus must have the capacity to hold a large volume of oxygen. For example, during exercise, a person may utilize 2–3 liters of oxygen per minute. Thus, for a 20-minute run, the apparatus must be able to contain at least 40–60 liters of oxygen. Finally, once subjects are on the apparatus, they cannot come off it until the final measure has been made. These limitations, plus the bulky size of the equipment and its proximity to the subject, have limited the use of closed-circuit spirometry for exercise studies.

2. Open-Circuit Spirometry

The open-circuit system has proven itself to be useful to measure energy use both at rest and during exercise. In this method, subjects do not rebreathe their own air. They simply breathe in room air and expire their air through a system that measures the total volume of air and the expired proportions of oxygen and carbon dioxide.[4-6] The difference between the inspired and expired is the oxygen uptake.

There are basically three major types of open-circuit systems:

1. A bag system
2. A computerized system
3. A portable system[8]

All three systems start with the subject's breathing through a mask or breathing valve that allows the expired air to be directed through the analyzers. All three types contain a meter to measure total air volume (ventilation meter, turbine, or pneumotach), an oxygen meter and a CO_2 meter. The bag system collects the volume of expired air in a large meteorological balloon or a standard rubberized Douglas bag.[6] The contents of the bag are measured for their volumes of oxygen and carbon dioxide, as well as the overall air volume. These values are then introduced into a formula to compute oxygen uptake. The computerized system takes the output from the three meters (expired oxygen, expired carbon dioxide, and ventilation) and computes the oxygen uptake.[8] The computerized system has the advantage of using instruments with much faster response time so that oxygen uptake can be computed on a breath-by-breath basis. Modern technology and microprocessors have resulted in miniaturizing the computerized systems to the point that they weigh less than 1 kg and can be worn on the back or abdomen; thus allowing freedom of movement. The portable units can also contain telemetry systems that allow investigators to obtain the energy expenditure data without being in direct contact with the subject. These portable systems allow researchers to obtain breath-by-breath information on energy expenditures of many activities with the person unimpeded.

All of the open-circuit systems have the same underlying assumptions as other indirect calorimetry systems; that is, the individual is not in a starvation state, protein makes up only a very small portion of the energy and can therefore be ignored, and the contribution of anaerobic metabolism to the energy production is quite small. However, the open-circuit systems do not generalize the energy production from a liter of oxygen. Instead, the open-circuit methods utilize the fact that carbohydrates and fats have different oxygen demands (VO_2) and carbon dioxide production (VCO_2) rates,[10] therefore allowing for differing energy rates (kcal/kJ) based on substrate utilization. Using open-circuit spirometry to measure energy expenditure requires that the person reach a steady state. This is because the VCO_2 and VO_2 represent substrate utilization only during steady state. In this state, the VCO_2 is usually less than the VO_2, so the relationship or ratio is always ≤ 1.0. However, any activity that produces considerable lactate acid will increase VCO_2, via the bicarbonate buffer equation ($H^+ + HCO_3^- \rightarrow H_2O + CO_2$). The increased CO_2 will increase the VCO_2 above what is expected for aerobic metabolism and reduce the ability to compute energy expenditure.[4-6] These are major limitations of indirect calorimetry.

a.   Computation of Energy Expenditure Using the Respiratory Exchange Ratio

The *respiratory exchange ratio* (RER), respiratory quotient (RQ), or simply the R value, is the ratio of VCO_2 to VO_2 uptake.[4-6] The RER does not take protein metabolism for energy into consideration; therefore, it is sometimes referred to as the nonprotein RER.[4,6] The RER for carbohydrate is 1.0, as the oxidation of a single glucose molecule requires 6 O_2 molecules and produces 6 CO_2 molecules, or a ratio of, 6/6 (CO_2/O_2), which equals 1.0. The reaction can be summarized by the following equation: $C_6H_{12}O_6 + 6O_2 \rightarrow 6CO_2 + 6 H_2O +$ energy. Conversely, the oxidation of a palmitic acid molecule, a typical fatty acid used for energy, uses 23 O_2 molecules and produces 16 CO_2 molecules (16/23 = 0.696), summarized by the following equation: $C_{16}H_{32}O_2 + 23O_2 \rightarrow 16CO_2 + 16H_2O +$ energy.

As the composition of the substrate used for energy changes from fat to glucose, the RER changes from 0.7 to 1.0. An individual consuming a 50/50 mixture of carbohydrates and fats has an RER of 0.85. In addition to revealing the source of energy, the RER also relates to the amount of caloric production per liter of O_2.[11] Carbohydrates produce 5.047 kcal/liter (21 kJ/L) of O_2 uptake, while fats only produce 4.686 kcal/liter (19.6 kJ/L) of O_2 uptake.

To measure energy expenditure, the O_2 uptake and CO_2 production per minute must be measured.[4,6] To accomplish this, six factors must be known: Inspired volume of air (V_I) per minute, inspired percent of O_2 (F_IO_2) and CO_2 (F_ICO_2), the expired air volume (V_E) per minute, and the expired percentages of O_2 (F_EO_2) and CO_2 (F_ECO_2). The ventilation, either V_I or V_E, is normally obtained from a gas meter, pneumotach or turbine. The F_IO_2 and F_ICO_2 are known (20.93% and 0.03%, respectively). Either V_I or V_E must be directly measured. The other volume can be calculated using the Haldane conversion.[6] The F_EO_2 and F_ECO_2 are obtained from monitoring expired air using O_2 and CO_2 meters. The following formulas can then be applied to compute the O_2 uptake (VO_2), CO_2 output (VCO_2) and obtain RER:

$$VO_2 = (V_I \times F_IO_2) - (V_E \times F_EO_2)$$
$$VCO_2 = (V_E \times F_ECO_2) - (V_I \times F_ICO_2)$$
$$RER = VCO_2/VO_2$$

RER on chart will give kcal/L O_2 (as well as percent carbohydrates and fats)

$$kcal/min = (kcal/L\ O_2) \times VO_2\ (L/min)$$
$$kJ/min = (kcal/min) \times 4.186\ kJ/kcal$$

Because barometric pressures, temperatures and relative humidity conditions vary in different locations, measurements of energy expenditure must be standardized.[6] Thus, researchers know that an O_2 uptake of 2 L/min in the desert below sea level is the same as 2 l/min in the high rain forests of a mountain range. To accomplish this, only the volume of air per minute need be corrected, because barometric pressure, temperature and relative humidity affect volume and not the percentage of the gases. The standard correction factor is to adjust barometric pressure to sea level (760 mmHg), temperature to 0°C, and relative humidity to 0%. This factor is known by the acronym *STPD*: standard temperature, pressure, and dryness.[6] Failure to apply the factor can result in a 7–15% error in the overall calculation of energy expenditure.

The O_2 uptake obtained from the above formulas results in the units of liters of O_2 per minute (L/min). This is considered the absolute VO_2. The O_2 uptake can also be expressed by taking into consideration body weight; milliliters of O_2 per kilogram body weight per minute (ml/kg/min). This is considered to be the relative VO_2. The absolute VO_2 is used to obtain overall energy expenditure. Individuals with larger muscle mass have larger absolute VO_2s. However, when trying to compare individuals of differing sizes, relative VO_2 is the preferred terminology. In 1936, D.B. Dill[12] proposed a system of expressing energy expenditure in increments of resting metabolic rate. Thus, the origin of the metabolic equivalent (*MET*). Research has suggested that an O_2 uptake of 3.5 ml/kg/min is an average resting value for an adult. Thus, the 3.5 ml/kg/min is referred to as one MET.[8,13] The MET has become a popular unit of measure in epidemiological studies of activity.

3. Doubly Labeled Water

Thus far, the methods described for measuring metabolic rate have limitations. They have the potential for precision, but some methods restrict movements while others are limited to gathering information during only minutes or hours of use. None of the methods relate well to nonsteady-state activity or very high intensity activity in which CO_2 output can become greater than O_2 uptake (anaerobic work). In an attempt to overcome these problems, a technique using doubly labeled water has been developed.[14-17] Doubly labeled water is an isotope of water in which both the hydrogen and O_2 are tagged, $^2H_2^{18}O$. The underlying principles of the technique are that the hydrogen from the doubly labeled water is eliminated as part of the water and the O_2 is eliminated both as part of the water and CO_2 molecule. Because there is equilibrium between the O_2 molecule in the water and the CO_2, it is possible to measure the CO_2 production by measuring the hydrogen and O_2 isotope in the body's water.[17] The energy expenditure is then computed based on total body water, daily CO_2 output, and isotope turnover in the urine. Subjects consume a dose of the labeled water. The dose is based on estimated total body water. The subjects simply go about their activities for a period of 5–7 days and the isotope turnover in the urine is measured by high-precision mass spectrometry. The overall error of this method is about 6%; however, considering this is spread over a week, the error is acceptable.[17]

The doubly labeled water method is based on six assumptions:[15,17]

1. The volume of water in which the $^2H_2^{18}O$ is diluted is constant. This is not quite true because eating and drinking behavior is episodic rather than constant and some individuals are losing or gaining weight. However, this difference turns out to be less than a 1–2% error.[17]

2. The fluxes of water and CO_2 are constant. Although this is not true due to the episodic nature of physical activity, eating and drinking, once again, the difference appears to be not quantitatively important.[17]

3. The body water compartments act as a single compartment with respect to the equilibration of isotopes. This assumption has proven to be controversial as the hydrogen has been noted to be more rapidly exchangeable than the O_2. Some investigators have then used dilution space correction factor rather than total body water.

4. The rate of tracer efflux exactly represents the rate of tracee efflux. The model has been adjusted for this.

5. No CO_2 or water enters the body through the skin or lungs. Because the aim is to measure the dietary water intake and CO_2 production,

any additional environmental sources would cause an error. Cigarette smoking can increase CO_2 intake, thus inducing a 3–6% increase in the estimate of energy expenditure. Although some exchange occurs in a nonsmoking person, once again the error is quantitatively unimportant.[17]

6. The food quotient, obtained from dietary intake, is used to estimate the dietary mix rather than the respiratory exchange ratio. This is important because the heat production (energy) per unit of CO_2 differs by about 30% when comparing carbohydrates and fats. The use of the food quotient introduces approximately a 3% error. This assumption does not account for alcohol intake or whether energy intake differs considerably from energy expenditure. The overall effect of the inaccuracies of these assumptions is to induce a 2–8% error depending upon dose and duration of the study.[14,16]

The major problem of the technique is the expense of equipment necessary for the isotope and total body water analyses and the expense of the dosages of $^2H_2{}^{18}O$. However, other problems have been reported. For example, Roberts et al.[18] completed an interlaboratory comparison using standards containing varying amounts of $^2H_2$ and ^{18}O. They found substantial variability between laboratories, including some physiologically impossible results. The differences were attributed to the quality of isotope analyses. Also, Speakman et al.[19] found that the error for estimating VCO_2 from doubly labeled water was not normally distributed and could result in an error for duplicate samples of 3–47%. In defense, this error could be reduced considerably by analyzing the samples in sets of five rather than two. Although these problems exist, $^2H_2{}^{18}O$ presently provides our best estimate of free-living energy expenditure.

C. Indirect Methods of Estimating Energy Expenditure

Because metabolic equipment is costly, requires considerable training to use, and is difficult to use for normal activities of life, indirect methods have been used in an attempt to estimate energy expenditure (EE). These methods include the use of heart rate monitors and motion sensors.

The use of heat rate to estimate EE has been explored because it is a relatively inexpensive method that allows the individual to be assessed in a free-living state.[20] In addition, it has the potential to provide the pattern of activity as well as the EE. The use of heart rate monitors to estimate EE requires planning and calibration. The subject first must undergo testing so that the resting and maximal heat rates are known, and a heart rate:EE relationship is developed. This usually requires the use of an ergometer to introduce the work and a spirometry system to measure the O_2 uptake and compute the EE. The subject then wears a heart rate monitor for a 24-hour period. The heart rates are downloaded to a computer and then averaged in 1- to 15-minute time segments. The average EE during that short time segment is then estimated by using the previously determined EE:heart rate relationship and multiplying that by the number of minutes of activity. This procedure is then used repeatedly and totaled until the entire 24-hour EE is obtained.

The major problem with this method is that not all heart rate increases are related to changes in metabolic rate.[20-22] Emotional stress and temperature changes are known to affect heart rate independent of metabolic rate. Thus, heart rates below 120 are not considered usable to determine EE.[22] In addition, heart rate represents metabolic rate only when a steady state of activity has occurred. Thus, during anaerobic activities, or activities that have considerable isometric component, in which heart rates are elevated above metabolic rate, the use of heart rate can skew the results. Finally, the heart rate may not be sufficiently sensitive to respond to short-term activities.[22] Therefore, it appears to be impractical to use heart rate to estimate metabolic rate. However, heart rate can be used to estimate minutes of moderate- to hard-intensity activities.[22]

Motion detectors have been used to estimate EE. These can be as simple as a pedometer or as complex as a three-dimensional accelerometer. Pedometers measure only ambulation and so are of limited value when calculating EE.[22,23] Accelerometers contain a piezoresistive microswitch that responds to motion. The units are small and usually worn on the hip. Some of these are designed to respond to movement in a single plane of motion (up–down) while others have the capability of responding in three dimensions. These units usually require a computer interface. The investigator enters the subject's age, sex, height and weight and resets the unit to zero (initializes the unit). The subject then wears the unit for a period of time, sometimes even up to 7 days. The motion counts are then downloaded to a computer. The accelerometer has a built-in EE prediction equation based on the motion counts, gender, age, height and weight. The accelerometer output can be divided up into segments as little as 1 minute, giving the ability to compute EE during a specific activity, as well as overall EE.

In adults, uni-axial accelerometers appear to slightly overpredict EE during those activities that involve ambulation, such as level walking or running.[13,24] However, they underpredict the energy cost of activities that involve arm movement or external work, such as stair climbing or hill walking.[12,24,25] In addition, the units are ineffective for measuring EE for activities that do not involve ambulation, such as swimming, cycling, weight lifting, or any seated activity. Tri-axial monitors appear to be slightly more accurate, but they still seem to have the same limitation as the uni-axial models with respect to evaluating intensity of activity, arm work or non-ambulatory activities.[22,26] In addition, the formulas to compute EE were derived from adult data, which is known to not directly apply to children.[27] Thus, motion detectors have a limited ability to estimate EE.

One final technique to estimate metabolic rate is stability of weight. If the weight is stable, then calorie intake equals calorie output. However, this serves only as a very crude estimate of overall EE.

III. Resting Energy Expenditure

Resting EE can be evaluated from two perspectives: the *basal metabolic rate,* or *BMR,* and the *resting metabolic rate,* or *RMR.* The *BMR* is also referred to as the basal energy expenditure and is the minimal amount of energy necessary to sustain life. The energy needed to maintain the heartbeat, respiration, cell metabolism, nerve transmission, constant body temperature, etc. Measuring the BMR requires that the person have no additional physiologic or psychologic stimulation, such as digestion, excess temperature regulation, psychological tension, or any form of physical activity or movement.[28] It is usually measured with the person resting supine, after at least 8 hours of sleep, and at least 12 hours after the last meal or exercise.[28] On the other hand, the RMR or resting energy expenditure (*REE*), is the EE required to maintain normal body functions at rest.[8,5] The REE is typically measured in the morning, after a normal night's sleep, with the individual lying down, or sitting, in a thermoneutral environment after a 12-hour fast, and not having exercised for 12 hours. The REE accounts for about two thirds of the daily EE. Because the two states are relatively close in definition, and because the difference between the BMR and the REE is less than 10%, both terms appear to be used interchangeably.[26] In fact, Schultz and Jequier[5] suggest that if the REE is measured in a postabsorptive condition, it is the same as BMR. However, they are really two differing states. True BMR is difficult to measure precisely and requires more controls than the REE. Therefore, rather than obtain the BMR, the REE is usually obtained. Both the BMR and the REE are usually expressed in kilocalories per hour (kcal/h) or kiloJoules per hour (kJ/h). The rate varies as much as ± 20% from one individual to another.[2,8]

A. Measurement of Resting Energy Expenditure

Any of the methods of calorimetry can be used to measure REE. However, the REE is usually obtained from two 5–7-minute continuous measures of VO_2 and VCO_2. In some cases, a single 15-minute collection period is used with the first 5 minutes of measurement discarded and last 10 minutes of measurement being averaged to obtain the REE.[28] The subject usually reclines in a supine position for approximately 30–45 minutes in a quiet, thermoneutral environment, sometimes covered with a light blanket. The mask or mouthpiece is put into place so that the subject is breathing through the apparatus during this initial rest period. This reduces any anxiety caused by the equipment. The subject is told not to sleep, but to remain fairly still. At the end of the initial 20–45 minutes of rest, the measurements are made.

The methods for measuring BMR need to be more restrictive to reduce subject awareness and anxiety and usually involve gas measurements obtained with the subject inside a transparent hood or using a room calorimeter.[5,28] In addition, the BMR measures are usually obtained over a 20–30-minute period rather than the two 5–7-minute measurements.[28]

B. Estimating Resting Energy Expenditure

Resting EE can be directly measured. However, the measurement takes considerable equipment, time and knowledge. Thus, methods have been derived to estimate REE based on indirect measures of weight, height and age. The simplest method is based on gender. Adult males will use 1.0 kcal/kg/h or 4.186 kJ/kg/h, while females will use 0.9 kcal/kg/h or 3.77 kJ/kg/h.[3,29] The person's weight (kilograms) is multiplied by the appropriate gender factor to obtain kcal/h. A variation on this simple method is to multiply the weight in pounds times ten. These methods are coarse and do not take into consideration age, size, muscle or fat mass, but can serve as an estimate of REE. Because REE declines with age, the World Health Organization (WHO) improved upon these simple prediction equations by developing six age-within-gender prediction equations.[29] These WHO equations correlate from 0.60–0.97 with reported direct measurements of REE (Table 9.1). Table 9.2 summarizes and compares the results obtained by using the four different analytical methods to estimate REE. As is evident from Table 9.2, there is a greater than 15% difference between methods of estimation and there is no simple way to determine which formula is most accurate for which person. Generally, equations based on gender, age, weight and height may be more accurate, usually within 10–15% of direct measures.[3] However, these formulas do not take into consideration extremes in muscle or fat mass. Thus, for the athlete who has larger muscle mass and less fat mass than a normal individual, the best means for obtaining REE appears to be some method of direct measurement.

C. Factors Affecting Resting Energy Expenditure

It is important to note that not all calories ingested are usable. The processes of digestion and absorption, as well as assimilation of substrate in the liver (proteins, glycogen) after feeding requires energy. This process is about 65–95% efficient, depending upon the type of food.[8] Therefore, 5–30% of the calories are given off in the form of heat.[5,30] These heat calories are referred to as *dietary-induced thermogenesis* or *specific dynamic action* (SDA). The dietary-induced thermogenesis varies by substrate. Carbohydrates increase REE about 4–5%, while fats increase REE by only about 2%. Conversely, protein increases REE by 20–30% and ethanol about 22%.[2,5] A typical mixed

TABLE 9.1

The World Health Organization Equations for Estimating Daily Resting Energy Expenditure Based on Age, Gender and Weight[29]

Age Range	Equation Males	Equation Females
0-3	$(60.9 \times wt) - 54$	$(61.0 \times wt) - 51$
3-10	$(22.7 \times wt) + 495$	$(22.5 \times wt) + 499$
10-18	$(17.5 \times wt) + 651$	$(12.2 \times wt) + 746$
18-30	$(15.3 \times wt) + 679$	$(14.7 \times wt) + 496$
30-60	$(11.6 \times wt) + 879$	$(8.7 \times wt) + 829$
>60	$(13.5 \times wt) + 487$	$(10.5 \times wt) + 596$

Resting energy expenditure (REE) = kcal/day
wt = weight in kilograms

TABLE 9.2

Examples of Computations Comparing Methods of Estimating Energy Needs

Male: 20 years old Height = 5'10" (1.78 m) Weight = 154 pounds (70 kg)	Female: 20 years old Height = 5'5" (1.65 m) Weight = 132 pounds (60 kg)
1. REE = $10 \times wt_{lbs}$ $10 \times 154 = $ **1540 kcal/d**	REE = $10 \times wt_{lbs}$ $10 \times 132 = $ **1320 kcal/d**
2. REE = 1.0 kcal/kg/h $1 \times 70 \times 24 = $ **1680 kcal/d**	REE = 0.9 kcal/kg/h $0.9 \times 60 \times 24 = $ **1296 kcal/d**
3. WHO equations based on age and gender $(15.3 \times wt) + 679$ $15.3 \times 70 + 679 = $ **1750 kcal/d**	 $(14.7 \times wt) + 496$ $14.7 \times 60 + 496 = $ **1378 kcal/d**
4. Equations based on gender, weight (wt = kg), height (ht = cm), and age (a = yr). $66.5 + (13.8 \times wt) + (5 \times ht) - (6.8 \times a)$ $66.5 + (13.8 \times 70) + (5 \times 179) - (6.8 \times 20)$ $66.5 + 966 + 895 - 136 = $ **1791.5 kcal/d**	 $655 + (9.6 \times wt) + (1.7 \times ht) - (4.7 \times a)$ $655 + (9.6 \times 60) + (1.7 \times 165) - (4.7 \times 20)$ $655 + 576 + 281 - 94 = $ **1488 kcal/d**

Comparison of the results of the four methods:

Method	Male Example	Female Example
1	1540 kcal/d	1320 kcal/d
2	1680 kcal/d	1296 kcal/d
3	1750 kcal/d	1378 kcal/d
4	1792 kcal/d	1488 kcal/d

meal would increase REE by about 5–10%. Dietary-induced thermogenesis usually peaks about an hour after eating and, if the meal is high in protein, the thermogenesis can last for a considerable amount of time (3–5 hours). The thermogenesis seems to be more dependent upon the feeding pattern than the total caloric intake, as feeding four meals produces a larger increase in thermogenesis than feeding one meal of the same caloric content.[30] However, gorging significantly elevates the thermogenesis[31,32] but the effect may not be as significant for obese individuals.[33]

Research has indicated that individuals who are overweight may have a blunted thermic effect on food. This is thought to be in some way related to their body fat.[34] However, the blunted effect appears to be relative to body weight (Kcal/kg or kJ/kg), as many overweight individuals actually have a greater muscle mass, which can increase the overall thermic effect (absolute Kcal or kJ). Endurance training may also lower the dietary-induced thermogenesis compared with untrained subjects.[35,36,37] The reduced thermogenesis could help conserve energy during periods of intense physical training. Other factors that may influence dietary-induced thermogenesis include genetics, caffeine, nicotine and diseases such as diabetes mellitus that affect insulin.[5]

The resting EE is directly influenced by the amount of metabolically active tissue, or lean body mass.[5] The National Research Council[29] reports that lean body mass accounts for about 80% of the variance in measuring REE. Failure to account for lean body mass can result in erroneous results. For example, publications have reported that the 24-hour EE of highly active subjects was greater than sedentary controls.[38,39] However, when the expenditure reported was based on lean body mass, the groups were found to be similar.

Although the lean body mass has a major influence on REE, the size of the individual will modify that relationship. Size is concerned with the height for a given weight.[29] Nutritionists define size using body mass index, a weight:height ratio ($wt_{kg}:ht_m^2$), whereas physiologists use the body surface area to mass ratio (AD/wt). Regardless of the units, the taller, thinner person will have a higher REE than the shorter heavier person of the same weight. This difference is related to the fact that the taller thinner person has more surface area through which heat is lost. Thus, the tall, lean person must produce more heat to maintain thermo-balance.

Age is also a significant factor affecting REE (Figure 9.1). The total resting EE of children is less than adults, generally < 75 kcal/h (314 kJ/h) vs. > 90 kcal/h 377 kJ/h).[29] However, expressed per unit of body weight, the expenditure of children is more than double that of an adult: 100 kcal/kg (418 kJ/h) vs. 30–37 kcal/kg (126–155 kJ/h).[29] The greater REE is related to growth and activity patterns. With regard to growth, the EE is quite small during the first year of life (approximately 1%). However, after that age, growth accounts for about 5 kcal/g of tissue gained.[40] In general, REE declines about 2% per year after growth has stopped.[41] Interestingly, lean body mass declines at a rate of about 2–3% per decade.[29] Thus, if the decline in lean body mass could be avoided, the age-related reduction in REE probably would not occur.[42] However, this age-related decline is actually quite small, amounting to only about 100–150 calories in 50 years.

Another factor proposed to be associated with REE is gender.[29,41] Figure 9.1 illustrates that there is little difference in the REE of boys and girls until about the age of 10 years. At approximately this time, pubescence starts and

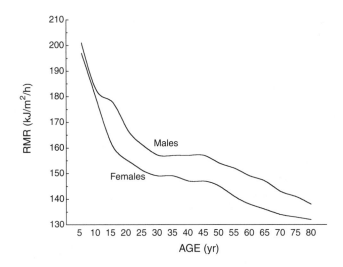

FIGURE 9.1

The relationship of age and gender to basal metabolic rate.[41] The data is corrected for body surface area.

the body composition of the genders begins to differentiate. The boys continue to gain in muscle mass, while the girls develop a greater proportion of body fat. This difference amounts to about a 10% greater REE in adult males. Thus, in general, women expend about 0.9 kcal/kg body weight/h. In contrast, men expend about 1 kcal/kg/h. This difference may not be a true gender difference but related to the greater body fat of females, or, conversely, to the greater muscle mass of males. This is verified by the fact that when metabolic rate is expressed per unit of fat-free mass (lean body weight), the comparative resting metabolic rates between men and women are very similar.[43]

Climate can be a factor that modifies REE. Both extremes in temperature can increase the REE. During acute cold exposure, REE can increase more than double.[44] This increase is a direct result of shivering in an attempt to maintain core temperature. Likewise, exposure to heat can elevate REE. This may be related to the increased sweat gland activity and circulatory demands from the heat. Chronic exposure to heat, as in living in the tropics, can result in a 5–20% increase in REE.[8] The increase is probably related to the adjustments in thermoregulation mentioned above or also possibly to the Q_{10} effect,[2] a general effect in which an elevation of temperature increases the rate of chemical reactions, including metabolism. Although REE may be increased during prolonged exposure to heat, the hot environment may reduce activity and, therefore, reduce overall caloric need.

Climatic effects on REE are relatively minor because most of the exposures to these extremes are limited in nature. Most humans residing in cooler climates live in heated, insulated houses or apartments, which reduces prolonged cold exposure. Further, the use of high-technology clothing and textiles reduces the direct effects of the cold during acute exposures. The same dwelling that provided insulation from the cold can be equipped with air conditioning that reduces prolonged exposure to high temperatures. Thus, climatic influences may be minimal in westernized cultures, but are of importance for many less developed societies.

The pattern of food intake not only affects the dietary-induced thermogenesis, but also can directly affect metabolic rate. Two weeks of overfeeding by 3000 kcal/d has been shown to increase REE, while 2 weeks of starvation (500 kcal/d) caused a reduction REE.[45] Conversely, dieting or underfeeding will lower REE and dietary thermogenesis.[5]

The hormones of thyroxin, epinephrine and insulin increase REE.[2,5,8] Thyroxin does so by increasing cell mitochondrial activity. Epinephrine increases metabolic rate via direct effects on glycolysis, as well as increasing muscle, respiratory and circulatory metabolic demands. Insulin, although primarily responsible for increasing the storage of glucose as glycogen, also increases the cellular metabolism of glucose, especially after consuming a meal.

Finally, exercise training appears to have an effect on REE (Figure 9.2). The effect of training on REE is controversial. Some studies have suggested that highly trained athletes have a greater REE per unit lean body mass than sedentary controls,[35,3841,46,47] while others disagree.[30,37,38,49,50] The disagreement may be related to differing methodologies that have not controlled for a carry-over effect of the previous exercise, which can persist up to 12–13 hours after prolonged strenuous exercise (3–5 h), the thermic effect of subsequent food intake, or the use of small sample sizes or cross-sectional samples.[5,35,37,38,44,47] Cross-sectional evidence also suggests that highly active males, world class endurance athletes, have a higher REE per unit lean body mass than moderately trained individuals.[48] At the other end of the spectrum, a 10-week exercise program in lean, initially sedentary females resulted in an elevation in REE.[51] Also, Trembley et al.[47] have shown that, in obese individuals, an 11-week training program increases the REE per unit of fat-free mass by approximately 8%. Thus, there is accumulating longitudinal data to support an increased REE with aerobic training. Also, the trained individuals usually have more lean body mass at a given weight, thus increasing absolute REE.[5]

IV. Energy for Work and Sport

The EE of daily life is greater than the REE and is dependent upon lifestyle and occupation. A typical sedentary adult (e.g., a receptionist) will need 140% of REE. A teacher will need 160% of REE, a nurse about 170% of REE, while a physical laborer (bricklayer) will need up to twice the REE.[3,29] This does not include the amount of exercise needed for an exercise program. Thus, EE during exercise needs to be superimposed on this daily need. For an adult who exercises about 30–45 minutes a day, the additional energy

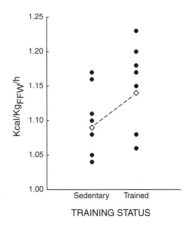

FIGURE 9.2

The effect of exercise training on the basal metabolic rate. The data presented with respect to lean body mass is a compilation of a number of studies.[35,37,47,48, 49,50] The open diamond ($\lozenge$) represents the mean response for all studies in that group.

demand will amount to only about 10–14% of the total caloric expenditure. However, for the athlete that exercises 3-5 hours a day the energy demand of the exercise alone can be greater than the total allowance for REE plus lifestyle needs. Table 9.3 summarizes the estimated additional energy needs of individuals training for specific sports.[52] These estimated energy needs should not be taken as absolutes, only as examples of additional caloric needs. Note that some sports, like recreational basketball, may require only slightly more than normal amounts of energy, while others, like the Tour de France cycle race, can require an enormous amount of additional energy. The actual energy demand of the exercise is based on the intensity and duration of the exercise. The type of activity and weight of the individual must also be taken into consideration (Table 9.4). The energy demands of activities that are weight bearing will be directly related to the weight whereas activities that are nonweight bearing, like bicycling, require fewer increments of energy as the individual's weight increases.[53] Thus, an obese person who wants to increase energy use is better off walking than riding a bicycle. In addition, the obese person actually utilizes more energy to walk at a given speed than a nonobese person. Conversely, the obese person riding a bicycle at the same speed uses just slightly more energy than a lean person.

A. Measurement of EE During Activity

EE during activity is usually measured by open-circuit spirometry. As previously mentioned, a computerized system appears to work best. Some of these systems are stationary and will work only with activities in which the participant strays little from the measurement device. Such systems have

TABLE 9.3

Estimates of the Energy Needs of Various Sports[52]

Sport	Additional Caloric Needs	Average Daily Caloric Intake
Basketball	300	2200
Dancers	1000	1500
Gymnasts	1400	1400
Football	2100	4000–5300
Runners (men)	1000	4400
Runners (women)	500	2397
Swimmers	500	2900
Tour de France	4000	6700
Triathletes	15-2000	4095
Wrestlers	200-1000	Varies with weight
Weightlifters	28-4600	3200-4700

TABLE 9.4

A Comparison of the Caloric Demands of Weight-Bearing (Running) and Nonweight-Bearing (Bicycling) Activities[8]

Body Weight	Running ~ 6 mph (9.6 km/h) kcal/min	~ Bicycling ~ 9 mph (14.5 km/h) kcal/min
110 lbs (50 Kg)	9.7	5.0
130 lbs (59 Kg)	11.4	5.9
150 lbs (68 Kg)	13.1	6.8
170 lbs (77 Kg)	14.9	7.7
190 lbs (86 Kg)	16.6	8.6

been used to measure energy cost of walking and running on treadmills, cycling on cycle ergometers, swimming using a swimming ergometer, rowing using a rowing ergometer, stair stepping using an escalator-type or step ergometer, or arm cranking using an arm ergometer. The treadmill allows the subject to walk or run at a specific pace while maintaining a central location. Thus, the subject is easily attached to the spirometry system. Although the treadmill simulates ambulation, it is not quite the same as normal walking or running. Studies have shown that there are differences in air resistance between treadmill and normal ambulation that may decrease the energy cost of ambulation on treadmill.[54,55] The same is true for cycle ergometers, they eliminate air resistance; however, the ergometer also eliminates the friction of the tires on the riding surface. With swimming and rowing ergometers, the problem is that they eliminate water resistance (drag forces, frontal resistance, and skin or surface friction).[56] Water resistance is considerable; therefore, the use of these ergometers may underestimate the true EE with these activities.

The bag technique of open-circuit spirometry has been used to measure O_2 uptake during ergometry work, as well as during actual cycling, swimming, rope skipping or household chores. Because the expired air bag is connected to the subject by a breathing tube, this technique requires that the researcher move with the subject, yet not impede any subject movements. In addition, the subject usually has to wear a mouthpiece and support the breathing tube during the collection period. The weight of the breathing tubing, breathing valve, and mouthpiece can be uncomfortable for the subject or cause additional effort to be expended to support the apparatus and maintain the mouthpiece in the mouth. Finally, the bags are typically not totally impermeable to gas exchange. Therefore, if a bag is used for a prolonged period of time (longer than 10–15 minutes), gases may diffuse and the results can be unreliable. Therefore, bag measurements are usually taken over periods of time lasting less than 10 minutes and the contents measured as quickly as possible at the end of the collection period. The bag method can be used successfully, but takes preparation, training, and good timing to obtain accurate data.[6,8]

The use of miniaturized portable systems has revolutionized our ability to obtain EE data during activities. The new systems are sufficiently small to be worn during activity, providing little impairment of motion and little additional weight. The systems have been used to measure EE of household chores, basketball, tennis, road cycling, and kayaking, among other activities. Some of these systems include a fairly good-sized memory or telemetry, which allows the investigator to obtain real-time data without being tethered to the subject.

Although these systems have proven to be accurate, there are some minor problems. The additional weight of the apparatus, usually about 1 kg, can increase the energy cost of the activities. The impact of the additional weight on an adult is negligible, because the system's weight may represent only < 2% of the body weight; however, for a child, the weight of the system can have a significant impact on the energy cost of the activity. It is also important that the systems be securely attached to the subject. If not, the system can impede motion, which will modify the energy cost. Most of these systems require that the subject wear a mask to measure expired gases, rather than the cumbersome breathing valve and mouthpiece. An improperly fitting mask can result in air leaks that can modify both the measured volume of air and the fractions of expired gases. Experience has also shown that the systems may lose their ability to function via telemetry if they are near an electric field such as a video display. Proper consideration and planning can eliminate these problems and allow the investigator to obtain accurate data.

V.   Estimating Daily Energy Expenditure

The total daily EE can be estimated by summing the REE, the daily activity factor, and the exercise program. For example, a 20-year-old woman who weighs 132 pounds (60 kg), works as a receptionist and takes a 45-minute aerobics class 5 days a week would have an REE of 1296 kcal/24 h (60 kg ×

0.9 kcal/kg/h × 24 h). Her daily activity would be an additional 390 kcal (REE × 30%). The aerobic program would expend about 275 kcals (6.1 kcal/ min × 45 min). Thus, on the days she exercises, her total EE amounts to 1961 kcal (1296 + 390 + 275), while her nonexercising days expend 1686 kcal (1296 + 390).

VI. Summary

The measurement of EE is a complex process that can be completed by several methods. Early studies employed direct calorimetry in which people were placed in a closed chamber and their heat production was directly measured. This method was based on the fact that the catabolism of substrate to produce energy directly results in the production of heat. Because direct calorimetry confines the movement of the subject, attempts have been made to develop portable systems. However, these systems are expensive and cumbersome, and still do not allow people to proceed with the activities of life. These limitations have led to the development of indirect calorimetry methods. These methods are based on the fact that the production of heat requires the use of O_2 and the production of CO_2. Therefore, measuring the O_2 uptake and CO_2 production will allow the investigator to compute the energy use. Indirect calorimetry has evolved to the point where systems are sufficiently small that subjects can exercise unimpeded, and metabolic measurements can occur. However, indirect calorimetry has a limited capacity to obtain data and has therefore been used mostly for measurements during short periods of time (e.g. minutes, hours). These indirect methods are not appropriate to obtain a measure of EE over a period of days. To overcome this limitation, a double-isotope method using $^2H_2^{18}O$ has been developed. This method is most applicable when measuring overall (total) EE over days; however, it will not work to measure the specific energy cost a given activity. Thus, it appears that indirect calorimetry is best for measuring specific activities, while the doubly labeled water is best to estimate overall daily energy use.

The resting EE (REE) can be defined as the minimal amount of energy necessary to sustain the human organism in a conscious resting state. The REE makes up about two thirds of daily EE. In general, the REE is dependent upon the amount of metabolically active tissue — lean body mass. However, other factors such as age, gender, size, climate, caloric intake, hormones, and exercise training will modify the REE. The amount of heat formed is dependent upon the substrate being digested, with protein producing more thermogenesis than either fats or carbohydrates. This dietary-induced thermogenesis is affected by the pattern of eating, the physical condition of the individual, and obesity.

Resting EE can be measured by a variety of means ranging from room calorimeters to simply measuring O_2 uptake (VO_2), which, using a mask, hood, or even a whole room, is the simplest means for obtaining an estimate of the EE. On the other hand, the measurement of EE during activity can be either quite simple or very complex depending upon the movements of the activity. At present, the best methods are through the use of portable, indirect calorimetry units. However, the measurement of EE from O_2 uptake requires that the activity can be completed in an aerobic state using fairly low- to moderate-intensity activities. Currently, we have a limited capability to measure energy cost of very high-intensity exercise, which results in the production of considerable lactic acid.

Ultimately, to compute the individual daily EE, three factors must be summed: 1) the REE for the 24-hr period, 2) the EE based on lifestyle (work or school), and 3) the EE from any exercise program.

References

1. Young, D.S., Implementation of SI units for clinical laboratory data. *Ann. Intern. Med.*, 106, 114, 1987.
2. Bell, G.H., Emslie-Smith, D., and Paterson, C.R., *Textbook of Physiology and Biochemistry*, Churchill Livingstone, New York, 1976, pp. 57-64.
3. Whitney, E.N. and Boyle, M.A., *Understanding Nutrition*, West Publishing Company, St. Paul, 1987, pp. 242-246.
4. Schutz, Y., The basis of direct and indirect calorimetry and their potentials. *Diabetes/Metabol. Rev.*, 11, 383, 1995.
5. Schutz, Y. and Jéquier, E., Resting energy expenditure, thermic effect of food, and total energy expenditure. In *Handbook of Obesity*, Bray, O.J., Bouchard, C., and James, W.P.T. Eds., Marcel Dekker, New York, 1998, pp.433-455.
6. Consolazio, C.F., Johnson, R.E., and Pecora, L.J., *Physiological Measurements of Metabolic Functions in Man*, McGraw-Hill, New York, 1963, pp.1-98.
7. Krogh, A. and Lindhard, J., The relative value of fat and carbohydrate as sources of muscular energy. *Biochem. J.*, 14, 290, 1920.
8. McArdle, W.D., Katch, F.I., and Katch, V.L., *Exercise Physiology: Energy, Nutrition and Human Performance*, Williams and Wilkins, Baltimore, 1996, pp.139-213.
9. Mellerowicz, H. and Smodlaka, V.N., *Ergometry: Basics of Medical Exercise Testing*, Urban and Schwarzenberg: Munich, 1981, pp.1-23.
10. Zuntz, N. and Schumburg, N.A.E.F., *Studien zu einer physiologie des macsches*. A. Hirschwald, Berlin, 1901.
11. Carpenter, T.M., *Tables, Factors and Formulas for Computing Respiratory Exchange and Biological Transformations of Energy*. Carnegie Institution of Washington, Washington, D.C., 1964, p.104.
12. Dill, D.B., The economy of muscular exercise. *Physiol. Rev.*, 16, 263, 1936.
13. Bassett, D.R. et al., Validity of four motion sensors in measuring moderate intensity physical activity. *Med. Sci. Sports Exerc.*, 32, S471, 2000.
14. Klein, P.D., James, W.P.T., Wong, W.W., Irving, C.S., Murgatroyd, P.R., Cabrera, M., Dallosso, H.M., Klein, E.R., and Nichols, B.L., Calorimetric validation of the doubly labeled water method for determination of energy expenditure in man. *Human Nutr. Clin. Nutr.*, 38C, 95, 1984.
15. Schoeller, D.A., Energy expenditure from doubly labeled water: some fundamental considerations in humans. *Am. J. Clin. Nutr.*, 38, 999, 1983.

16. Schoeller, D.A. and Webb, P., Five-day comparison of doubly labeled water method with respiratory gas exchange. *Am. J. Clin. Nutr.*, 40, 153, 1984.
17. Schoeller, D.A., Measurement of energy expenditure in free-living humans by using doubly labeled water. *J. Nutr.*, 118, 1278, 1988.
18. Roberts, S.B., Dietz, W., Sharp, T., Dallal, G.E., and Hill, J.O., Multiple laboratory comparison of the doubly labeled water technique. *Obes. Res.* 3(Suppl 1), 3, 1995.
19. Speakman, J.R., Estimation of the precision in DLW studies using the two-point methodology. *Obes. Res.* 3(Suppl 1), 31, 1995.
20. Wareham, N.J., Hennings, S.J., Prentice, A.M. and Day, N.E., Feasibility of heart-rate monitoring to estimate total level and pattern of energy expenditure in a population-based epidemiological study: the Ely Young Cohort Feasibility Study 1994-5. *Br. J. Nutr.*, 78, 889, 1997.
21. Major P., Subtle physical activity poses a challenge to the study of heart rate. *Physiol. Behav.*, 63, 381, 1997.
22. Ott, A. E., Pate, R.R., Trost, S.G., Ward, D.S. and Saunders, R. The use of uniaxial and triaxial accelerometers to measure children's free play physical activity. *Pediatr. Exerc. Sci.*, 12, 360, 2000.
23. Bassett, D.R., Ainsworth, B.E., Leggett, S.R., Mathien, C.A., Main, J.A., Hunter, D.C. and Duncan, G.E., Accuracy of five electronic pedometers for measuring distance walked. *Med. Sci. Sports Exerc.*, 28, 1071, 1996.
24. Nichols, J.F., Morgan, C.G., Sarkin, J.A., Sallis, J.F. and Calfas, K.J., Validity, reliability, and calibration of the Tritrac accelerometer as a measure of physical activity. *Med. Sci. Sports Exerc.*, 31, 908, 1999.
25. Jakicic, J.M., Winter, C., Lagally, K., Ho, J., Robertson, R.J. and Wing, R.R., The accuracy of the TriTrac-R3D accelerometer to estimate energy expenditure. *Med. Sci. Sports Exerc.*, 31, 747, 1999.
26. Matthews, C.E. and Freedson, P.S., Field trial of a three-dimensional activity monitor: comparison with self report. *Med. Sci. Sports Exerc.*, 27, 1071, 1995.
27. McMurray, R.G. et al., Effects of gender, age and developmental stage on energy expenditure: the EEPAY Study, presented at the 21st Symposium of the European Group of Pediatric Work Physiology, Corsendonk Priory, Belgium, September 12-16, 2001.
28. *Burszstein, S., Elwyn, D.H., Askanazi, J. and Kinney, J.M., Energy Metabolism, Indirect Calorimetry, and Nutrition.* Williams and Wilkins, Baltimore, 1989.
29. National Research Council. *Recommended Dietary Allowances.* (10th ed.), National Academy Press, Washington D.C., 1989.
30. LeBlanc, J. and Mercier, I., Components of postprandial thermogenesis in relation to meal frequency in humans. *Can. J. Physiol. Pharm.*, 71, 879, 1993.
31. Miller, D.S., Gluttony 2: Thermogenesis in overeating man. *Am. J. Clin. Nutr.*, 20, 1233, 1967.
32. Verboeket-Van de Venne, W.P.H.G., Westertrep, K.R., and Kester, A.D.M., Effect of the pattern of food intake on human energy metabolism. *Br. J. Nutr.*, 70, 103, 1993.
33. Zahorska-Markiewicz, B., Thermic effects of food and exercise in obesity. *Eur. J. Appl. Physiol.*, 44, 231, 1980.
34. Shetty, P.S., Postprandial thermogenesis in obesity. *Clin. Sci.*, 60, 519, 1980.
35. Poehlman, E.T., Melby, C.L. and Badylek, S.F., Resting metabolic rate and postprandial thermogenesis in highly trained and untrained males. *Am. J. Clin. Nutr.*, 47, 793, 1988.
36. Thorbek, G., Chwalibog, A., Jakobsen, K. and Henckel, S., Heat production and quantitative oxidation of nutrients by physically active humans. *Ann. Nutr. Metabol.*, 38, 8, 1994.

37. Davis, J.R., Tagiaferro, A.R., Kertzer R., Gerardo, T., Nichols, J. and Wheeler, J., Variation in dietary-induced thermogenesis and body fatness with aerobic capacity. *Eur. J. Appl. Physiol.* 50, 319, 1983.

38. Horton, T.J. and Geissler, C.A., Effects of habitual exercise on daily energy expenditure and metabolic rate during standardized activity. *Am. J. Clin. Nutr.*, 59,13, 1994.

39. Toth, M.J. and Poehlman, E.T., Effect of exercise on daily energy expenditure. *Nutr. Rev.* 54, S140, 1996.

40. Roberts, S.B. and Young, V.R., Energy cost of fat and protein deposition in the human infant. *Am. J. Clin. Nutr.*, 48, 951, 1988.

41. Altman, P.L. and Dittmer, D.S., Metabolism. *Fed. Am. Soc. Exper. Biol.*, Bethesda, 1968.

42. Poehlman, E.T., Berke, E.M., Joseph, J.R., Gardner, A.W., Katzman-Rooks, S.M. and Goran, M.I., Influence of aerobic capacity, body composition and thyroid hormones on the age-related decline in resting metabolic rate. *Metabolism*, 41, 915, 1992.

43. Keys, A., Taylor, H.L., and Grande, F., Basal metabolism and age of adult men. *Metabolism*, 22, 579, 1973.

44. Jacobs, I., Martineau, L. and Vallerand, A.L., Thermoregulatory thermogenesis in humans during cold exposure, in *Exercise and Sport Science Reviews,* Holloszy, J.O. Ed., 22, 221, 1994.

45. Lammert, O. and Hansen, E.S., Effects of excessive caloric intake and caloric restriction on body weight and energy expenditure at rest and light exercise. *Acta Physiol. Scand.*, 114, 135, 1982.

46. Horton, E.S., Metabolic aspects of exercise and weight reduction. *Med. Sci. Sports Exerc.*, 18, 10, 1986.

47. Tremblay, A.E., Fontaine, E., Poehlman, E.T., Mitchell, D., Perron, L. and Bouchard, C., The effect of exercise training on resting metabolic rate in lean and moderately obese individuals. *Int. J. Obes.* 10, 511, 1986.

48. Poehlman, E.T., Melby, C.L., Badylak, S.F. and Calles, J., Aerobic fitness and resting energy expenditure in young adult males. *Metabol.* 38, 85, 1989.

49. Wilmore, J.H., Stanforth, P.R., Hudspeth, L.A., Gagnon, J., Warwick Daw, E., Leon, A.C., Rao, D.C., Skinner, J.S. and Bouchard, C., Alterations in resting metabolic rate as a consequence of 20 weeks of endurance training: the Heritage Family Study. *Am. J. Clin. Nutr.* 68, 66, 1998.

50. Dolezal, B.A. and Potteiger, J.A., Concurrent resistance and endurance training influence basal metabolic rate in nondieting individuals. *J. Appl. Physiol.* 85, 695, 1998.

51. Lawson, S., Webster, J.D., Pacy, P.J. and Garrow, J.S.,Effect of a 10-week aerobic exercise program on metabolic rate, body composition and fitness in lean sedentary females. *Brit. J. Clin. Pract.* 41, 684, 1987.

52. Short, S.H. and Short W.R., Four-year study of university athletes' dietary intake. *J. Am. Diet. Assoc.*, 82, 632, 1983.

53. Swain, D.P., The influence of body mass in endurance bicycling. *Med. Sci. Sports Exerc.*, 26, 58, 1994.

54. Herk, H., Mader, A., Hess, G., Mucke, S., Muller, R. and Hollmann, W., Justification of the 4-mmol/l lactate threshold. *Int. J. Sports Med.*, 6, 117, 1985.

55. McMurray, R.G., Berry, M.J., Vann, R.T., Hardy, C.J. and Sheps, D.S., The effect of running in an outdoor environment on plasma beta endorphin. *Ann. Sports. Med.*, 3, 230, 1988.

56. Councilman, J.E. *The Science of Swimming*, Prentice Hall, Englewood Cliffs, 1968, pp. 1-5.

10

Field Assessment of Physical Activity and Energy Expenditure among Athletes

Michael J. LaMonte and Barbara E. Ainsworth

CONTENTS

I.   Introduction

Regular, moderate to high-intensity physical activity confers substantial health-related[1] and performance-related[2] benefits. The specific activity-related physiologic adaptations and the degree to which these adaptations occur is dependent on the interaction of the frequency, duration and intensity of the activity being performed.[3] This interaction is often quantified as *"energy expenditure"* (EE). It should be noted that total daily EE is the sum of energy expended at rest (resting metabolic rate), while eating and digesting a meal (thermic effect of food), during and after bouts of physical activity (activity-related EE).[4] However, although resting metabolic rate may account for the largest percentage of total daily EE (~55–70%), differences in physical activity-related EE represent the largest source of variability in the energy requirements of a given individual as well as among groups of individuals.[4] A recent position statement on nutrition and athletic performance emphasized the relation between energy intake and activity-related EE to enhance athletic performance, maintain total and lean body mass, govern metabolic and endocrine factors associated with the regulation of energy stores and to enhance recovery between exercise bouts.[5]

To appropriately match athletes' energy intake with their EE, valid measures are needed to precisely quantify and track physical activity and exercise patterns and their associated energy costs. Because physical activity is a complex multidimensional behavior, precise measurement remains a challenge for researchers and practitioners, especially among free-living individuals.[6,7] Feasibility considerations both in terms of expense and administrative burden result in the need for low-cost reliable indirect methods of assessing activity-related EE as part of a holistic approach to meeting the energy requirements of athletes. The objective of this chapter is to review current methods used to quantify free-living physical activity-related EE. First, important terminology will be introduced as an entree to the presentation of a conceptual framework that will guide the discussion on measuring physical activity and EE. Following will be a discussion of measurement techniques with an emphasis on field methods that can be used to assess activity-related EE among athletic populations.

II.   Definitions

Before a specified construct (e.g., cardiorespiratory fitness) can be operationalized into a measurable variable (e.g., maximal oxygen consumption, VO_{2max}, measured in units of mL $\cdot$ O_2 $\cdot$ kg^{-1} $\cdot$ min^{-1}) for research or exercise training purposes, precise conceptual definitions must be established for the construct of interest.[8] Conceptually different terms pertaining to the measurement of physical activity and EE have often been used interchangeably by researchers and practitioners. This has resulted in confusion, inconsistent study designs, limitations to interstudy comparisons and a lack of standardized measurement practices.[3,9,10] Attempts to standardize terminology have been made.[10,11] These efforts were aimed at developing a universal framework from which definitions can be drawn to aid in operationalizing constructs into measurable study variables and within which more precise data interpretations and comparisons can be made among studies that relate physical activity to health or performance variables. Table 10.1 presents several definitions of terms related to the measurement of physical activity and EE.

It is important to recognize that physical activity and EE are not synonymous terms. Physical activity is a behavioral process characterizing body movement that results from skeletal muscle contraction, of which a product is EE.[7] Several types or categories of physical activity exist (Figure 10.1) and likely overlap to some extent, depending on an individual's purpose for performing the activity. For example, a brisk walk to and from the store may be a form of transportation for one individual, whereas the same brisk walk may be part of a planned exercise program aimed at managing blood pressure for another. Exercise training and competitive sport compose a subcategory of physical activity that is systematically structured for the primary objective of enhancing one or more dimension of physical fitness or sport-specific skills to optimize an individual's sport-related performance. Because the subcategories of physical activity overlap, they are very difficult to measure as independent categories.[9] Additional categorization of physical activities can be based on the intensity or rate of EE attributed to a specific activity.[12-15] Activities can be self-rated as *light, moderate,* or *vigorous* intensity,[16] or activities can be described according to objective published intensity categories.[12-15] Hence, physical activity may be classified by purpose, such as sports, occupation and home care, or by intensity, as in light, moderate and vigorous. Seasonal and day-to-day intra-individual variation in physical activity patterns[17-19] and discordance between self-rated and actual activity intensity[16,20] have been shown to affect the precision of measuring activity and EE. Further, because the subcategories of physical activity have different meanings according to sex, race-ethnicity and cultural perspectives,[21,22] self-report activity instruments must reflect the specific demographics and lifestyle of the targeted population. Accordingly, these issues should be considered when choosing a method of assessing physical activity and its related EE. It is critical to consider all sources of daily habitual physical activity to precisely quantify activity-related EE to accurately meet an individual's energy requirements.

Physical activity is typically quantified in terms of its frequency (number of bouts) and its duration (e.g., minutes per bout). The resulting EE is a direct function of all metabolic processes involved with the exchange of energy required to support the skeletal muscle contraction associated with a given physical activity. Energy expenditure reflects the intensity or metabolic cost of a given physical activity and is a product of the frequency, duration and

TABLE 10.1

Definitions of Terms Related to the Measurement of Energy Expenditure and
Physical Activity

Energy	The capacity to do work.
Energy Expenditure	The exchange of energy required to perform biological work.
Physical Activity	Bodily movement that is produced by the contraction of skeletal muscle and that substantially increases energy expenditure.
Physical Fitness	A set of attributes (e.g., muscle strength and endurance, cardiorespiratory fitness, flexibility, etc.) that people have to achieve that relate to the ability to perform physical activity.
Exercise	Planned, structured, and repetitive bodily movement done to improve or maintain one or more components of physical fitness. Exercise is a specific sub-category of physical activity.
Calorimetry	Methods used to calculate the rate and quantity of energy expenditure when the body is at rest and during physical activity.
Calorie	A unit of energy that reflects the amount of heat required to raise the temperature of 1 gram of water by $1°C$.
Kilocalories (kcal)	1,000 calories, 4.184 kilojoules.
Kilojoules (kJ)	The unit of energy in the International System of Units. 1,000 Joules, 0.238 kcal.
Metabolic Equivalent (MET)	A unit used to estimate the metabolic cost (oxygen consumption) of physical activity. One MET equals the resting metabolic rate of approximately 3.5 ml $O_2 \cdot kg^{-1} \cdot min^{-1}$, or, 1 $kcal \cdot kg^{-1} \cdot hr^{-1}$.
Duration	The dimension of physical activity referring to the amount of time an activity is performed.
Frequency	The dimension of physical activity referring to how often an activity is performed.
Intensity	The dimension of physical activity referring to the rate of energy expenditure while the activity is performed.
Hours/Minutes	Typical units of time used in quantifying the rate of energy expenditure or the period of physical activity measurement (e.g., kcal per minute or $kcal \cdot min^{-1}$).
MET-minutes	The rate of energy expenditure expressed as METS per minute, which is calculated by multiplying the minutes a specific activity is performed by the corresponding energy cost of the activity.
MET-hours	The rate of energy expenditure expressed as METS per hour, which is calculated by multiplying the hours a specific activity is performed by the corresponding energy cost of the activity.
Unitless Indices	A unitless number that is computed as an ordinal measure of physical activity or energy expenditure.
Dose-Response	A relationship where increasing levels or "doses" of physical activity result in corresponding changes in the expected levels of the defined health parameter.

Sources: Brooks, Fahey, and White, 1996, pp.15-25 [28]; Caspersen, Powell, and Christenson, 1985 [30]; Corbin, PangraZi & Franks, 2000 [33]; Montoye, Kemper, Saris, and Washburn, 1996, pp. 3-14 [68].

energy cost of the specific activity. For example, if a 55 kg female runner completes a 45-minute tempo run at a 6-min/mile pace (4 min/km), her EE would be about 660 kcal based on the following computation: frequency (1) × duration (45 min) × the energy cost of running a 6-min/mile pace (~ 0.267 $kcal \cdot kg^{-1} \cdot min^{-1}$). [23] The previous calculation determined the *gross* EE for

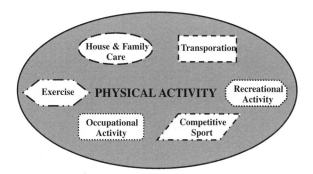

FIGURE10.1
Physical activity and its related subcategories.

running 45 minutes at a 6-min/mile pace (4 min/km). This value, however, reflects both the activity-related and resting EE.[24] To account for only the energy expended during the running activity, one must compute the *net* EE. To do so, the amount of energy assumed to be expended to sustain resting metabolic functions within the specified activity duration must be subtracted from the gross EE. A 55 kg individual has a resting EE of about 55 kcal $\cdot$ hr^{-1} or 0.92 kcal $\cdot$ min^{-1}. Therefore, the amount of energy expended within the 45-min running bout attributed to resting metabolism would be about 41.2 kcal (0.92 $\times$ 45). After subtracting this value from the previously computed gross EE of 660 kcal, a net EE of about 619 kcal would be attributed to the 45 minutes of running activity. Net EE should be used when comparing the energy cost of one activity to another and when comparing activity-related EEs between individuals.[24]

Another important consideration pertaining to quantifying activity-related EE is the use of absolute vs. relative scales to index the energy cost of specific activities. Although several factors may influence EE on a relative scale (e.g., age, body size, fitness level), if one assumes a fairly constant human mechanical efficiency to perform physical work (~23%),[25] then absolute EE is generally constant for a given activity. Therefore, it is possible to standardize methods of assigning energy costs to specific activities for the purpose of assessing activity-related EE among large populations of free-living individuals. Factors such as age, sex and fitness level will undoubtedly influence the precision by which a standardized activity-specific absolute energy cost reflects a given individual's relative intensity level (e.g., percentage of actual maximal capacity).[26] For example, a 3.5-mph (5.6 km/hr) walk carries an absolute energy cost of 3.8 kcal $\cdot$ kg^{-1} $\cdot$ hr^{-1}.[13] For a young healthy individual with a maximal capacity of about 12 kcal $\cdot$ kg^{-1} $\cdot$ hr^{-1} the relative intensity is about 32% of maximal capacity; whereas, for an older individual with a maximal capacity of 7 kcal $\cdot$ kg^{-1} $\cdot$ hr^{-1} the relative intensity is about 55%. The issue of absolute vs. relative intensity is probably more important when prescribing exercise or when categorizing individuals into intensity-specific levels of activity (e.g., moderately vs. vigorously active). Feasibility considerations related to individualized measures of relative EE limit assessment methods among large free-living populations to the use of absolute energy cost scales. However, because EE is closely related to body size, it is essential to account for this factor when quantifying activity-related EE.[27] It is therefore preferable to express EE per unit of body mass, for example, as kcal per kilogram of body mass per minute (kcal $\cdot$ kg^{-1} $\cdot$ min^{-1}). Returning to the 55 kg female runner who completes a 45-minute run at a 6-min/mile pace (4 min/km), the absolute net EE was 619 kcal, whereas the net EE relative to this individual's body mass would be about 11.25 kcal $\cdot$ kg^{-1} during the 45-minute bout of running activity. A 75 kg runner who completes the same running task would have an absolute net EE of 844.75 kcal, but when expressed per kg of body weight, the EE is the same (11.26 kcal $\cdot$ kg^{-1}) as that computed for the lighter runner.

An alternative unit of quantifying activity-related EE is the metabolic equivalent, or MET.[12] The MET represents the ratio of work to resting metabolic rate.[27] It is accepted that resting EE is approximately 1 MET, which is equivalent to 3.5 mL O$_2$ $\cdot$ kg^{-1} $\cdot$ min^{-1}, or about 1 kcal $\cdot$ kg^{-1} $\cdot$ hr^{-1}.[27] To compute the MET level of a given physical activity, multiply by the duration (e.g., minutes) for which the activity was performed. This results in the MET-minute. This index quantifies the rate at which energy is expended for the duration an activity is performed, while accounting simultaneously for body size and resting metabolism.[12,28,29] To standardize the quantification of EE and reduce potential sources of extraneous variation in physical activity research, a systematic approach to assigning MET levels of EE to specific physical activities has been published.[12,13] The *Compendium of Physical Activities*[12,13] provides researchers and practitioners with a standardized linkage between specific activities, their purpose and their estimated energy cost expressed in METs. A sample entry from the Compendium is listed below:

CODE	MET	ACTIVITY	EXAMPLES
12120	16	Running	running, 10 mph (6 min/mile)

Column 1 shows a five-digit code that indexes the general class or purpose of the activity. In this example, 12 refers to running and 120 refers specifically to running a 6 min/mile (4 min/km) pace. Column 2 shows the energy cost of the activity in METs. Columns 3 and 4 show the type of activity (running) and a specific example related with the activity code.

Much of the original work to standardize the energy cost of physical activity was calibrated for a 60 kg person.[12] Therefore, the conversion between MET minutes and kcal of EE is approximated by multiplying MET minutes by the quotient of an individual's body mass divided by 60.[12] For a 60 kg person, MET minutes is equivalent to kcal; for persons who weigh more than 60 kg, the caloric equivalent will be slightly higher and, for those weighing less than 60 kg, the caloric equivalent will be slightly lower than the MET-minute value. The caloric equivalent of 150 MET-minutes of walking for a 70 kg person is about 75 kcal, for a 60 kg person the caloric equivalent is about 150 kcal and for a 50 kg person, about 125 kcal. Returning to the 55 kg runner, completing the 45-min bout of running at 6-min/mile (4 min/km) pace would result in 720 MET-minutes (16 MET activity $\times$ 45 minutes), or 660 kcal (720 MET-min $\times$ [55/60]).

Defining and standardizing terms associated with physical activity measurement is a critical step in reducing unwanted sources of variation and producing unbiased estimates of activity-related EE.[12,13,27,28] It should be apparent from the previous discussion that, although the use of a standardized compendium to index activity-specific energy costs results in potentially large differences between individuals in terms of absolute net EE, after accounting for body size, EE estimates for a given activity are quite small. The *Compendium of Physical Activities* may not resolve every issue related with individual vs. population-based assessment of activity-related EE. It does, however, provide a standardized measurement method for use in research and practical settings, which should enhance the consistency of EE assessment in terms of precision and reproducibility.

III. Conceptual Framework for Quantifying Energy Expenditure

To incorporate the terminology described above into a framework that can guide the measurement of EE under laboratory and field conditions, it could be argued that the construct of interest within the activity-EE measurement paradigm might best be defined as *"movement."* Movement can be operationalized into two measurable variables: physical activity (a behavior) and EE (the energy cost of the behavior) (Figure 10.2). Direct and indirect measures exist for both physical activity and EE. However, because researchers and practitioners are ultimately interested in matching energy intake with EE, researchers typically extrapolate activity measures to units of EE prior to evaluating potential effects on energy balance. Energy expenditure is often estimated from physical activity questionnaires or other indirect measures that reflect patterns of activities in various settings. Indirect measures of activity or EE may provide acceptable estimates of actual EE, depending on the degree of concordance with more direct measures of EE. Following is a review of methods to assess physical activity and EE, with emphasis placed on direct and indirect techniques that can be used to quantify EE among free-living athletic populations. Laboratory-based methods for assessing physical activity and EE are covered elsewhere in this volume. Comprehensive reviews of free-living and laboratory methods used to assess activity-related EE can be found elsewhere. [6,7,27,30-32]

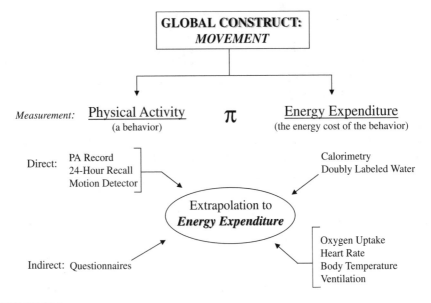

FIGURE 10.2
Conceptual framework for defining and assessing physical activity and energy expenditure. Adapted with permission from M.J. LaMonte and B.E. Ainsworth, Quantification of Energy Expenditure and Physical Activity in the Context of Dose Response, *Med. Sci. Sports Exerc.* 2001; 33(6 suppl): 5370–5378.

IV.   Methods of Assessing Physical Activity and Energy Expenditure

The primary objective of measuring activity-related EE is to obtain a reliable and accurate estimate of the energy cost for a given activity or series of activities. The EE score can then be applied within the context of designing and tracking exercise training and nutrition programs to optimize athletic performance (e.g., endurance, power, muscular strength). The practical application of linking physical activity and EE is predicated upon precise measures of both variables. Several direct and indirect methods exist to assess physical activity and EE in laboratory and field settings.[6,7,9,27] Table 10.2 lists the most common measurement techniques.

Direct measures of physical activity include the use of physical activity records, logs, 24-hour recalls and mechanical or electronic motion sensors to obtain detailed information pertaining to the frequency, duration and pattern of physical activities performed over a defined observation period. Indirect physical activity measures involve the use of questionnaires that require respondents to recall their usual activity habits during a period in the far or recent past. Indirect methods typically provide less detail than direct physical activity measures, but offer substantially less administrative burden and cost.

TABLE 10.2

Methods of Assessing Physical Activity and Energy Expenditure

	Dimension Measured	Units	Technical/ Administrative Burden
Direct Measures			
Observation	Physical Activity	Frequency, Duration, Type	Moderate
Room Calorimetry	Energy Expenditure	kcal of heat production	High
Doubly Labeled Water	Energy Expenditure	kcal from CO_2 production	High
Biochemical Forces	Energy Expenditure	kcal from $\dot{V}O_2$ – force curves	High
Acceleration Vectors (e.g., Accelerometry)	Physical Activity	Frequency, Duration	
	Energy Expenditure	kcal, METs from $\dot{V}O_2$ regressions	Moderate
Motion Sensors (e.g., Pedometry)			
PA Records or Diaries, Recall Interviews	Physical Activity	Frequency, Duration, Type	High
	Energy Expenditure	kcal, METs from Compendium of Physical Activities [ref 9]	High
Indirect Measures			
Indirect Calorimetry	Energy Expenditure	kcal, METs from CO_2 production	High
Physiologic Measures (e.g., Heart Rate)	Energy Expenditure	kcal, METs from relation with $\dot{V}O_2$	Moderate
PA Surveys or Questionnaires	Physical Activity	Frequency, Duration, Type	Low
	Energy Expenditure	kcal, METs from Compendium of Physical Activities [ref 12,13]	
Surrogate Reports (e.g., Energy Intake)	Energy Expenditure	kcal, assumes weight stable	Low

Precise measures of EE are difficult without the use of expensive laboratory procedures involving metabolic chambers or radioactive isotope tracers [6,27]. Activity-related EE can be estimated indirectly from field measures of physiologic variables or physical activity,[7,9] however, indirect assessment of EE (e.g., motion sensors, heart rate) has yet to be refined for application outside the context of controlled research settings.

A. Measuring Energy Expenditure

The complex biochemical processes that drive the transfer of metabolic energy required for skeletal muscle contraction during physical activity result in a large amount of heat energy.[33] The rate of heat production is directly proportional to the net activity-related EE, therefore, EE can be precisely quantified by measuring body heat at rest or during exercise.[34] The oxidation of food substrate is a primary source of energy production at rest, during and following physical activity. Therefore, activity-related EE can be estimated by measuring the fractional concentrations of expired CO_2 and O_2 during physical activity and calculating EE based on some assumptions about the energy cost of substrate oxidation.[34] Laboratory methods for direct measures of heat production (e.g., room calorimetry) and ventilatory gas exchange (e.g., indirect calorimetry) have been described elsewhere in this volume. Following is an overview of field methods used to assess activity-related EE in a variety of settings.

1. Direct Measures of Energy Expenditure

a. Doubly Labeled Water (DLW)

Energy expenditure estimated from DLW is based on the rate of metabolic carbon dioxide production ($\dot{V}CO_2$).[35,36] The DLW solution consists of the stable water isotopes ^2H_2O and $H_2^{18}O$ and is administered according to body size. Urinary isotope excretion is tracked using an isotope-ratio mass spectrometer prior to dosing, shortly after dosing and over several days thereafter. Labeled hydrogen (^2H_2O) is excreted as water alone, while labeled oxygen ($H_2^{18}O$) is lost as water and CO_2 ($C^{18}O_2$) through the carbonic anhydrase system. The difference in the isotope turnover rates provides a measure of metabolic $\dot{V}CO_2$.[36] Oxygen uptake ($\dot{V}O_2$) and total body EE are extrapolated from measured $\dot{V}CO_2$ and an estimate of the respiratory quotient (RQ) based on established equations.[37] Under steady-state conditions, RQ reflects the relative percentage of carbohydrate and fat oxidation and is calculated as $\dot{V}CO_2/\dot{V}O_2$. Inherent error will exist in DLW EE estimates when RQ is estimated and when measurements are made under non-steady-state conditions such as exercise.[27]

Differences in EE estimates between DLW and indirect calorimetry measures have been as high as 20%.[38-41] Discrepancies between DLW and indirect calorimetry may reflect a greater amount of activity-related EE under free-living conditions than can be simulated and measured under controlled laboratory conditions. Although DLW provides precise estimates of free-living EE over prolonged periods (e.g., weeks), this technique is limited to studies of total EE and does not differentiate the duration, frequency or intensity of specific physical activity. A "physical activity level" index (PAL) has been computed as the DLW total daily EE divided by measured or estimated resting metabolic rate.[42] However, the lack of information as to the type, duration and frequency of activities resulting in the expended energy, as well potential errors with estimating resting metabolic rate, challenge the utility of the PAL. The expense of the isotopes and mass spectrometry analysis may limit this method of assessing EE exclusively to research settings.

b. Labeled Bicarbonate

The labeled bicarbonate ($NaH^{14}CO_3$) method is very similar to DLW and has been used to measure free-living total daily EE over shorter observation periods (e.g., days) than in studies of DLW.[43] A known amount of isotope is infused at a constant rate that will eventually be diluted by the body's CO_2 pool. Labeled carbons are recovered from expired air, blood, urine or saliva. Metabolic $\dot{V}CO_2$ is determined from the degree to which the isotope was diluted. Total EE can be calculated from $\dot{V}CO_2$ based on assumptions made about RQ. Controlled experimental studies of this method have demonstrated EE estimates within < 6% of that measured in a respiratory chamber.[43,44] Labeled bicarbonate measures of EE are limited by similar concerns as described for the DLW method.

2. Indirect Measures of Energy Expenditure

a. Oxygen Uptake

Activity-related EE measured with indirect calorimetry procedures is based on assumed relations between oxygen uptake and the caloric cost of substrate oxidation.[27,33,34] Based on the gas concentrations and volume of expired air, rates of carbon dioxide production ($\dot{V}CO_2$) and oxygen uptake ($\dot{V}O_2$) can be determined. RQ is typically estimated by the respiratory exchange ratio (RER) as $\dot{V}CO_2/\dot{V}O_2$. Then, $\dot{V}O_2$ and RQ can be used to estimate EE in kcal according to Weir's equation:[45]

Equation 1: $EE \ (kcal) = \dot{V}O_2 \ (3.9 + 1.1 \ RQ)$.

Differences between actual and estimated RQ can result because of unreliable assumptions regarding the caloric cost of specific substrate oxidation, bicarbonate buffering of metabolic CO_2 during exercise and post-exercise oxygen consumption kinetics. Therefore, measured RQ, which involves urinary nitrogen collection,[34] is required for precise estimates of activity-related EE using indirect calorimetry methods.

It is likely that free-living activity patterns are altered during laboratory simulations, methods for performing indirect calorimetry outside the laboratory setting. These techniques are based on the same principles described above and utilize small, portable indirect calorimeters that integrate O_2 and CO_2 analyzers, a ventilation flow-volume meter and a microcomputer to process expired air collected through a fitted hood, face mask or mouthpiece.[46] Devices such as the Cosmed K4b^2 have allowed for field assessment of $\dot{V}O_2$ and thus, measures of gross activity-related EE during a variety of free-living activities.[47,48] Cost issues, the necessity of wearing cumbersome and obtrusive instrumentation, the potential for altered patterns of physical activity and lack of testing under a variety of field settings, limit the usefulness of this approach to measuring free-living activity-related EE outside of the research setting.

b.   Heart Rate (HR)

Activity-related EE has been estimated from HR based on the assumption of a strong linear relation between HR and $\dot{V}O_2$.[49,50] However, variation in the HR-$\dot{V}O_2$ relationship during low and very high-intensity PA and considerable between-person HR-$\dot{V}O_2$ variability,[51,52] have led some researchers to recommend using individual HR-$\dot{V}O_2$ calibration curves to estimate activity-related EE.[52,53] One such method requires establishing a heart rate "threshold" prior to estimating activity-related EE from the HR-$\dot{V}O_2$ calibration curve.[54] This threshold is referred to as the "FLEX HR" and is determined from laboratory-based indirect calorimetry studies at various work intensities. Activities eliciting an HR below the FLEX HR are assigned an activity-related energy cost based on resting EE. Activities eliciting an HR above the FLEX HR are assigned an activity-related energy cost using the individual HR-$\dot{V}O_2$ calibration curve. Other techniques have been used to estimate activity-related EE from the HR response during physical activity.[52,55,56]

Correlations of 0.53 to 0.73 have been reported between total EE estimated from DLW and HR values based on individual HR-$\dot{V}O_2$ calibrations.[57] Although activity-related EE estimates based on individual HR-$\dot{V}O_2$ curves correlate reasonably well with an objective EE measure such as DLW, measurement variability is high. Livingstone et al.[54] reported difference scores of –22% to +52% between total EE estimated from DLW and FLEX HR. Recently, however, Strath et al.[56] showed a strong correlation between activity-related EE estimated from HR reserve and indirect calorimetry (r = .87, SEE = .76 METs) among adults performing moderate-intensity lifestyle activities. Energy expenditure estimates based on relative vs. absolute HR measures may reduce between-person sources of variation related with age, sex and fitness level, which may improve the precision of estimating activity-related EE from HR responses during physical activity.

The HR-$\dot{V}O_2$ relationship is not linear during low and very high-intensity activity.[31,51] Because many daily activities are low to moderate intensity,[13] HR monitoring may not provide precise estimates of habitual daily activity-related EE under free-living conditions. Imprecise estimates of activity-related EE may also be attributed to several factors that influence HR without having substantial effects on oxygen uptake, such as day-to-day HR variability, body temperature, size of the active muscle mass (e.g., upper vs. lower body), type of exercise (static vs. dynamic), stress and medication.[7,27,31] The need to develop individual HR-$\dot{V}O_2$ calibration curves and instrumentation costs ($150 per unit) make HR monitoring a less suitable surrogate activity-related EE outside the research setting. HR measurements may best be utilized as part of an integrated monitoring system rather than as a single measure of activity-related EE among free-living individuals.[58]

c.   Body Temperature and Ventilation

Because a close relationship between EE and core body temperature and ventilation has been reported under laboratory conditions,[27] continuous monitoring of these variables could provide a means of extrapolating activity-related EE under certain conditions. However, body temperature and ventilation measures of EE may be limited by time requirements, several confounding factors and inconvenient measurement techniques.[7] Similar to HR, these measurements may best be utilized as part of an integrated monitoring system rather than as single measures of activity-related EE among free-living individuals.[58]

B. Measuring Physical Activity

Several methods are available to measure free-living physical activity levels using methods that range in precision from crude categorization of activity status (e.g., sedentary vs. active) to detailed descriptions of activities (e.g., type, duration, frequency) and their estimated energy cost (e.g., MET-min · d^{-1}). Below is an overview of some direct and indirect methods that have been used to assess physical activity in various settings.

1. Direct Measures of Physical Activity

a. Physical Activity Records

Physical activity records are detailed accounts of activity types and patterns recorded in diary format during a defined period of time.[6] Their level of detail ranges from recording each activity and its associated duration[59] to recording activities performed at specified time intervals (e.g., every 15 minutes).[60] The physical activity record is about as big as a pocket-size book. Respondents record information about the type (e.g., sleep, running, weightlifting), purpose (e.g., exercise, transportation), duration (e.g., minutes), self-rated intensity (light, moderate, vigorous) and body position (reclining, sitting, standing, walking) for every activity completed within a defined observation period (typically 24 hr). Seasonal records (e.g., winter, summer) can be kept to obtain information about habitual physical activity levels and patterns and related seasonal variations in these behaviors.[18,19] Because entries are recorded in the activity record at the time the behavior is executed, there is little concern over the effects of recall bias on the precision of quantifying activity-related EE. Figure 10.3a illustrates a sample page from a completed physical activity record including codes from the *Compendium of Physical Activities* that would be used to assign an energy cost to each activity for scoring purposes. Once scored, the physical activity record provides a detailed account of the minutes spent and estimated energy expended in various types, intensities and patterns of physical activity. The physical activity record is a highly objective and reproducible method[61] of tracking the specific types (e.g., walking, running, occupation) and patterns (e.g., single continuous bouts, sporadic intermittent bouts) of activity that account for individual or population (e.g., entire sport teams) activity-related EE. For example, an athlete thought to be in chronic negative energy balance could complete a series of physical activity records over a defined time frame, from which estimates of total daily EE as well as activity-specific EE can be obtained. It may be discovered that the athlete in question is expending a large amount of energy in non-sport activities (e.g., occupational or recreational activity) that are not being met with a compensatory increase in energy intake. Using data from the activity record, nutritional counseling and training modifications can be implemented to reestablish energy balance in this athlete.

Physical activity records have been used in field settings to obtain comprehensive detailed accounts of free-living physical activities and related EE.[16,38,59,61-66] The precision of a physical activity record's measurement of free-living EE has been studied. Conway et al.[38] reported a difference of only 7.9 ± 3.2% between a 7-day physical activity record and doubly labeled water estimates of free-living activity-related EE in men. Richardson et al.[67] observed moderate to strong age-adjusted correlations (r = 0.35 – 0.68) between total MET-min per day of EE from the physical activity record and an electronic accelerometer among free-living men and women. Physical activity records have also been used to study activity patterns among free-living individuals. Ainsworth et al.[59,63] characterized the types and patterns of physical activity and related EE among Caucasian, African-American and Native-American women living in the southeastern and southwestern regions of the U.S. as part of the NIH-funded Women's Health Initiative.[68] Data from the physical activity record were then used to develop population-specific physical activity surveys that would precisely measure habitual daily activity-related EE among these population sub-groups of women.[63] Focus groups[22] or individual debriefings pertaining to recorded information have been used to enhance the richness and interpretation of data gleaned from physical activity records. Together, these methods can be used to obtain information required to identify athletes at risk for overtraining,[2,69] chronic energy imbalance[5] and related declines in athletic performance and overall health status.[2,4,5,70]

Similar to their dietary counterpart aimed at assessing energy intake,[71] physical activity records provide a very detailed and comprehensive method of assessing an important determinant of energy balance. As with dietary records, feasibility is limited by cost, the potential for altered behavior and administrative burden on the practitioner and participant. For these reasons, physical activity records may best be suited for use with individuals considered to be at high risk for energy imbalance or as a criterion measure for validating simpler field surveys of physical activity and related EE.

b. Physical Activity Logs

A modified version of the physical record is the physical activity log. These instruments aim to provide detailed accounts of habitual daily activities, their associated duration and EE.[6] The activity log is structured as a checklist of activities specific to the target population's usual activity patterns.[6,22,72] The Bouchard Physical Activity Log[60] is designed for respondents to check the type and intensity of activity they are performing every 15 minutes during a specific period. The Ainsworth Physical Activity Log[63,71] is a modifiable form that includes a list of 20 to 50 activities that reflect population-specific PA interests (Figure 10.3b). At the end of the day, respondents complete the single-page checklist by identifying the type and duration of activities performed that day. Activity-related EE is computed by assigning intensity values from the *Compendium of Physical Activities* to each activity selected by the respondent. The log takes only a few minutes to complete and can be quickly scored to provide information about the type, time and estimated energy cost of physical activities performed during specified periods (e.g., 7 days). Summary scores for daily activity-related EE (e.g., MET-min · d^{-1}), or for specific categories of activity (e.g., exercise or sport, sleep, occupation) can be tracked for individual or groups of athletes. Because the log is completed at the end of the day, the degree of recall bias associated with this method of quantifying activity-related EE is likely higher than with the physical activity record.

Physical activity logs may be more convenient to complete and process than physical activity records as they are less time consuming for the respondent and contain less information for data processing. Alternatively, activity logs may underestimate actual activity-related EE if participants engage in activities other than those listed on the log.

c. Physical Activity Recalls

Physical activity recalls are typically conducted as interviews (telephone or in person) and are aimed at detailing an individual's activity level during the past 24 hours or longer.[6] Activity recalls are similar to physical activity records in that they can identify the type, duration, purpose and related EE of activities performed during the recall frame. The physical activity recall was developed after methods used in 24-hr dietary recalls and takes from 20 to 45 minutes to complete.[71,73] Multiple random 24-hr activity recalls have recently been used to profile activity patterns and estimate EE among adults in a 1-year cohort study of blood lipid variability.[73] The range of test-retest reliability coefficients was very large and the magnitude of the coefficients was moderate at best (R = 0.22 to 0.58). Criterion validity correlations between total MET-hr · d^{-1} from the 24-hr recalls and activity data from an electronic accelerometer were r = 0.74 and r = 0.32 for men and women, respectively. Based on the feasibility, reasonable reliability and validity, minimal participant effort and potential reductions in response bias and altered activity patterns during assessment, the researchers advocated using the 24-hr recalls to assess activity-related EE among free-living populations. However, this method may not be suitable in populations with limited telephone access, may be hampered by individuals who are unwilling or unable to complete the phone interview and may utilize a time frame (e.g., past 24 hr) that does not capture an individual's true habitual PA pattern or level. On the other hand, this method may be useful during tapering periods of the

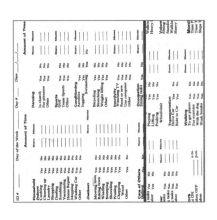

TIME BEGAN	POSITION (circle one)	DESCRIPTION (What are you doing?)	HOW HARD? (circle one)	Activity Group (circle one)	(leave blank) CODE	MINS
8:05 AM PM	Recline Sit Stand Walk	walk in house to fix breakfast	Light Moderate Vigorous	SC HH PAR TRANS OCC WALK INAC LG EC MISC	17150	1
8:06 AM PM	Recline Sit Stand Walk	fix breakfast	Light Moderate Vigorous	SC HH PAR TRANS OCC WALK INAC LG EC MISC	05050	4
8:10 AM PM	Recline Sit Stand Walk	eat breakfast	Light Moderate Vigorous	SC HH PAR TRANS OCC WALK INAC LG EC MISC	13030	5
8:15 AM PM	Recline Sit Stand Walk	gather things to leave home	Light Moderate Vigorous	SC HH PAR TRANS OCC WALK INAC LG EC MISC	09071	3
8:18 AM PM	Recline Sit Stand Walk	walk to car	Light Moderate Vigorous	SC HH PAR TRANS OCC WALK INAC LG EC MISC	17161	2
8:20 AM PM	Recline Sit Stand Walk	drive car to work	Light Moderate Vigorous	SC HH PAR TRANS OCC WALK INAC LG EC MISC	16010	

A. Physical Activity Record

B. Physical Activity Log

C. Yamax Digiwalker   D. CSA Accelerometer   E. Caltrac Accelerometer   F. Tritrac Accelerometer

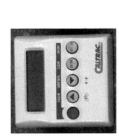

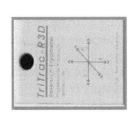

FIGURE 10.3

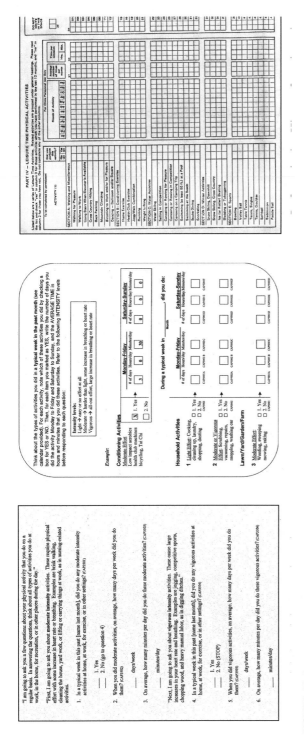

FIGURE 10.3

Direct and indirect methods of assessing physical activity. Adapted by permission from B.E. Ainsworth, M.J. LaMonte, and C.E. Tudor-Locke, Physical activity, in *Obesity: Etiology, Assessment, Treatment, and Prevention*, edited by R. Anderson, Champaign, IL, in press.

yearly training plan, where small acute changes in an athlete's total exercise volume and its associated energy requirements might be highly influential on performance in an upcoming competition.

d. Motion Detectors

The use of mechanical and electronic motion detectors as a direct measure of free-living physical activity has become increasingly popular.[7,74,75] Energy expenditure is often extrapolated from the activity data under the assumption that movement (or acceleration) of the limbs and torso is closely related to whole-body activity-related EE.[31] There are several types of motion detectors that differ in cost, technology and data output (Figure 10.3c–f).

Pedometers. Pedometers are small, inexpensive devices (~$20) used to directly quantify walking activity in terms of accumulated steps per unit time (e.g., per day).[6,8] Because mechanical pedometers have relied on relatively crude spring-loaded mechanisms to register steps, these devices were found to have unacceptable accuracy and reliability due to stretching of the springs and lack of a suitable calibration mechanism.[27,76,77] Recently developed electronic pedometers (e.g., Yamax Digiwalker) are smaller and may be more reliable than earlier models. These devices are worn at the waist and are triggered by the vertical forces of foot-strike that cause a horizontal spring-suspended lever arm to move up and down. Movement of the lever arm opens and closes an electrical circuit. Each time the circuit closes, a "step" is counted. Step registration, in theory, should reflect only the vertical forces of footstrike, however, any vertical force through the hip area (e.g., sitting down hard onto a chair) can trigger the device. An estimate of distance walked is obtained by calibrating the pedometer to an individual's stride length during a short walking trial over a known distance.

Pedometers have demonstrated reasonable precision for use in research and clinical settings where walking is the primary type of PA.[46,75,78-80] Correlations of $r = 0.84 - 0.93$[79] and $r = 0.48 - 0.80$[47] have been reported between pedometer steps per day and EE estimates from electronic accelerometers. Investigators have also shown pedometer steps per day to be moderately correlated with measured oxygen uptake ($r = 0.49$[47]) and self-reported total daily activity-related EE ($r = 0.21 - 0.49$[63,75]). A major limitation to using pedometers as an objective field measure of activity-related EE is that pedometers lack temporal information on the type, duration and intensity of activities performed while steps were being recorded.[7,31] Although some pedometers include an estimate of net EE based on an assumed relation of about 100 kcal per mile walked, empirical data is lacking as to the precision of these estimates compared with measured EE. Furthermore, EE from activities that require both upper- and lower-body muscle activity would be greatly underestimated under this assumption.

Because researchers recommend using the "raw steps" data as opposed to estimated EE to represent ambulatory activity,[81] pedometry may not be a suitable method of assessing activity-related EE among athletes. Pedometers may, however, serve as an inexpensive method of monitoring ambulatory activity among athletes who are rehabilitating sport-related injuries wherein walking is a major part of the rehabilitation, or is being restricted due to the specific nature of the injury. Used in conjunction with a detailed self-report of physical activity (e.g., activity log), pedometers may provide a simple cost-effective way to monitor both the quantity and quality of certain types of physical activity.

Accelerometers. Accelerometers are battery operated electronic motion sensors that, in theory, measure the rate and magnitude of that which the body's center of mass displaces during movement. Solid state technology integrates and sums the absolute value and frequency of acceleration forces over a defined observation period. Data is output as an activity "count." Regression equations have been developed from controlled laboratory experiments to allow for the estimation of activity-related EE from the integral of accelerometer count.[82-86] Accelerometers are typically worn at the waist and measure movement in single (uniaxial — Caltrac, CSA) or multiple planes (triaxial — Tritrac) by way of piezoelectric signaling. Activity or EE data is either displayed for hand recording (Caltrac) or stored in solid-state memory for computer downloading and processing at a later time (CSA, Tritrac).

The Caltrac accelerometer (Muscle Dynamics Fitness Network, Torrence, CA) was first described in the early 1980s by Montoye et al.[84] To assess activity-related EE, the device first estimates resting EE using information programmed in by the user as follows (Hemokinetics, Inc., Madison, WI):

Equation 2:   Men: kcal · min^{-1} ([473 × Wt lbs] + [982 × Ht in] – [531 × Age] + 4686)/100,000

Equation 3:   Women: kcal · min^{-1} ([331 × Wt lbs] + [351 × Ht in] – [352 × Age] + 49,854)/100,000

Using the activity counts recorded during movement and assuming 5 kcal for every 1 L oxygen uptake, activity-related EE is estimated from oxygen uptake (VO$_2$) using the following equation [84]:

Using the activity counts recorded during movement, and assuming 5 kcal for every 1 L oxygen uptake, activate-related EE is estimated from oxygen uptake (VO$_2$) using the following equation:[84]

Equation 4: $\dot{V}O_2$ (ml · kg^{-1} · min^{-1}) = 8.2 + 0.08 (counts · min^{-1})

Equation 5:   kcal = 5 × ($\dot{V}O_2$ [ml · kg^{-1} · min^{-1}] × body mass (kg)/1000)

The activity-related EE is continuously added to the resting EE value and summed across the specified observation period to yield a value of total or *gross* EE. Net activity-related EE can be approximated by dividing gross EE by the estimated resting metabolic rate (Equations 1 and 2). MET-min · d^{-1} of activity-related EE can be computed by dividing the net kcal/day value by 1440 min · d^{-1}. To quantify physical activity in terms of movement counts rather than kcal of EE, Caltrac count data can be obtained by entering the following constants into the resting metabolic rate equation: weight = 25, height = 36, age = 99 and gender = 0.[87] Caltrac cannot store data and, because it cannot be programmed for interval-based time sampling, only total daily activity counts or EE can be measured.

The reliability and validity of the Caltrac has been established in a variety of settings.[27,28,46,65,66,84,88] One-, 6- and 13-month age-sex adjusted test-retest correlations of 0.69, 0.84 and 0.79, respectively, were reported for Caltrac total EE among free-living men and women.[28] Strong correlations between Caltrac total EE and measured VO_2 (pooled r = 0.74, SEE = 6.6 ml · kg^{-1} · min^{-1}) and high test-retest reproducibility (r = 0.93 to 0.98) were reported in the original work of Montoye et al.[84] In another study, Caltrac and VO_2 were highly correlated (r = 0.89) but no relation between Caltrac and treadmill grade (r = 0.02) was observed.[87] The latter observation illustrates the inability of accelerometers to detect changes in the energy cost of activities due to increased resistance to movement.[7,53,87] More recently, a moderate correlation (r_{pooled} = 0.58) but large variation in quantitative estimates of EE were observed between the Caltrac and VO_2 during a variety of field and laboratory activities.[47]

The Computer Science and Applications (CSA; Shalimar, FL) accelerometer has become increasingly popular for field studies physical activity and EE because of its small size and ability for time-interval sampling and data storage. Unlike the Caltrac, the CSA must be computer initialized. Data are presented as counts per unit sampling time and regression equations have been developed to estimate EE from raw CSA count data.[82,83,86] These equations were generated from controlled studies of treadmill exercise or limited simulations of lifestyle physical activities. The most common equations are those developed by Freedson et al.,[82,87] which are preprogrammed into the CSA unit:

Equation 6:   METs = 1.439008 + (0.000795 × counts · min^{-1})

Equation 7:   kcal · min^{-1} = (0.00094 × counts · min^{-1}) + (0.1346 x mass in kg)

The precision of each equation was R^2 = 0.82 (SEE = 1.12 METs) for METs and R^2 = 0.82 (SEE = 1.4 kcal · min^{-1}) for kilocalories during treadmill exercise at 80, 106 and 162 m · min^{-1}.[82]

Several studies have recently assessed the ability of the CSA to assess activity-related EE.[47,72,74,83,86,87,89] CSA counts have varied significantly with monitor placement at three different ipsilateral hip locations.[74] Melanson and Freedson [87] showed CSA counts/min^{-1} were correlated with VO_2 during treadmill walking (r = 0.82), but unrelated with treadmill grade (r = 0.03). CSA counts · min^{-1} were sensitive to changes in ambulatory velocity across three walking speeds (p < 0.0001), but interinstrument reliability was substantially lower during slower (53 m · min^{-1}, R = 0.55) vs. faster (107 m $\cdot$ min^{-1}, R = 0.91).[89] Correlations between VO$_2$ and CSA counts/min^{-1} have been stronger during controlled laboratory activity (e.g., r = 0.80 to 0.95)[74,87] than during simulated or actual field conditions of lifestyle activities (e.g., r = 0.40 to 0.60).[72,74] Hendelman et al.[83] showed large differences (e.g., 30–57%) between measured and predicted METs for a variety of daily lifestyle activities. Regression equations used to estimate EE from lifestyle activities have shown lower precision (R^2 = 0.32–0.35, SEE = 0.96–1.2 METs)[83,86] compared with equations derived from controlled laboratory activity (R^2 = 0.82-0.89, SEE = 1.1 METs).[82,89] Discrepancies in the time spent (e.g., min $\cdot$ d^{-1}) in defined EE categories were large between detailed physical activity logs and CSA data based on cutpoints derived from three different regression equations.[72]

The Tritrac (Hemokinetics Inc., Madison, WI) is a triaxial accelerometer that provides count data for the anterior-posterior, medial-lateral and vertical planes, as well as an integrated vector magnitude (Vmag) of counts for all three planes combined. Energy expenditure can be estimated through regression equations that account for body mass and resting EE. Resting EE is calculated as follows:[85]

Equation 8: Men: (0.00473 × wt kg) + (0.00971 × ht cm) – (0.00513 × age yr) + 0.04687

Equation 9: Women: (0.00331 × wt kg) + (0.00352 × ht cm) – (0.00353 × age yr) + 0.49854

A regression equation (R^2 = 0.90, SEE = 0.014 kcal $\cdot$ kg^{-1} $\cdot$ min^{-1} has been developed during treadmill walking and running to estimate activity-related EE from the Tritrac Vmag:[85]

Equation 10: kcal $\cdot$ kg^{-1} $\cdot$ min^{-1} = 0.018673 + (0.000029051 × Vmag $\cdot$ min^{-1})

Oddly, the preceding regression equation predicts EE using a triaxial monitor based on experimental activity that results in acceleration from essentially one plane (e.g., vertical). Measurement in three planes should theoretically account for more sources of body movement and therefore provide more precise estimates of activity-related EE, particularly under lifestyle conditions. Studies have shown that triaxial devices have only slightly better correlations with both laboratory (r$_{Triaxial}$ = 0.84–0.93 vs. r$_{uniaxial}$ = 0.76–0.85) and lifestyle activity (r$_{Triaxial}$ = 0.59–0.62 vs. r$_{uniaxial}$ = 0.48–0.59)-related EE.[74,83]

Although data from accelerometers can be used to assess frequency, duration and intensity of physical activity, the specific type of physical activity is unknown. Accelerometers tend to overestimate walking-related EE and underestimate lifestyle activity-related EE. Furthermore, activity-related EE owed to the upper extremities or increased resistance to body movement (e.g., uphill walking) is not accounted for. Subject compliance issues, potentially altered physical activity patterns and the cost of the more sophisticated instruments (uniaxial ~ \$300, triaxial ~ \$550 per unit) limit the practicality of using electronic accelerometers to measure activity-related EE among free-living athletes. If used together with a detailed activity log, accelerometers may be useful to quantify physical activity patterns and their related EE for an athlete at high risk for energy imbalance.

2. Indirect Measures of Physical Activity

a. Physical Activity Questionnaires

Self-report questionnaires are the most frequently used method of assessing physical activity levels among free-living individuals. Based on their level of detail and subject burden, activity questionnaires are generally classified as global, recall and quantitative history instruments.[6,27] Table 10.3 provides a list of questionnaires that have been used to estimate physical activity and EE in various studies. Most, if not all, of the questionnaires listed in Table 10.3 were designed for use in population-based epidemiological studies of heart disease or other health outcomes. To date, there has been no self-reported physical activity questionnaire designed specifically for athletic populations.

Global Questionnaires. Global activity questionnaires are typically one to four items long and provide an estimate of an individual's general physical activity level (Figure10.3g). They are short and easy to complete, but global questionnaires provide little detail on specific types and patterns of physical activity. Therefore, global questionnaires allow for only simple classifications of activity status (e.g., active vs. inactive)[90,91] and do not allow for precise assessment of activity-related EE. Global questionnaires are preferred in physical activity surveillance systems[92] where sample sizes are very large, administrative time is limited and the goal for assessment may be to merely classify respondents as inactive, irregularly active, or regularly active at levels recommended for health benefits. The accuracy and reproducibility of global activity instruments have been reported.[28,72,93] Age-adjusted test-retest correlations of 0.90 and 0.81 for men and women, respectively, and an age–sex-adjusted coefficient of determination of 0.29 between the activity score and maximal aerobic capacity have been reported for a two-point (e.g., active vs. inactive) global activity question.[93] Lack of detail on the type, frequency, duration and intensity of physical activity render global question-naires inadequate for estimating activity-related EE.

Recall Questionnaires. Recall instruments are more burdensome (10–20 items) to complete than their global counterparts, but these questionnaires ask for details on the frequency, duration and types of PA performed during the past day, week, or month (Figure 10.3h). Scoring systems vary among recall questionnaires, ranging from simple ordinal scales (e.g., 1–5 representing low to high levels of PA),[94] to comprehensive summary scores of continuous data (e.g., kcal, kJ, or MET-min $\cdot$ d^{-1}).[63,95,96] The advantage of the latter measure is the ability to quantify time spent (e.g., min $\cdot$ d^{-1}) per-forming specific physical activities, as well as their related EE.

Recall surveys have demonstrated acceptable levels of accuracy and repeatability.[28,62,63,66,95,97] One-month test-retest correlations for activity-related EE computed from self-reported walking, stair climbing and sport activity were 0.61 and 0.75 for men and women, respectively, who completed the College Alumnus questionnaire.[97] Criterion validity correlations between activity-related EE and Caltrac accelerometer METs · d^{-1} and kcal · d^{-1} were 0.29 and 0.17, respectively, for all participants. Richardson et al. [66] observed age-adjusted test-retest correlations of 0.60 and 0.36 for total MET-min · d^{-1} of EE among men and women, respectively, who completed the Stanford 7-Day Activity Recall twice over 26 days apart. Age-adjusted criterion validity correlations for total daily EE between the 7-day recall and the Caltrac accelerometer were 0.54 and 0.20 for men and women, respectively and, between the 7-day recall and 48-hr physical activity records were 0.58 and 0.32 for men and women, respectively. Recall surveys typically do a poor job of assessing nonoccupational, nonleisure activity-related EE,[7,28,63] which may be particularly relevant sources of health-related EE among women and minorities[22,98] and may partly explain the lower correlations between self-reported and objectively measured activity levels among women.[63] Ainsworth et al.[62,63] have reported data from a comprehensive Typical Week Physical Activity Survey administered to middle-aged minority women. This survey (Figure10.3h) is very detailed and requires respondents to recall frequency and duration of several types of activities including items for house and family care, exercise and sport and occupation. Age-adjusted test-retest correlations were 0.43 to 0.68 summary scores for total, light, moderate and vigorous MET-min · d^{-1} of activity-related EE, and age-adjusted criterion validity correlations were 0.45 to 0.54 between detailed physical activity records and logs and the activity summary scores. Despite being one of the most detailed and comprehensive recall questionnaires, the validity and reliability characteristics of the Typical Week Activity Survey[62,63] are similar or better than other more frequently used recall questionnaires.[66,94-96]

There are two primary limitations to physical activity recall instruments. First, the activity estimate is subject to errors in recall that may result in biased measures of activity-related EE.[99-101] This bias seems to be intensity-related in that recall error is typically highest for light and moderate intensity physical activities that are more habitual in nature (e.g., walking, house-work).[28,66,63,73,100] This may be particularly relevant when trying to quantify activity-related EE among athletic populations who have little trouble remembering planned bouts of vigorous sports activity, but pay little attention to other sources of habitual daily EE (e.g., walking on campus or at work) that may contribute substantially to an individual's total energy requirements. Second, the structure of the instrument may not include relevant population-specific sources of activity-related EE, which would likely lead to an underrepresentation of an individual's actual physical activity level and related EE.[7,9]

Quantitative History Questionnaires. Quantitative histories (Figure10.3i) are detailed (e.g., > 20 items) records of the frequency and duration of leisure-

TABLE 10.3

Self-Report Questionnaires Used to Quantify Levels of Physical Activity and Energy Expenditure in Free-Living Populations

Method/Questionnaire[a]	Type of Activity[b]	Recall Time Frame	Burden[c]	Expression of PA Score[d,e]	Author
Global:					
NSPHPC	TOTAL (relative to peers)	General	Low	5-point Qualitative Scale	Slater et al. 1987[107]
				2-point Qualitative Scale	Belloc et al. 1972[90]
Lipid Research Clinics	JOB, EX	Usual day	Low	2-point Qualitative Scale	Siscovick et al. 1988[91]
BRFSS	JOB, NON-JOB, EX			4-point Qualitative Scale	Ainsworth et al. 1993[93]
	JOB, EX, SP, LEIS, HH, CARE	Usual day	Low	3-point Qualitative Scale	Macera et al. 2000[92]
Recall Questionnaires:					
Baecke	JOB, SP, LEIS	General	Moderate	5-point Ordinal Scale	Baecke et al. 1982[94]
Seven Day Recall	EX, LEIS	Past 7 days	Moderate	$kcal \cdot kg^{-1} \cdot d^{-1}$	Blair et al. 1985[95]
College Alumnus	EX, SP, LEIS	Past 7 days	Moderate	$kcal \cdot wk^{-1}$	Paffenbarger, 1986[96]
Typical Week Survey	JOB, EX, SP, LEIS, TRAN, HH, YRD, CARE, VOL, TOTAL	Typical week in past month	Moderate	$MET \cdot min \cdot d^{-1}$	Ainsworth et al. 2000[62]
					Ainsworth et al. 2001[63]

Quantitative History:

MN LTPA	EX, SP, LEIS, HH	High	AMI·d⁻¹	Taylor et al., 1978[102]
Tecumseh Occupation	JOB, TRAN	Moderate	MET·hr·wk⁻¹	Montoye, 1971[103]
Historical PA	SP, LEIS	High	Ordinal Scale in hr·wk⁻¹ and kcal·wk⁻¹	Kriska et al. 1988[104]

Note: Table 3 is adapted by permission from B.E. Ainsworth, H.J. Montoye and A.S. Leon, 1994. Methods of assessing physical activity during leisure and work, in *Physical Activity, Fitness, and Health*, edited by C. Bouchard, R. Shephard, and T. Stephens (Champaign, IL: Human Kinetics), 148-149, and M.J. LaMonte and B.E. Ainsworth, Quantifying energy expenditure and physical activity in the context of dose response. *Med. Sci. Sports Exerc.*, 2001; 33(6 suppl): 5370–5378.

a   NSPHPC, National Survey of Personal Health Practices & Consequences; BRFSS, Behavioral Risk Factor Surveillance System; MN LTPA, Minnesota LTPA; Tecumseh LTPA, Tecumseh, Michigan LTPA; LTPA, leisure-time physical activity.

b   JOB, occupational; EX, exercise; SP, sport; TRAN, transportation; LEIS, leisure; HH, household; YRD, yard work; CARE, care giving; VOL, volunteer; TOTAL, total physical activity.

c   Administrative burden including cost, time to administer/respond, data management/processing time.

d   MET, Metabolic Equivalent; AMI, Activity Metabolic Index; kcal, Kilocalorie; kJ, Kilojoule; kg, Kilogram.

e   Qualitative Scale refers to categories such as "More Active versus Less Active," or :"Sedentary versus Active." Ordinal Scale refers to an ordered range of numbers (e.g., 1-5) used to rank activity status (e.g., low to high).

time or occupational physical activities over the past year[102,103] or lifetime.[104] Activity scores are usually expressed as a continuous variable (e.g., kcal $\cdot$ kg^{-1} $\cdot$ wk^{-1}), allowing for the evaluation of activity-related EE. The most frequently used quantitative history is the Minnesota Leisure Time Physical Activity Questionnaire (MNLTPA),[102] which uses a 1-year recall frame to identify the frequency (events per year) and average duration (hr:min per event) of 74 activity items in categories of walking, conditioning, hunting and fishing, water, winter, sports, home repair and household maintenance activities. Richardson et al. [67] reported age-adjusted 1-year test-retest correlations for total, light, moderate and heavy MET-min $\cdot$ d^{-1} of activity-related EE of 0.69, 0.60, 0.32 and 0.71, respectively, among adults responding to the MNLTPA. These investigators also showed age-adjusted criterion validity correlations of 0.75, 0.72, 0.70 and 0.75 between MNLTPA and 4-week activity history summary scores of total, light, moderate and heavy MET-min $\cdot$ d^{-1}.

Similar to the "remote diet recall" used to assess past dietary habits,[71] quantitative activity histories are useful in settings where investigators and practitioners are interested in detailing activity-related EE patterns over long periods of time (e.g., 12 months). The intensive administrative burden (e.g., 60 min) and recall effort required by the respondent limits the feasibility of these instruments.

b. Body Composition

Body composition is known to vary with energy intake and activity-related EE.[4,5,70,105] Measures of body composition include body weight, percent body fat, fat-free mass, bone mineral density, patterns of fat deposition, skinfolds and girth measurements.[57] Generally, higher levels of physical activity are associated with more favorable body composition measures.[28,106] Studies of self-reported free-living physical activity show the highest correlations between vigorous activity (> 6 METs or > 7 kcal $\cdot$ min^{-1}) and body composition measures.[28] Measures of body composition represent only a crude surrogate of activity-related EE, as information pertaining to the type, frequency and duration of specific activities is not available from these measures. Simple measures of body composition (e.g., body weight, regional skinfold thickness) may be useful as a global indicator of activity-related EE, however, the high costs and administrative burden associated with more sophisticated body composition measures (e.g., hydrostatic weighing, DEXA scans) limits their use essentially to research settings. Because body composition is influenced by both energy intake and EE, body composition measures may best serve as a surrogate of energy balance as opposed to an independent measure of energy intake or EE.

V. Summary

Many direct and indirect methods are available to measure physical activity and its related EE under free-living conditions. These measurements exist along a continuum of precision, cost and administrative burden. Sophisticated laboratory measures of EE are not feasible for studying large numbers of individuals under free-living conditions, but may be appropriate to evaluate individual athletes thought to be at high risk for energy imbalance and the related consequences on performance and health parameters. The utility of direct laboratory procedures for measuring EE as a means of validating field techniques for assessing activity-related EE, however, should not be understated.

Field measures are often used to assess activity-related EE with an acknowledged trade-off between precision and practicality. Each method is limited by between- and within-person variation in the measured variable, as well as ancillary factors that may confound each method's true association with activity-related EE. Portable indirect calorimeters may be the most accurate indirect method for assessing activity-related EE in the field, but costs, restricted movement and potential alteration in usual behavior limit using this technique as the gold-standard field measure. Development of small, nonobtrusive integrated systems that employ multiple indirect measures of activity-related EE (e.g., HR, body temperature, ventilation, acceleration, steps) may improve the accuracy and feasibility of estimating EE under field conditions. Physical activity records and questionnaires are the least expensive and least burdensome methods that allow for detailed assessment of activity-related EE under free-living conditions, although how well an instrument represents population-specific activity behaviors and recall biases are concerns. Use of standardized methods for assigning energy costs to self-reported (e.g., activity log, recall questionnaire) or objectively measured (e.g., accelerometer), free-living physical activities will improve the accuracy and reproducibility of these field measures.

References

1. U.S. Department of Health and Human Services. Physical activity and health: a report of the Surgeon General. Atlanta, GA: U.S. Department of Health and Human Services, Centers for Disease Control and Prevention, National Center for Chronic Disease Prevention and Health Promotion. 1996.
2. Pate, R.R. and Branch, J.D., Training for endurance sport, *Med. Sci. Sport. Exerc.*, 24(9 Suppl), S340, 1992.
3. Haskell, W.L., Dose-response issues from a biological perspective, in *Physical Activity, Fitness and Health. A Consensus of Current Knowledge*, Bouchard, C., Shephard, R.J. and Stephens, T., Eds., Human Kinetics, Champaign, IL, 1994, 1030.
4. Hill, J.O., Melby, C., Johnson, S.L. and Peters, J.C., Physical activity and energy requirements, *Am. J. Clin. Nutr.*, 62(suppl), 1059S, 1995.

5. American College of Sports Medicine, American Dietetic Association and Dietitians of Canada, Nutrition and athletic performance, *Med. Sci. Sports Exerc.*, 32, 2130, 2000.
6. Ainsworth, B.E., Montoye, H.J. and Leon, A.S., Methods of assessing physical activity during leisure and work, in *Physical Activity, Fitness and Health. A Consensus of Current Knowledge*, Bouchard, C., Shephard, R.J. and Stephens, T., Eds., Human Kinetics, Champaign, IL, 1994, 146.
7. LaMonte, M.J. and Ainsworth, B.E., Quantifying EE and physical activity in the context of dose response, *Med. Sci. Sports. Exerc.*, 2001: 33(6 suppl): 5370–5378.
8. Thomas, J.R. and Nelson, J.K., Research methods in physical activity, 3rd ed., Human Kinetics, Champaign, IL, 1996.
9. Ainsworth, B.E. Practical assessment of physical activity, in *Barrow and McGee's Practical Measurement and Assessment*, 5 ed., Tritscher, K. Ed., Lippincott, Williams and Wilkins, Baltimore, MD, 2000, 475.
10. Caspersen, C.J., Powell, K.E. and Christenson, G.M., Physical activity, exercise and physical fitness: Definitions and distinctions for health-related research, Public Health Reports, 100, 126, 1985.
11. Corbin, C.B., Pangrazi, R.P. and Franks, B.D., Definitions: Health, fitness and physical activity, *Research Digest*, Series 3, 1, 2000.
12. Ainsworth, B.E., Haskell, W.L., Leon, A.S., Jacobs, D.R., Montoye, H.J., Sallis, J.F. and Paffenbarger, R.S., Compendium of physical activities: classification of energy costs of human physical activities. *Med. Sci. Sports Exerc.*, 25, 71, 1993.
13. Ainsworth, B.E., Haskell, W.L., Whitt, M.C., Irwin, M.L., Swartz, A.M., Strath, S.J., O'Brien, W.L., Bassett, D.R., Schmitz, K.H., Emplaincourt, P.O., Jacobs, D.R. and Leon, A.S., Compendium of physical activities: an update of activity codes and MET intensities, *Med. Sci. Sports. Exerc.*, 32(Suppl), S498, 2000.
14. American College of Sports Medicine, The recommended quantity and quality of exercise for developing and maintaining cardiorespiratory and muscular fitness and flexibility in healthy adults, *Med. Sci. Sports Exerc.*, 30, 975, 1998.
15. Pate, R.R., Pratt, M., Blair, S.N., Haskell, W.L., Macera, C.A., Bouchard, C., Buchner, D., Ettinger, W., Heath, G.W., King, A.C., Kriska, A., Leon, A.S., Marcus, B.H., Morris, J., Paffenbarger, R.S., Patrick, K., Pollock, M.L., Rippe, J.M., Sallis, J.F. and Wilmore, J.H., Physical activity and public health. A recommendation from the Centers for Disease Control and Prevention and the American College of Sports Medicine. *J. Am. Med. Assoc.*, 273, 402, 1995.
16. Stolarczyk, L.M., Addy, C.L., Ainsworth, B.E., Chang, C. and Heyward, V., Accuracy of self-reported physical activity intensity in minority women. *Med. Sci. Sports Exerc.*, 30(5 Suppl), S10, 1998.
17. Gretebeck, R.J. and Montoye, H.J., Variability of some objective measures of physical activity, *Med. Sci. Sports Exerc.*, 24, 1167, 1992.
18. Levin, S., Jacobs, D.R., Ainsworth, B.E., Richardson, M.T. and Leon, A.S., Intra-individual variation and estimates of usual physical activity, *Ann. Epidemiol.*, 9, 481, 1999.
19. Uitenbroek, D.G., Seasonal variation in leisure time physical activity, *Med. Sci. Sports Exerc.*, 25, 755, 1993.
20. Robertson, R.J., Caspersen, C.J., Allison, T.G., Skrinar, G.S., Abbott, R.A. and Metz, K.F., Differentiated perceptions of exertion and energy cost of young women while carrying loads, *Eur. J. Appl. Physiol.*, 49, 69, 1982.
21. Ainsworth, B.E., Richardson, M.T., Jacobs, D.R. and Leon, A.S., Gender differences in physical activity, *Women Sports Phys. Activ. J.*, 1, 1, 1993.
22. Henderson, K.A. and Ainsworth, B.E., Sociocultural perspectives on physical activity on the lives of older African American and American Indian women: A Cross-Cultural Activity Participation Study, *Women & Health*, 31, 1, 2000.
23. McArdle, W.D., Katch, F.I. and Katch, V.L. Exercise physiology. Energy, nutrition and human performance, 3rd ed., Lea & Febiger, Philadelphia, 1991.

24. Howley, E.T., You asked for it. Question authority, *ACSM's Health & Fitness J.*, 3, 12, 1999.
25. Sparrow, W.A., Ed., *Energetics of Human Activity*, Human Kinetics, Champaign, IL, 2001.
26. Arroll, B. and Beaglehole, R., Potential misclassification in studies of physical activity, *Med. Sci. Sports Exerc.*, 23, 1176, 1991.
27. Montoye, H.J., Kemper, H.C.G., Saris, W.H.M. and Washburn, R.A., *Measuring Physical Activity and Energy Expenditure*, Human Kinetics, Champaign, IL, 1996, 3.
28. Jacobs, D.R., Ainsworth, B.E., Hartman, T.J. and Leon, A.S., A simultaneous evaluation of 10 commonly used physical activity questionnaires, *Med. Sci. Sports Exerc.*, 25, 81, 1993.
29. Sallis, J.F., Haskell, W.L., Wood, P.D., Fortmann, S.P., Rogers, T., Blair, S.N. and Paffenbarger, R.S., Physical activity assessment in the five-city project, *Am. J. Epidemiol.*, 121, 91, 1985.
30. Bassett, D.R., Validity and Reliability in objective monitoring of physical activity, *Res. Q. Exerc. Sport.*, 71, 30, 2000.
31. Freedson, P.S. and Miller, K., Objective monitoring of physical activity using motion sensors and heart rate, *Res. Q. Exerc. Sport.*, 71, 21, 2000.
32. Washburn, R.A. and Montoye, H.J., The assessment of physical activity by questionnaire, *Am. J. Epidemiol.*, 123, 563, 1986.
33. Brooks, G.A., Fahey, T.D. and White, T.P., *Exercise Physiology. Human Bioenergetics and its Application*, 2nd ed., Mayfield Publishing, Mountain View, CA, 1996.
34. Ferrannini, E., The theoretical bases of indirect calorimetry: a review, *Metabol.*, 37, 287, 1988.
35. Lifson, N., Gordon, G.B. and McClintock, R. Measurement of carbon dioxide production by means of D_2O^{18}, *J. Appl. Physiol.*, 7, 704, 1955.
36. Speakman, J.R., The history and theory of the doubly labeled water technique, *Am. J. Clin. Nutr.*, 68, 932S, 1998.
37. Black, A.E., Prentice, A.M. and Coward, W.A., Use of food quotients to predict respiratory quotients for the doubly labeled water method of measuring EE, *Human Nutr.: Clin Nutr.*, 40C, 381, 1986.
38. Conway, J.M., Seale, J.R., Irwin, M.L., Jacobs, D.R. and Ainsworth, B.E., Ability of 7-day physical activity diaries and recalls to estimate free-living EE, *Obes. Res.*, 7(Suppl 1), 107S, 1999.
39. Schulz, S., Westersterp, K. and Bruck, K., Comparison of EE by the doubly labeled water technique with energy intake, heart rate and activity recording in man, *Am. J. Clin. Nutr.*, 49, 1146, 1989.
40. Seale, J.L., Rumpler, W.V., Conway, J.M. and Miles, C.W., Comparison of doubly labeled water, intake balance and direct- and indirect-calorimetry methods for measuring EE in adult men, *Am. J. Clin. Nutr.*, 52, 66, 1990.
41. Westersterp, K.R., Brouns, F., Saris, W.H.M. and Ten Hoor, F., Comparison of doubly labeled water with respirometry at low- and high-activity levels. *J. Appl. Physiol.*, 65, 53, 1988.
42. Black, A.E., Coward, W.A., Cole, T.J. and Prentice, A.M., Human EE in affluent societies: an analysis of 574 doubly labelled water measurements, *Eur. J. Clin. Nutr.*, 50, 72, 1996.
43. Elia, M., Fuller, N.J. and Murgatroyd, P.R., Measurement of bicarbonate turnover in humans: applicability to estimation of EE, *Am. J. Physiol.*, 263, E676, 1992.
44. Elia, M., Jones, M.G., Jennings, G., Poppitt, S.D., Fuller, N.J., Murgatroyd, P.R. and Jebb, S.A., Estimating EE from specific activity of urine urea during lengthy subcutaneous $NaH^{14}CO3$ infusion, *Am. J. Appl. Physiol.*, 269, E172, 1995.
45. Weir, J.B., New methods for calculating metabolic rate with special reference to protein metabolism, *J. Physiol.*, 109, 1, 1949.
46. Davis, J.A., Direct determination of aerobic power, in *Physiological Assessment of Human Fitness*, Maud, P. and Foster, C., Eds., Human Kinetics, Champaign, 1996, 9.

47. Bassett, D.R., Ainsworth, B.E., Swartz, A.M., Strath, S.J., O'Brien, W.L. and King, G.A., Validity of four motion sensors in measuring moderate intensity physical activity, *Med. Sci. Sports Exerc.*, 32 (9 Suppl), S471, 2000.

48. King, G.A., McLaughlin, J.E., Howley, E.T., Bassett, D.R. and Ainsworth, B.E., Validation of Aerosport KB1-C portable metabolic system, *Int. J. Sports Med.*, 20, 304, 1999.

49. Berggren, G. and Chritensen, E.H., Heart rate and body temperature as indices of metabolic rate during work, *Arbeitsphysiologie*, 14, 255, 1950.

50. Wilmore, J.H. and Haskell, W.L., Use of the heart rate-EE relationship in the individualized prescription of exercise, *Am. J. Clin. Nutr.*, 24, 1186, 1971.

51. Christensen, C.C., Frey, H.M.M., Foenstelien, E., Aadland, E. and Rafsum, H.E., A critical review of EE estimates based on individual O_2 consumption/heart rate curves and average daily heart rate, *Am. J. Clin. Nutr.*, 37, 468, 1983.

52. Washburn, R.A. and Montoye, H.J., Validity of heart rate as a measure of daily EE, *Exerc. Physiol.*, 2, 161, 1986.

53. Haskell, W.L., Yee, M.C., Evans, A. and Irby, P.J., Simultaneous measurement of heart rate and body motion to quantitate physical activity, *Med. Sci. Sports Exerc.*, 25, 109, 1993.

54. Livingstone, M.B., Prentice, A.M., Coward, W.A., Ceesay, S.M., Strain, J.J., McKenna, P.G., Nevin, G.B., Barker, M.E. and Hickey, R.J., Simultaneous measurement of free-living EE by the doubly labeled water method and heart-rate monitoring, *Am. J. Clin. Nutr.*, 52, 59, 1990.

55. Andrews, R.B., Net heart rate as a substitute for respiratory calorimetry, *Am. J. Clin. Nutr.*, 24, 1139, 1971.

56. Strath, S.J., Swartz, A.M., Bassett, D.R., O'Brien, W.L., King, G.A. and Ainsworth, B.E., Evaluation of heart rate as a method for assessing moderate intensity physical activity, *Med. Sci. Sports Exerc.*, 32 (9 Suppl), S465, 2000.

57. Roche, A.F., Heymsfield, S.B and Lohman, T.G., Eds., *Human Body Composition*, Human Kinetics, Champaign, IL., 1996.

58. Healey, J., Future possibilities in electronic monitoring of physical activity, *Res. Q. Exerc. Sport*, 71, 137, 2000.

59. Ainsworth, B.E., Irwin, M.L., Addy, C.L., Whitt, M.C. and Stolarczyk, L.M., Moderate physical activity patterns of minority women: The Cross-Cultural Activity Participation Study, *J. Women's Health*, 8, 805, 1999.

60. Bouchard, C., Tremblay, A., Leblanc, C., Lortie, G., Savard, R. and Theriault, G., A method to assess EE in children and adults, *Am. J. Clin. Nutr.*, 37, 461, 1983.

61. LaMonte, M.J., Durstine, J.L., Addy, C.L., Irwin, M.L. and Ainsworth, B.E., Physical activity, physical fitness and Framingham 10-year risk score: The Cross-Cultural Activity Participation Study, *J. Cardiopulm. Rehab.*, 21, 1, 2001.

62. Ainsworth, B.E., LaMonte, M.J., Drowatzky, K.L., Cooper, R.S., Thompson, R.W., Irwin, M.L., Whitt, M.C. and Gilman, M., Evaluation of the CAPS Typical Week Physical Activity Survey among minority women, in *Proc. Community Prevention Res. in Women's Health Conference*, 17, Bethesda, MD: National Institutes of Health, 2000.

63. Ainsworth, B.E., LaMonte, M.J., Whitt, M.C., Irwin, M.L., Drowatzky, K.L., Addy, C.L. and Durstine, J.L., Evaluation of a questionnaire to measure moderate physical activity in ethnically diverse women, *J. Clin. Epidemiol.*, in press, 2001.

64. Fogelholm, M., Assessment of EE in overweight women, *Med. Sci. Sports Exer.*, 30, 1191, 1998.

65. Richardson, M.T., Leon, A.S., Jacobs, D.R., Ainsworth, B.E. and Serfass, R., Ability of the Caltrac accelerometer to assess daily physical activity levels, *J. Cardio. Rehab.*, 15, 107, 1995.

66. Richardson, M.T., Ainsworth, B.E., Jacobs, D.R. and Leon, A.S., Validation of the Stanford 7-day recall to assess habitual physical activity, *Ann. Epidemiol.*, 11, 145, 2001.

67. Richardson, M.T., Leon, A.S., Jacobs, D.R., Ainsworth, B.E. and Serfass, R., Comprehensive evaluation of the Minnesota Leisure Time Physical Activity questionnaire. *J. Clin. Epidemiol.*, 47, 271, 1994.

68. Finnegan, L.P. The NIH's Women's Health Initiative: its evolution and expected contributions to women's health,. *Am. J. Prev. Med.*, 12, 292, 1996.

69. Lehman, M., Foster, C. and Keul, J., Overtraining in endurance athletes: a brief review, *Med. Sci. Sports Exerc.*, 25, 854, 1993.

70. Brownell, K.D., Steen, S. and Wilmore, J.H., Weight regulation practices in athletes: analysis of metabolic and health effects, Med. Sci. Sports Exerc., 19, 546, 1987.

71. Willett, W.C., *Nutritional Epidemiology*, 2nd ed., Oxford Press, New York, 1998.

72. Ainsworth, B.E., Bassett, D.R., Strath, S.J., Swartz, A.M., O'Brien, W.L., Thompson, R.W., Jones, D.A., Macera, C.A., Kimsey, C.D., Comparison of three methods for measuring the time spent in physical activity, *Med. Sci. Sports Exerc.*, 32, 9 (Suppl), S457, 2000.

73. Matthews, C.E., Freedson, P.S., Hebert, J.R., Stanek, E.J., Merriam, P.A. and Ockene, I.S., Comparing physical activity assessment methods in the Seasonal Variation of Blood Cholesterol Study, *Med. Sci. Sports Exerc.*, 32, 976, 2000.

74. Welk, G.J., Blair, S.N., Wood, K., Jones, S. and Thompson, R.W., A comparative evaluation of three accelerometry-based physical activity monitors, *Med. Sci. Sports Exerc.*, 32 (9 Supl), S489, 2000.

75. Welk, G.J., Differding, J.A., Thompson, R.W., Blair, S.N., Dziura, J. and Hart, P., The utility of the Digi-Walker step counter to assess daily physical activity patterns, *Med. Sci. Sports Exer.*, 32 (9 Suppl), S481, 2000.

76. Bassey, E.J., Dallosso, H.M., Fentem, P.H., Irving, J.M. and Patrick, J.M., Validation of a simple mechanical accelerometer (pedometer) for the estimation of walking activity, *Eur. J. Appl. Physiol.*, 56, 323, 1987.

77. Gayle, R., Montoye, H.J. and Philpot, J., Accuracy of pedometers for measuring distance walked, *Res. Q. Exer. Sport*, 48, 632, 1977.

78. Bassett, D.R., Ainsworth, B.E., Leggett, S.R., Mathien, C.A., Main, J.A., Hunter, D.C. and Duncan, G.E., Accuracy of five electronic pedometers for measuring distance walked, *Med. Sci. Sports Exerc.*, 28, 1071, 1996.

79. Leenders, N.Y.J.M., Sherman, W.M. and Nagarja, H.N., Comparisons of four methods of estimating physical activity in adult women, *Med. Sci. Sports Exerc.*, 32, 1320, 2000.

80. Nelson, T.E., Leenders, N.Y.J. and Sherman, W.M., Comparison of activity monitors worn during treadmill walking, *Med. Sci. Sports Exer.*, 30 (5 Suppl), S11, 1998.

81. Tudor-Locke, C.E. and Myers, A.M., Methodological considerations for researchers and practitioners using pedometers to measure physical (ambulatory) activity, *Res. Q. Exerc. Sport*, 72, 1, 2001.

82. Freedson, P.S., Melanson, E. and Sirard, J., Calibration of the Computer Science and Applications, Inc. accelerometer. *Med. Sci. Sports Exerc.*, 30, 777, 1998.

83. Hendelman, D., Miller, K., Bagget, C., Debold, E. and Freedson, P., Validity of accelerometry for the assessment of moderate intensity physical activity in the field. *Med. Sci. Sports Exerc.*, 32 (9 Supl), S442, 2000.

84. Montoye, H.J., Washburn, R., Servais, S., Ertl, A., Webster, J.G. and Nagle, F.J., Estimation of EE by a portable accelerometer. *Med. Sci. Sports Exerc.*, 15, 403, 1983.

85. Nichols, J.F., Morgan, C.G., Sarkin, J.A., Sallis, J.F. and Calfas, K.J., Validity, reliability and calibration of the Tritrac accelerometer as a measure of physical activity. *Med. Sci. Sports Exerc.*, 31, 908, 1999.

86. Swartz, A.M., Strath, S.J., Bassett, D.R., O'Brien, W.L., King, G.A. and Ainsworth, B.E., Estimation of EE using CSA accelerometers at hip and waist sites. Med. Sci. Sports Exerc., 32 (9 Suppl), S450, 2000.

87. Melanson, E. and Freedson, P., Validity of the Computer Science and Applications, Inc. (CSA) activity monitor. *Med. Sci. Sports Exerc.*, 27, 934, 1995.

88. Pambianco, G., Wing, R.R. and Robertson, R., Accuracy and reliability of the Caltrac accelerometer for estimating EE. *Med. Sci. Sports Exerc.*, 22, 858, 1990.

89. Nichols, J.F., Morgan, C.G., Chabot, L.E., Sallis, J.F. and Calfas, K.J., Assessment of physical activity with the Computer Science and Applications, Inc., accelerometer: laboratory vs. field validation, *Res. Q. Exerc. Sport*, 71, 36, 2000.

90. Belloc, N.B. and Breslow, L., Relationship of physical health status and health practices. *Prev. Med.*, 1, 409, 1972.

91. Siscovick, D.S., Ekelund, L.G., Hyde, J.S., Johnson, J.L., Gordon, D.J. and La-Rosa, J.C., Physical activity and coronary heart disease among asymptomatic hypercholesterolemic men. *Am. J. Public Health*, 78, 1428, 1988.

92. Macera, C.A. and Pratt, M., Public health surveillance of physical activity. *Res. Q. Exerc. Sport*, 71, 97, 2000.

93. Ainsworth, B.E., Jacobs, D.R. and Leon, A.S., Validity and reliability of self-reported physical activity status: the Lipid-Research Clinics questionnaire, *Med. Sci. Sports Exerc.*, 25, 92, 1993.

94. Baecke, J.A.H., Burema, J. and Frijters, J.E.R., A short questionnaire for the measurement of habitual physical activity in epidemiological studies, *Am. J. Clin. Nutr.*, 36, 936, 1982.

95. Blair, S.N., Haskell, W.L., Ho, P., Paffenbarger, R.S., Vranizan, K.M., Farquhar, J.W. and Wood, P.D., Assessment of habitual physical activity by a seven-day recall in a community survey and controlled experiments, *Am. J. Epidemiol.*, 122, 794, 1985.

96. Paffenbarger, R.S., Hyde, R.T., Wing, A.L. and Hsieh, C.C., Physical activity, all-cause mortality and longevity of college alumni. *New Eng. J. Med.*, 314, 605, 1986.

97. Ainsworth, B.E., Leon, A.S., Richardson, M.T., Jacobs, D.R. and Paffenbarger, R.S., Accuracy of the College Alumnus Physical Activity Questionnaire. *J. Clin. Epidemiol.*, 46, 1403, 1993.

98. Weller I. and Corey, P., The impact of excluding non-leisure EE on the relation between physical activity and mortality in women, *Epidemiol.*, 9, 632, 1998.

99. Baranowski, T., Validity and reliability of self-report measures of physical activity: An information-processing perspective, *Res. Q. Exerc. Sport*, 59, 314, 1988.

100. Durante, R. and Ainsworth, B.E., The recall of physical activity: using a cognitive model of the question-answering process, *Med. Sci. Sports Exerc.*, 28, 1282, 1996.

101. Lichtman, S.W., Pisarska, K., Raynes Berman, E.R., Pestone, M., Dowling, V., Offenbacher, E., Weisel, H., Heshka, S., Matthews, D.E. and Heymsfield, S.B., Discrepancy between self-reported and actual caloric intake and exercise in obese subjects, *New Eng. J. Med.*, 327, 1893, 1992.

102. Taylor, H.L., Jacobs, D.R., Schucker, B., Knudsen, J., Leon, A.S. and De Backer, G., A questionnaire for the assessment of leisure time physical activities. *J. Chronic Disease*, 31, 741, 1978.

103. Montoye, H.J., Estimation of habitual physical activity by questionnaire and interview, *Am. J. Clin. Nutr.*, 24, 1113, 1971.

104. Kriska, A.M. et al., The assessment of historical physical activity and its relation to adult bone parameters, *Am. J. Epidemiol.*, 127, 1053, 1988.

105. Ravussin, E., Energy expenditure and body weight, in *Eating Disorders and Obesity*, Brownell, K.D. and Fairburn, C.G., Eds., Guilford, New York, 1995, 32.

106. Kriska, A.M., Sandler, R.B., Cauley, J.A., LaPorte, R.E., Hom, D.L. and Pambianco, G., The interrelationships of physical activity, physical fitness and body composition measurements, *Med. Sci. Sports Exerc.*, 19, 564, 1987.

107. Slater, C.H., Green, L.W., Vernon, S.W. and Keith, V.M., Problems in estimating the prevalence of physical activity from national surveys, *Prev. Med.*, 16, 107, 1987.

Section Five

Biochemical Assessment of Athletes

11

Assessment of Lipid Status in Athletes

Scott A. Lear and Gregory P. Bondy

CONTENTS

I. Introduction

One of the many benefits enjoyed by athletes who participate in regular activity and exercise is the effect on lipid metabolism and the resultant favorable changes in serum lipids. Common assessment of serum lipids consists of a full lipid profile, which includes total cholesterol (TC), low density lipoprotein cholesterol (LDL-C), high density lipoprotein cholesterol (HDL-C) (which assesses cholesterol present in all HDL subparticles such as HDL_2 and HDL_3) and triglycerides (TG). Other lipid parameters that may be of use in an assessment are apolipoprotein B (apo B), apolipoprotein A (apo A) and LDL particle size. Emerging evidence has also indicated effects

0-8493-0927-1/02/$0.00+$1.50
© 2002 by CRC Press LLC

of exercise on lipoprotein lipase (LPL) and hepatic lipase (HL), (Lp(a)), oxidized LDL-C (ox-LDL-C), lecithin-cholesterol acyltransferase (LCAT) and cholesterol ester transfer protein (CETP). Athletes and individuals who exercise regularly commonly present with a more favourable lipid profile than their inactive counterparts.[1-4] However, cross-sectional studies such as these do not establish a cause and effect. Understanding the chronic and acute affects of exercise on lipids is important when assessing these variables in athletes. Things that also need to be considered are the effects of change in plasma volume that occur as a result of chronic and acute exercise and possible lipid oxidation that may result from ultra-endurance activities. This chapter will begin with a brief overview of lipid metabolism and then discuss the changes that occur in lipids due to both chronic and acute exercise participation as it pertains to the athlete, as well as recommended methods of clinical assessment and special considerations for assessing serum lipids in athletes.

II.   Lipid Metabolism

Due to the hydrophobic nature of cholesterol, triglycerides and other lipids, their transport within plasma is conducted by heterogeneous lipoprotein particles. In general, these lipoprotein particles consist of a hydrophobic core of cholesterol esters and triglycerides surrounded by a hydrophilic complex of cholesterol, phospholipids and proteins. The various lipoproteins are named according to their density and composition: chylomicron, very low density lipoprotein (VLDL), intermediate density lipoprotein (IDL), low density lipoprotein (LDL) and high density lipoprotein (HDL). As the lipoproteins become smaller, their density increases due to the removal of triglycerides, resulting in a greater proportion of cholesterol and protein content. Metabolism of plasma lipoproteins consists of three main pathways: exogenous and endogenous pathways and reverse cholesterol transport. The exogenous pathway begins by the transport of lipids and cholesterol absorbed in the intestine, which are packaged into chylomicrons by the epithelial cells. The chylomicrons travel to the liver to deliver lipids for packaging into other lipoprotein particles. Along the way, triglycerides in the chylomicrons may undergo hydrolysis into free fatty acids (FFA) by LPL circulating in the plasma and attached to capillary walls. The FFA are used by the surrounding cells as an energy substrate. As a result, the chylomicron particles become smaller and smaller as they travel through the circulation and eventually become chylomicron remnant particles. Excess membrane material from these particles may then slough off and enter into the HDL particle pool, while the remaining chylomicron remnants are taken up by the liver. The endogenous pathway is a mirror of the exogenous pathway, which transports cholesterol and triglycerides from the liver to the peripheral cells. The liver packages cholesterol and triglycerides into the apo B-containing VLDL particle. As the VLDL circulates through the plasma, the triglycerides undergo hydrolysis, resulting in IDL particles and then LDL particles. Again, excess membrane from the decreasing particles falls apart and enters the HDL particle pool. All along this path, the VLDL, IDL and LDL particles may be taken up by the liver. The reverse cholesterol is named for its role in removing cholesterol from peripheral tissues to the liver for excretion with bile. In this pathway, the apolipoprotein AI accepts cholesterol released from peripheral cells via the ABC-1 transporter forming nascent HDL, which matures via a reaction with LCAT, thereby modifying HDL_3 particles to HDL_2 particles. The mature HDL particle is transported to the liver and eventually excreted in bile.

A. Metabolism of Lipids during Exercise

The importance of lipid metabolism becomes clearly apparent as the majority of energy used at rest and during mild to moderate exercise is provided by the catabolism of TG and FFA. As described previously, TG are transported to the peripheral working muscles via chylomicrons and VLDL particles. The TG then undergo hydrolysis by LPL at the site of the working muscles. The resulting FFA are then taken up by the muscles, transported to the mitochondria and metabolized via the beta-oxidation pathway to produce ATP for skeletal muscle contraction. Chylomicrons and VLDL particles also transport TG to peripheral adipose tissues. Again the TG are hydrolyzed by LPL so that the FFA can pass into the adipocytes and combine with glycerol to be stored as TG to be used for energy at a later time. While TG from circulating lipoproteins provide FFA for energy substrate utilization, the majority of FFA consumed during exercise are provided by FFA bound to albumin or freely circulating in the plasma. The FFA-albumin complex binds to the fatty acid binding receptor on the muscle cell and the FFA are released into the muscle cell to be transported to the mitochondria to be metabolized. The pool of circulating FFA are mainly the result of mobilized adipose stores of TG.

III. Effects of Exercise on Lipids

A. Cross-Sectional Studies

The idea that exercise can result in an improved lipid profile came from early cross-sectional studies of athletes, individuals who regularly exercise and sedentary men and women. Athletes, when compared with sedentary age-matched men and women, have lower TC, LDL-C, TG and VLDL and higher HDL-C.[1-4] These differences tend to be more pronounced and consistent with regards to HDL-C and TG. When further analyzed, athletes tend to have higher LPL activity and lower HL activity than sedentary controls; this may account, in part, for the differences in lipoprotein particles.[5]

A number of cross-sectional studies have investigated the association between exercise volume and serum lipids. Lakka et al.[6] investigated the relationship between physical activity participation and serum lipids in a cross-sectional study of 2492 middle-aged men. The authors reported a positive relationship between HDL-C and activity levels and an inverse relationship between TG and activity levels. When HDL-C was further analyzed by HDL particle subspecies (HDL_2 and HDL_3), the relationship with physical activity was similar to that observed with HDL-C. Using a different measure of exercise volume, namely kilometers of a week's running, Williams[7] reported that HDL-C levels were associated with kilometers run per week in 1837 recreational female runners. This finding was later confirmed in a similar group of male runners.[8] However, when the relationship between physical fitness, a marker of exercise participation and serum lipids was analyzed, little or no apparent associations were found.[9,10] It is difficult to determine from the aforementioned studies whether exercise itself leads to an improved lipid profile or if those with an improved lipid profile tend to participate in regular exercise. This can be answered only through well-conducted, prospective randomized control trials.

B. Effects of Chronic Exercise

Numerous studies have been conducted to investigate the effects of exercise on serum lipids. These studies have utilized various populations of men and women (pre- and postmenopausal) including those with normal lipid profiles, different types of dyslipidemias, primary and secondary prevention, as well as those with ideal and elevated body weight. Despite the reporting of a wealth of studies, many are fraught with methodological errors that make it difficult to draw definitive conclusions. These include the absence of a nonexercise control group, low sample size or a nonrandomized control group. Variations in the exercise interventions utilized, such as mode, duration, frequency and intensity of exercise, also make comparisons between studies a challenge. In addition, the presence or absence of weight loss further complicates matters. This section will highlight some of the randomized studies reported to date and the implications of their findings; more detailed investigations can be found in other reviews.[11-13]

Williams et al.[14] conducted one of the earliest randomized controlled trials on the effects of exercise in sedentary men. Eighty-one healthy sedentary men were recruited and randomized to either a 1-year exercise intervention or control. The exercise consisted of running initially three times per week and progressing to 5 days per week for 45 minutes. After 1 year, VO_{2max} increased and percent body fat decreased to a significantly greater extent in the intervention group compared with control. There were no significant differences with respect to serum lipids between the two groups. Despite these results, the authors reported that the volume of exercise assessed as miles run per week was negatively correlated with change in TC and LDL-C and positively correlated with HDL-C. They speculated that the average number of miles run per week for the exercise intervention was not enough to illicit a significant improvement in serum lipids and that a threshold of 10 miles (16 kilometers) run per week may be required to observe increases in HDL-C.

These same investigators later studied a group of 155 overweight sedentary men.[15] Study subjects were randomized to one of three groups: weight loss by supervised exercise, diet or control. After 1 year, participants in the exercise and diet group underwent significant weight loss. While those in the diet group lost more weight than those in the exercise group, changes in body fat mass were similar. As expected, VO_{2max} increased significantly in the exercise group only. Reductions in TG and the TC/HDL-C ratio and increases in HDL-C, HDL_2 and HDL_3 were all significantly greater in both the exercise and diet groups compared with controls. There were no differences with respect to TC and LDL-C among the three groups and no differences between the exercise and diet groups. In later analysis, LDL particle diameter increased significantly in the exercise and diet groups compared with control, reflecting more buoyant and less atherogenic LDL particles.[16] The investigators also reported that HL activity decreased significantly in both of the intervention groups.[17] It is likely that the changes in HL contributed to the observed changes in TG and HDL-C. Overall, these results suggest that the changes in serum lipids were due mainly to weight loss regardless of whether it occurred from exercise or dietary changes in initially overweight men.

Another investigation looked at the effects on exercise in men and women with dyslipidemia. Men and postmenopausal women with low HDL-C and high LDL-C were randomly assigned to four groups: diet only, exercise only, diet and exercise and control, and followed for 1 year.[18] Data were analyzed separately for each gender. Exercising men significantly increased their VO_{2max} but underwent no changes in weight. There were nonsignificant reductions in TC, LDL-C, TG and apo B and an increase in HDL-C. Reductions in TC, LDL-C and apo B were more pronounced in the diet-only group and significant only in the diet and exercise combined group, who also experienced the greatest amount of weight loss. Results for the postmenopausal women were similar — significant reductions in TC and LDL-C were observed only in the exercise and diet combined group, who also experienced greater weight loss than the other groups. While not significant, the most pronounced increase in HDL-C occurred in the exercise-only groups, regardless of gender.

Most of the above studies investigated men; how exercise affects serum lipids in women may be different, due to their higher premenopausal serum lipids, which decline after menopause. Two studies have investigated the effect of exercise on serum lipids in pre- and postmenopausal women.[19,20] Both of these studies consisted of 12 weeks of exercise without a nonexercise control group. The first study investigated 25 pre- and 25 postmenopausal women.[19] The authors reported significant weight loss in both groups but no significant change in serum lipids except for a decrease in HDL-C in postmenopausal women. The other study also reported no significant changes with respect to serum lipids after 12 weeks of exercise in either 21 pre- or 16 postmenopausal women.[20] There was no change in weight and no interaction regarding menopausal status and serum lipid changes. However, it is difficult to extrapolate these results due to the small sample sizes, the short length of the interventions and lack of control group.

The differences in designs of these studies (sample size, intervention type and length, etc.) and the populations investigated make comparisons between the studies difficult. To this end, Halbert et al.[21] conducted a meta-analysis of 31 randomized controlled trials of exercise with a mean length of 25.7 weeks (range 9 to 52 weeks). Overall, the exercise intervention resulted in small but significant decreases in TC, LDL-C and TG of 0.10 mmol/L, 0.10 mmol/L and 0.08 mmol/L respectively and a significant increase in HDL-C of 0.05 mmol/L. There where no significant relationships between serum lipid changes and the intensity or the frequency of the exercise intervention, however, there was a consistent trend toward greater changes in serum lipids for those exercise interventions of three times per week compared with those with more than three exercise sessions per week. It is difficult to determine why less frequent exercise resulted in greater lipid changes from the data reported. The authors' final conclusion was that exercise did result in significant beneficial changes in serum lipids. A second review of 51 exercise interventions, 28 of which were randomized controlled trials, concluded that the majority of the studies supported the hypothesis that exercise exerts beneficial changes in serum lipids, with the strongest finding being an increase in HDL-C.[11]

The reported changes in TG and HDL particles are believed to be due to changes that occur in LPL and HL activity. This was confirmed in a study of eight sedentary men undergoing stationary bicycling five times per week, which revealed a 22% increase in LPL and a reciprocal decrease in HL of approximately 15%.[22] This occurred in the presence of significantly greater levels of HDL-C and lower TG levels compared with baseline. Results from Simsolo et al.[23] also support this finding. These investigators reported a significant reduction in muscle LPL activity, following 2 weeks of exercise cessation in 16 athletes.

To date, no single study has conclusively demonstrated an effect of exercise on serum lipids. Many of the studies conducted used small sample sizes, various exercise frequencies and intensities and an exercise intervention of no more than 12 months. However, overall, these studies suggest an effect of exercise on serum lipids that results in an increase in HDL-C and a decrease in TC, LDL-C and TG in previously sedentary men and women. It is unclear whether changes in serum lipids require concomitant weight loss, as many of the studies observed significant reductions in weight. Many of these studies did not try to control for changes in energy expenditure and maintenance of baseline weight. It is reasonable to assume that more prolonged exercise participation is associated with greater changes in serum lipids[7] and that cessation of exercise results in a reversal of these changes. Many of the noted changes in lipoproteins can be attributed to changes in LPL and HL activities.

Athletes tend to be leaner, exercise more frequently and over a period of several years. It is possible that this extra exercise stimulus in athletes may be responsible for the greater differences observed in cross-sectional studies comparing athletes with sedentary controls than reported in the aforementioned prospective studies. As it is unlikely that a study would be conducted to replicate, in sedentary volunteers, the high volume of exercise that athletes practice, investigations of current athletes who abstain from exercise for a specified period may be of value. A study of 24 male cyclists who underwent 2 months of training cessation compared with their peak training period reported a significant increase in body weight and TG with a significant decrease in VO_{2max}, HDL-C, HDL_2, HDL_3 and apo A.[24]

C. Effects of Acute Exercise

As TG and FFA are major energy substrates during exercise, one would expect that exercise also exerts an acute effect on serum lipids. Characterizing this effect is important when determining the appropriate timing for serum lipid assessment in actively exercising athletes. As with investigations of chronic exercise, numerous studies of acute exercise have been conducted. These too are wide ranging in their methodology and study populations and, therefore, results. Only those studies that have been conducted with scientific rigor and corrected for changes in plasma volume will be highlighted and drawn upon for recommendations for lipid assessment in athletes.

An early study of nine male cyclists and 10 sedentary men of similar age investigated the effect of a 60-minute exercise session on a stationary bicycle at each individual's anaerobic threshold as determined from an earlier maximal exercise test.[25] The nine cyclists also participated in an additional session of 2 hours 1 week later. Alcohol consumption and exercise were abstained from for 4 and 3 days prior to each exercise session respectively. No other dietary changes were undertaken and the authors did not indicate if fasting occurred prior to each test. When corrected for changes in plasma volume, there were no significant changes in TC, LDL-C, HDL-C or TG immediately following or within 72 hours of the 60-minute exercise session for either the cyclists or sedentary men compared with immediately before the exercise. There was, however, a trend toward reduced TG of 17% and 22% for the cyclists and sedentary men, respectively, 24 hours following the 60-minute exercise session. This was accentuated following the 2-hour exercise session in the cyclists — TG were significantly lower after 24 hours than the pre-exercise levels (by 33%). The TG levels returned to baseline within 48 hours.

The authors concluded that there is a dose-response effect of exercise duration with reductions in TG levels.

Klein et al.[26] investigated the effects of a 30-minute exercise session in six untrained men following a meal high in fat. Following a 12-hour fast, subjects ingested a high-fat meal adjusted for body size. Blood samples were drawn before the meal and 4, 6 and 8 hours after. On the following day, the protocol was repeated with the addition of a 30-minute exercise session 1 hour after the high fat meal. For both days, TG levels increased at 4, 6 and 8 hours after the high-fat meal compared with the baseline fasting levels. However, the increase in TG levels following exercise was significantly lower for all of these time periods compared with those on the previous day without exercise. These results indicate that exercise attenuates the increase in TG levels due to a high-fat meal. This is consistent with the previous results indicating TG levels are reduced after acute exercise.

As differences in the duration of exercise may reflect either exercise intensity or kcals (kcal) utilized or both, controlling one of these variables may provide additional insight. To investigate the effect of exercise intensity, 39 sedentary men with elevated TC levels (> 6.00 mmol/L) were randomized to perform stationary cycling at either 60% or 80% of their previously assessed VO_{2max} until a total of 350 kcal had been expended.[27] Subjects began the exercise sessions following a 12-hour fast, at which time serum lipids were assessed as well as immediately following the exercise and 24 and 48 hours after. As expected, the duration of the two exercise intensities was different, 35 ± 7 and 59 ± 12 minutes for the 80% and 60% intensity sessions, respectively. The investigators combined the results of the entire cohort, as they reported no effect of exercise intensity on serum lipid changes. TC and LDL-C each fell by approximately 4% immediately following the exercise and rose to over 5% of the baseline levels after 48 hours, HDL-C levels were immediately elevated by nearly 10% and remained elevated at 48 hours post-exercise (due to elevations in both HDL_2 and HDL_3) and TG levels did not change immediately following the exercise but were 18% and 15% lower at 24 and 48 hours post-exercise, respectively. Apo B also increased at 24 hours and remained elevated after 48 hours. These results suggest that, as long as energy expenditure remains constant, exercise intensity does not influence the acute exercise effects on serum lipids conducted within 1 hour. Of note was the inability of 15 of the subjects in the higher intensity group to complete the exercise in one continuous bout, instead they were allowed to rest and complete the exercise in intervals. This may have affected the results of the higher intensity group and attenuated the differences between the two groups. As exercise intensity dictates the type and proportion of the various energy substrates utilized, the intermittent periods of rest likely affected the energy substrates used, making the session not truly reflective of a continuous bout of exercise. It also would have been preferable to use individual subjects as their own control and have them undergo two separate exercise sessions; this would remove possible interindividual differences with respect to response to exercise. While it is difficult to truly determine the effects of the different exercise intensity, the results suggest that the changes observed in serum lipids may take longer than 48 hours to resolve.

Elevation in HDL-C levels was also observed in a group of nine competitive male cyclists following a 70-minute exercise session.[28] The subjects were instructed to exercise (stationary cycling) for a 60-minute period at 70% VO_{2max} followed by a maximal effort for the duration of the session. This was designed to reflect what commonly occurs during a bicycle race. Each subject completed the test twice, separated by 1 week. Regular diet and activity patterns were allowed between the two sessions. Blood samples were taken before, during and immediately after the exercise session. As expected, there were no differences observed between the two exercise sessions and so the results were combined. Levels of HDL-C were significantly elevated immediately following exercise compared with the baseline levels. No significant changes in TC and TG were apparent.

In contrast, Ferguson et al.[29] investigated the effects of different amounts of energy expenditure from exercise at a constant exercise intensity. Eleven men who participated in regular exercise for the previous year underwent four different exercise sessions to achieve 800, 1100, 1300 and 1500 kcal of expended energy. All exercise sessions were conducted at an intensity of 70% of previously determined VO_{2max} and separated by 2 weeks, during which the subjects were to maintain their regular dietary and exercise habits. Blood samples were collected after a 12-hour fast the day before each exercise session, immediately before and after the session and 24 and 48 hours after. Based on food records collected during the days surrounding the exercise sessions, no variability in eating habits was observed. Both TG and VLDL-C were significantly lower 24 hours after exercise compared with immediately before for all four exercise sessions. For all but the 1500 kcal exercise session, TG and VLDL-C levels had returned to baseline at 48 hours. LDL-C levels were reduced immediately following the exercise session for the 1300 and 1500 sessions only and remained lower at 24 hours in the 1500 kcal session. HDL-C levels were elevated immediately following all exercise sessions, but this was significant only for the longest session (1500 kcal). After 24 hours, HDL-C levels increased and were significant for the 1100, 1300 and 1500 sessions and remained elevated at 48 hours for the 1500 kcal session. This was mainly due to increases in HDL_2 particles and possibly the significant increases in LPL activity observed 24 hours after exercise for the same three exercise sessions. The elevated LPL activity was even apparent after 48 hours in the 1500 kcal session. Significant increases in LDL-C occurred immediately following the 1300 and 1500 sessions. This well-conducted study identified a clear dose-dependent relationship between the caloric expenditure of an acute bout of exercise and changes in serum lipids while controlling for exercise intensity and dietary intake. The authors suggested that the changes observed in TG and HDL-C were mediated by the increased LPL activity, as LPL hydrolyses TG, which in turn would provide substrate for HDL-C production. These results indicate that an exercise bout of 1100 kcal is required to result in significant serum lipid changes that may last for 48 hours.

To extend the investigation of prolonged acute exercise, 39 men and women were studied before and after an acute bout of ultra-endurance exercise (an Ironman triathlon).[30] The average participant completed the exercise session in a mean of 753 ± 128 minutes. Because of the nature of the event, nonfasting baseline blood samples were collected 24 hours prior to the exercise. Compared with baseline, TC, LDL-C, apo B and TG were reduced by 9%, 11%, 10% and 39% respectively. There was also a nonsignificant increase in HDL-C by 3%. Even though the authors did not report any changes in weight, one would expect that, over a period of approximately 12.5 hours, most participants would lose weight through fluid and fat loss. The large decrease in TG levels is expected as the duration of the exercise session and its intensity would require fat as the major energy substrate. These findings are in contrast to previous studies that observed immediate increases in HDL-C and delayed decreases in TG levels due to acute exercise. The absence of a delay in decreasing TG is most likely due to the extreme duration of the exercise. A possible confounding factor that was not addressed by the authors, is the fact that all of these individuals would be consuming high-energy foods during the exercise to replenish their energy stores. Depending on the macronutrients of these foods, this may also have contributed to the dramatic changes in TG levels. The results of this study demonstrate that, under extreme exercise conditions, TG levels and, to a lesser extent, TC, LDL-C and apo B levels, decrease. While an exercise bout of this duration is not common, it does indicate that a longer bout of exercise will result in greater TG changes.

All but one of the above-cited studies were restricted to men and the one that included women did not distinguish by gender. Investigations of the acute effects of exercise and serum lipids in women need to be separately conducted, as many more variables must be accounted for, such as menopausal status, stage of the menstrual cycle, oral contraceptives, among others, as these all affect serum lipid levels.

Skinner et al.[31] studied the effects of completing a marathon in 12 female athletes (average time of completion was 254 ± 28 minutes). Compared with baseline serum lipids assessed 1 hour prior to the start of the race, TC significantly increased by 10.6% and HDL-C significantly increased by 22.8% immediately following the marathon. There was a nonsignificant decrease with respect to VLDL-C levels and no change in LDL-C levels; TG levels or weight changes were not reported. The authors also reported no significant changes in the composition of the HDL particles. The increase in TC is most likely due to the increase in HDL-C. The increase in HDL-C is consistent with studies in men, although this occurred to a much greater extent in the women. Of note is that five of the subjects were using oral contraceptives at the time, which are known to influence serum lipids.[32] While the authors reported no difference in the results between those using oral contraceptives and those who were not, it is possible that the small sample size may have limited this observation. The author also did not control for possible variations in the menstrual cycle of the subjects, which also affects serum lipids.[33]

Another study investigated 11 pre- and 10 postmenopausal women.[34] All subjects were sedentary but otherwise healthy and none were known to be using oral contraceptives. The investigators studied two isocaloric bouts of exercise (350 kcal) at two different intensities: 50% and 70% VO_{2max}, determined from an initial maximal exercise test. The exercise sessions were conducted during the early follicular phase of the menstrual cycle for the premenopausal women based on self-report. The order of the two exercise sessions was randomly determined and they were held approximately 1 month apart to control for menstrual cycle variation. Baseline serum lipids were assessed 24 hours prior, immediately after and 24 and 48 hours after the exercise sessions. All samples were taken under fasting conditions. All subjects were provided a defined diet and asked to maintain their weight throughout the study. With respect to the premenopausal women, TC and LDL-C were significantly lower following each exercise session compared with baseline levels and the decreases in TC and LDL-C were much greater following the higher intensity exercise session. In contrast, TG levels increased significantly by nearly 7% immediately after the exercise sessions and there were no differences between the intensities. All levels returned to baseline within 24 hours. Levels of HDL-C, HDL_2 and HDL_3 remained similar to baseline. In the postmenopausal women, LDL-C levels increased after the low intensity exercise session and decreased following the high intensity exercise session and the difference between these changes was significant. A similar observation was noted in TG levels, which decreased after the low intensity exercise session and increased following the high intensity exercise session; again, the difference between these changes was significant. All levels returned to baseline within 24 hours. There were no differences in TC, HDL-C and HDL_3 levels, but HDL_2 levels were significantly higher immediately following both exercise sessions. As expected, the postmenopausal women were older, had greater body mass index and lower exercise capacity compared with the premenopausal subjects; no other comparisons were provided between the two groups. The authors concluded that the intensity of the exercise does affect the changes in TC and LDL-C immediately following exercise in women. The changes in TC and LDL-C observed in this study are consistent with those reported by the same authors in a similar study in men undergoing a 350 kcal exercise bout as mentioned above.[27] In contrast, the study in men did not report a difference in the effects based on exercise intensity and TG actually decreased immediately following the exercise sessions. It is possible that men and women may have opposing results with respect to TG changes following acute exercise. Despite being a well controlled study, the small sample size may limit definitive conclusions to be drawn.

A more recent study investigated the effect of exercise duration on serum lipids.[35] The authors studied seven healthy sedentary premenopausal women following both a 30- and 60-minute bout of exercise conducted at 60% of pre-determined VO_{2max}. None of the women had previously taken oral contraceptives or had any weight changes greater than 1 kg during the previous year. Both exercise sessions were completed during the follicular phase of the menstrual cycle as determined by basal temperature. All subjects stayed on a metabolic ward during the experimental procedures and dietary intake was kept constant. Baseline serum lipids were assessed following a 12-hour fast and immediately prior to exercise. Subsequent samples were collected as follows: immediately, 30 minutes, 1 hour, 2 hours and 24 hours after the exercise sessions. The two exercise sessions were held 3 days apart and assigned in a random order. There were no significant changes in any of the lipid variables assessed over the various time points for both exercise durations compared with baseline. There was however, a nonsignificant decrease in TG levels that was more pronounced following the 60-minute exercise session and remained lower for all time periods. Again, this study may have been limited by the low number of study subjects.

While a number of the previous studies investigated the effects of acute exercise on LPL activity, very few have reported on changes to hepatic lipase activity. A study of 12 male runners assessed fasting hepatic lipase activity 24 hours prior to (baseline), 6 hours after and 24 hours after a bout of exercise expending 800 kcal.[36] HDL-C and HDL$_3$ levels were significantly higher 24 hours after the exercise session than before and this was coincident with a significant increase in LPL and a decrease in HL activities. However, these results were not corroborated in a more recent study of acute exercise in sedentary men with normal and elevated levels of cholesterol.[37] These authors investigated a bout of 500 kcal of treadmill running and reported significant increases in HDL-C and HDL$_3$ along with decreased TG levels 24 hours after the exercise bout compared with 24 hours prior; these lasted for 48 hours. There were no significant changes in HL activity but LPL activity was increased significantly at 24 and 48 hours after the exercise session. It is possible that the exercise bout was not a sufficient stimulus to change HL activity. The inclusion of hypercholesterolemic subjects may also have affected the results, as it is likely that these individuals already have an altered lipid metabolism. These results suggest that acute exercise may modify HL activity and is possibly implicated in the resultant lipoprotein changes observed, however, changes in LPL activity likely have a much more predominant role.

Studies of men, both sedentary and previously trained, indicate that TG levels decrease in the days following activity and HDL-C increases immediately following exercise and may be elevated for up to 24 hours. Some studies observed immediate decreases to TC and LDL-C as well, but this was less consistent. The changes in TG and HDL-C appear to be mediated through changes in LPL and HL and longer exercise bouts result in greater changes observed over a longer duration following the activity. Investigations with women are less clear, due to the influence of hormones on serum lipids and the much smaller sample sizes of these investigations. Of the studies reviewed, no consistent alteration in serum lipids is apparent, however, it is likely that exercise does exert some influence on serum lipids that may last for 24 hours. It is unclear from the current studies on women whether exercise intensity affects the lipid changes.

D. Effects of Exercise on Other Lipid Parameters

A number of other parameters of lipid metabolism have been investigated with respect to their response to exercise: Lp(a), ox-LDL-C, LCAT and CETP. Levels of evidence for each vary, and definitive conclusions have not been reached for all. This section will describe some of the available literature to date and provide some perspective.

The Lp(a) particle is a lipoprotein that shares some characteristics with the LDL particle such as a LDL-like core and an apo B protein. The Lp(a) particle is different in that it is also linked to an apo (a) protein. Interest in the Lp(a) particle and exercise arises from its implication as a risk factor for coronary artery disease.[38] Two review articles concluded that there is a consistent lack of association between moderate exercise and Lp(a) levels.[39,40] Their conclusions were based on similar levels of Lp(a) between athletes and nonathletes and the lack of changes in levels following either a chronic or acute exercise intervention in sedentary and athletic individuals. Two studies did, however, show a difference in Lp(a) levels following a more intense exercise regimen. The first study investigated 36 sedentary men and women who trained for 9 months for a 21 km running race.[41] At the end of the training session, Lp(a) levels were significantly higher than baseline for both men and women. This study did not have a control group to compare with. The second study investigated 219 men and women with a number of coronary artery disease risk factors in four different groups: diet alone, exercise alone, diet and exercise, and control for 1 year.[42] The exercise intervention consisted of 1 hour of exercise three times per week at 60% to 80% of measured peak heart rate. The investigators reported a significant increase in Lp(a) levels for the exercise and diet and exercise-only groups compared with baseline levels. These two studies suggest that more structured regular exercise for a long period of time may modestly increase Lp(a) levels. Neither of the increases in Lp(a) levels were considered to put the individuals at increased cardiovascular risk. It has been suggested that the increased levels may be the result of adaptations to regular muscle cell damage.[40]

Interest in the oxidation of LDL particles has been studied due to increased plasma free radical concentration that occurs with intense exercise training.[43] This led to speculation that regular exercise may increase the concentration of circulating ox-LDL and thereby impart an increased cardiovascular risk. However, this has not been borne out in recent investigations. Compared with sedentary controls of similar age and body mass index (BMI), trained runners actually had a significantly lower susceptibility for LDL oxidation as determined by *in vitro* methods.[44] This was also observed in comparisons between groups of adolescent women who participated in gymnastics or running to controls.[45] The authors did not report the measure of ox-LDL alone, but noted a significantly lower ratio of ox-LDL:LDL particles in the group of gymnasts compared with controls that remained significant after adjusting for BMI differences. The lack of a significant difference between the controls and the runners was thought to be a result of a lower amount of exercise participation in the runners (compared with the runners, the gymnasts participated in nearly double the weekly amount of exercise). Only one study to date has investigated the effects of an exercise intervention on ox-LDL in sedentary men and women.[46] A total of 104 sedentary men and women completed a 10-month exercise program that resulted in a significant increase in VO_{2max} of 19% and a decrease in weight. The amount of circulating ox-LDL decreased significantly by 23% and 26% for men and women respectively. While there was no significant change in the antioxidant potential of LDL particles, the ratio of the antioxidant potential of LDL to LDL-C increased significantly in men and women. Despite a significant increase in VO_{2max} and decrease in weight, these changes did not correlate with changes in ox-LDL suggesting a possible independent mechanism. These results indicate that chronic exercise may lead to decreased ox-LDL particles, but it does not provide insight into the potential of prolonged exercise, which is most commonly associated with increased free radical production. A study of 39 men and women found the susceptibility of lipids to oxidation to decrease significantly immediately following completion of an Ironman triathlon compared with baseline levels assessed 2 days prior to the event.[30] This occurred regardless of prior antioxidant dietary supplementation. Taken together, these studies suggest that participation in regular exercise does not lead to increased levels of ox-LD particles and, in fact, indicates that exercise may actually reduce the amount of circulation of ox-LDL and the susceptibility of LDL particles to be oxidized.

Two enzymes involved with lipid metabolism, CETP and LCAT, have also been investigated to elucidate the mechanisms behind the changes in the various lipid parameters. Investigation of 57 men and women who had undergone a 9-month exercise regimen revealed that CETP concentration significantly decreased in both men and women as a result of the exercise intervention.[47] Although not corrected for possible increases in plasma volume that occur with exercise, the decreased CETP concentration is consistent with the increases observed in HDL-C. With respect to LCAT, also involved in the modification of HDL particles, a 1-year exercise program did not result in any significant changes in LCAT mass compared with the randomly assigned control group.[48] This result is not surprising, given that there were no significant changes in any of the serum lipids assessed. A study of a group of sedentary and a group of trained healthy men found that, following a maximal exercise stress test to exhaustion, LCAT activity increased significantly immediately after exercise compared with pre-exercise values in both groups.[49] This occurred coincident with increases in HDL-C. As LCAT is involved in the maturation of HDL_3 to HDL_2, one would expect that an increased LCAT activity would result in greater HDL_2 particles, as discussed previously — exercise is associated with increased HDL_2 particles. With only a few research studies reporting assessment of CETP and LCAT with respect to exercise, implicating changes in these enzymes to those in the various lipoproteins is difficult. However, based on these studies, there is cursory evidence that changes in CETP and LCAT are consistent with increased HDL-C levels.

IV. Influence of the Menstrual Cycle on Lipids

A number of studies have investigated the association between the phases of the menstrual cycle and serum lipid levels. A study of 54 healthy women compared serum lipids during the luteal and follicular phase of the menstrual cycle.[50] The authors reported that TC, LDL-C and apo B were significantly lower during the luteal phase compared with the follicular phase, while HDL-C and TG were unchanged. A later well controlled study investigated 16 healthy women during one full menstrual cycle while maintaining a diet of 30% kcal from fat.[33] TC and LDL-C were reported to be lower and HDL-C levels higher during the luteal phase compared with the follicular phase. Changes in serum lipid levels were associated with changes in endogenous sex hormones. While it is apparent that serum lipid levels change throughout the female menstrual cycle, this is generally not considered with respect to timing of lipid assessment.

An important factor to consider when interpreting serum lipid levels in women is their menstrual status. Premenopausal women tend to have lower TC, LDL-C and TG with higher HDL-C levels compared with men at a similar age. However, once menstruation ceases, these differences are less pronounced, such that postmenopausal women have higher TC, LDL-C and TG and lower HDL-C than premenopausal women independent of age.[51,52]

V. Female Athletes with Amenorrhea

Women presenting with amenorrhea tend to have lower levels of estrogen, lower percent body fat and a more adverse lipid profile than controls. Compared with sedentary controls, the prevalence of amenorrhea is much higher in female athletes.[53,54] A number of studies investigating whether amenorrhea secondary to exercise has negative effects on serum lipids have reported either no difference in serum lipids,[58] a nonsignificant trend toward a more adverse lipid profile[56] or significant adverse differences in lipid profile among female athletes with amenorrhea.[55,57] The studies that reported no significant differences used small sample sizes and similar BMI and percent body fat between the eumenorrheic and amenorrheic female athletes. The largest study conducted compared 24 amenorrheic female athletes with 31 regularly menstruating controls.[57] The amenorrheic individuals were slightly younger and had significantly higher TC, LDL-C, TG, HDL-C and HDL$_2$ levels than the controls. This was coincident with significantly lower estradiol and progesterone levels as well as lower BMI, dietary fat content and a higher training volume in the women with amenorrhea. The serum lipids of the amenorrheic women were also noted to be much higher than those reported in the Lipid Research Clinics population for women of the same age. Due to the elevated HDL-C level in the amenorrheic women, the TC/HDL-C ratio was similar between groups. A smaller study reported significantly higher LDL-C levels in eight female athletes with amenorrhea than in nine regularly menstruating athletes.[55] There were no differences between the two groups with respect to HDL-C levels, BMI, VO$_{2max}$ or percent body fat. The women with amenorrhea did, however, consume significantly fewer dietary calories. The cause of amenorrhea in this population is unclear, but its presence has been consistently associated with lower estradiol and progesterone levels as well as lower dietary fat and caloric intake.[55-57] Further research needs to be conducted on this subject, but these studies indicate that the presence of amenorrhea secondary to exercise may adversely affect serum lipids. Therefore, assessment of serum lipids in female athletes must take this into consideration.

VI. Methodological Considerations Prior to Lipid Assessment

A number of factors (physiological and environmental) can dramatically alter circulating lipid levels and must be considered to determine when to assess serum lipids and how to interpret the results. These factors include exercise, menstrual status, weight change, age, alcohol, fasting, smoking and drugs. As discussed in detail in earlier sections of this chapter, regular exercise can result in decreased TC, LDL-C, TG and apo B and increases in HDL-C and apo A. Evidence suggests that this can occur due to an acute bout of exercise and regular exercise participation. Therefore, analysis of lipids should be avoided within 48 hours of a strenuous bout of exercise. A female's menstrual status may also influence lipid levels as discussed above, but these variations are minimal and should not influence when analyses are conducted. Lipid analysis should also be avoided in subjects who are actively losing weight, as weight loss can dramatically affect LDL-C, HDL-C and TG levels; lipids should be assessed once weight loss has finished. Age is another factor that can influence lipid levels; as one ages, lipid levels may slowly increase.[59] Recent alcohol intake can result in elevation of TG levels.[60] To avoid the effects of alcohol on TG, subjects should abstain from alcohol for at least 48 hours before a blood sample is drawn. To properly interpret a comprehensive lipid profile, blood samples should be obtained after an overnight fast of 12 hours. Fasting is required to interpret the TG levels and also to permit the determination of LDL-C. In general, TC and HDL-C levels are not affected by the fasting state. During the 12-hour fast, subjects are permitted to drink water only. Smoking is a major factor that has shown to lower HDL-C levels.[61] Several drugs also known to cause hypertriglyceridemia include B-blockers, glucocorticoids, exogenous estrogens and retinoids. It is not recommended that these medications be discontinued prior to assessing lipids. Use of anabolic steroids can adversely affect lipid levels such that TC, LDL-C and TG are elevated and HDL-C is reduced.[62] While timing of lipid assessment need only take into consideration exercise, weight loss, alcohol and fasting status, it is important to capture numerous other variables to properly interpret the results.

Lipid analysis is normally conducted in serum. Blood samples should be centrifuged and serum separated within 1 hour of being drawn. Serum samples may be stored up to 1 week at 4°C prior to analysis. Serum can also be stored frozen at –70°C indefinitely but frozen samples should not be used for lipid particle sizing assays.

VII. Methods

Methods should be standardized to Centers of Disease Control (CDC) – Cholesterol Reference Method Laboratory Network using appropriate calibrators and internal controls. Analysis performance should be monitored using CDC redeemed external quality control samples. Total cholesterol, HDL-C and TG are measured using automated enzymatic assays, which use a series of linked enzyme reactions to generate metabolic products that are used to produce a colored product from a chromogen (dye). The colored product generated is measured spectrophotometrically. Total cholesterol enzyme-based reagents include cholesterol esterase, cholesterol oxidase and peroxidase. Cholesterol esterase is used to liberate cholesterol and fatty acids from cholesterol esters. Cholesterol from this reaction is then used to generate H_2O_2 using cholesterol oxidase. The H_2O_2 produced by this reaction is used to generate a colored product from a chromogen. A commonly used chromogen is 4-aminoantipyrine. HDL-C is measured by precipitating non-HDL cholesterol with heparin and then measuring the TC remaining in the extracted serum. Most laboratories measure LDL-C indirectly, using the Friedewald equation:[63]

$$LDL\text{-}C = TC - HDL\text{-}C - TG/5 \qquad (mg/dL)$$

$$LDL\text{-}C = TC - HDL\text{-}C - TG/2.22 \qquad (mmol/L)$$

This equation is valid if the TG levels are less than 5 mmol/L. In those subjects with TG above 5 mmol/L, LDL-C can be measured directly. Triglyceride enzyme-based assays use a lipase to hydrolyse triglycerides to glycerol and fatty acids. Glycerol kinase is then used to phosphorylate the glycerol liberated by the lipase reaction. Glycerol phosphate is then used to generate the formation of a colored product (commonly quinone-imine). The amount of colored product is monitored spectrophotometrically.

LDL and HDL particle size is most commonly measured using sizing gel protein electrophoresis. A number of reference laboratories may also use nuclear magnetic resonance to determine LDL and HDL particle size. Apo B and apo A levels are measured in routine laboratories, commonly using automated nephelometric assays. Apo B and apo A levels can also be measured by immunoassays such as radial immunodiffusion and radioimmuno assays. These assays are generally performed manually and can be done in small laboratories. Lp(a) is measured by immunoassays, including manual radioimmunoassy and automated nonisotropic immunoassay analyses. Commercially available radioimmunoassay kits are available for the assessment of Lp(a).

Assays for LPL and HL have not been standardized and are available only at reference laboratories. Samples for LPL and HL activity and mass are obtained 5 minutes following the infusion of 60,000 units per kg weight of heparin. Standardized protocols must be followed to collect and process samples, which also must be frozen rapidly to avoid loss of activity and mass.

Assessment of ox-LDL, LCAT and CETP require specialized assays and are not widely available other than in research settings.

VIII.   Lipid Level Recommendations

Several national and international organizations have established guidelines and recommendations for lipid levels. For simplicity, reference will be made to the most recent recommendations from the National Cholesterol Education Program recently released.[64] Measurement of a full lipid profile (TC, LDL-C, HDL-C and TG) is recommended beginning at age 20 and then every 5 years after for cardiovascular risk factor screening. Table 11.1 outlines the classification of the various lipid parameters. In addition to assessing the standard lipid profile, calculation of the TC/HDL-C ration is also recommended, as this ratio has been demonstrated to have the greatest predictive power with respect to cardiovascular mortality.[65] A TC/HDL-C ratio below 4 is considered optimal, while a ratio above 5 is considered to be high.[66] Generally, assessment of other lipid parameters (apo B, apo A, Lp(a), particle size, LPL, HL, etc.) is not recommended for cardiovascular risk screening. However, in certain individuals with preexisting disease, assessment of these additional parameters may be of use in determining attributable risk, such as those with normal lipid levels or in those believed to have a genetic predisposition to adverse lipid levels.

TABLE 11.1

Classification of TC, LDL-C, HDL-C and TG by the NCEP[64]

Total Cholesterol (mg/dL)

< 200	Desirable
200–239	Borderline high
≥ 239	High

LDL-C (mg/dL)

< 100	Optimal
100–129	Near optimal/above optimal
130–159	Borderline high
160–189	High
≥ 190	Very high

HDL-C (mg/dL)

< 40	Low
≥ 60	High

Triglycerides (mg/dL)

< 150	Normal
150–199	Borderline high
200–499	High
≥ 500	Very high

IX.   Summary

Based on the numerous investigations, it is well accepted that men and women who exercise regularly have a more favorable lipid profile compared with sedentary men and women of a similar age. However, these studies have not been able to address the question as to whether regular exercise is responsible for these observed differences. While not all investigations of sedentary men and women undergoing a regular exercise routine have conclusively demonstrated improvements in serum lipids, there is consistent evidence that HDL-C levels increase while TC, LDL-C and TG levels decrease compared with either pre-exercise levels or with nonexercising controls. Many of these studies also noted concomitant reductions in weight, predominantly due to fat loss. Changes in weight make it difficult to determine if lipid changes are directly due to exercise or indirectly due to exercise-related weight loss. Those studies that have observed weight loss generally report greater changes in serum lipid levels. However, none of these studies have reported changes in lipids to the extent that they approach those levels of athletes. This is likely because the exercise interventions are not able to replicate the intensity, frequency and duration of the exercise practices of athletes. As a result of these observed effects of chronic exercise, studies also investigated the effects of acute exercise. Despite a lack of consistent results due to inconsistencies in methodology across the different studies, acute exercise exerts an immediate effect on lipid levels that may persist for up to 48 hours. These changes consist of decreased TC, LDL-C and TG and increased HDL-C demonstrated in men, with changes in lipids in women not as clear as a result of the limited studies available. Evidence also suggests that the longer the duration of the activity or the greater the number of calories expended, the greater the change.

Assessment of serum lipids (TC, LDL-C, HDL-C and TG) in athletes is recommended to begin at age 20 for the purpose of screening for cardiovascular risk and then every 5 years thereafter. Prior to assessment, it is important that individuals abstain from alcohol for a 48-hour period and from food for 12 hours and it is suggested that they abstain from strenuous exercise in the 48 hours preceding the assessment. Factors that must be taken into consideration when interpreting the results include medication use, menopausal status, age and smoking status.

Despite the great number of studies that have investigated exercise and lipids, there are still some unanswered questions. Future research should be directed at investigations of chronic exercise on lipids while controlling for weight changes, the effect of varying intensities of exercise on both chronic and acute changes as well as investigations on women using larger sample sizes.

References

1. Vodak, P.A., Wood, P.D., Haskell, W.L. and Williams, P.T., HDL-cholesterol and other plasma lipid and lipoprotein concentrations in middle-aged male and female tennis players, *Metabolism* 29 (8), 745, 1980.
2. Berg, A., Keul, J., Ringwald, G., Deus, B. and Wybitul, K., Physical performance and serum cholesterol fractions in healthy young men, *Clin Chim Acta* 106 (3), 325, 1980.
3. Ericsson, M., Johnson, O., Tollin, C., Furberg, B., Backman, C. and Angquist, K., Serum lipoproteins, apolipoproteins and intravenous fat tolerance in young athletes, *Scand J Rehabil Med* 14 (4), 209, 1982.
4. Thompson, P.D., Cullinane, E.M., Sady, S.P., Flynn, M.M., Chenevert, C.B. and Herbert, P.N.,High density lipoprotein metabolism in endurance athletes and sedentary men, *Circulation* 84 (1), 140, 1991.
5. Williams, P.T., Krauss, R.M., Wood, P.D., Lindgren, F.T., Giotas, C. and Vranizan, K.M.,Lipoprotein subfractions of runners and sedentary men, *Metabolism* 35 (1), 45, 1986.
6. Lakka, T.A. and Salonen, J.T., Physical activity and serum lipids: a cross-sectional population study in eastern Finnish men, *Am J Epidemiol* 136 (7), 806, 1992.

7. Williams, P.T., High-density lipoprotein cholesterol and other risk factors for coronary heart disease in female runners, *N Engl J Med* 334 (20), 1298, 1996.

8. Williams, P.T., Relationship of distance run per week to coronary heart disease risk factors in 8283 male runners. The National Runners' Health Study, Arch *Intern Med* 157 (2), 191, 1997.

9. MacAuley, D., McCrum, E.E., Stott, G., Evans, A.E., Duly, E., Trinick, T.R., Sweeney, K. and Boreham, C.A.,Physical fitness, lipids and apolipoproteins in the Northern Ireland Health and Activity Survey, *Med Sci Sports Exerc* 29 (9), 1187, 1997.

10. Kostka, T., Lacour, J.R., Berthouze, S.E. and Bonnefoy, M., Relationship of physical activity and fitness to lipid and lipoprotein (a) in elderly subjects, *Med Sci Sports Exerc* 31 (8), 1183, 1999.

11. Leon, A.S. and Sanchez, O.A., Response of blood lipids to exercise training alone or combined with dietary intervention, *Med Sci Sports Exerc* 33 (6 Suppl), S502, 2001.

12. Kokkinos, P.F. and Fernhall, B., Physical activity and high density lipoprotein cholesterol levels: what is the relationship?, *Sports Med* 28 (5), 307, 1999.

13. Despres, J.P. and Lamarche, B., Low-intensity endurance exercise training, plasma lipoproteins and the risk of coronary heart disease, *J Intern Med* 236 (1), 7, 1994.

14. Williams, P.T., Wood, P.D., Haskell, W.L. and Vranizan, K., The effects of running mileage and duration on plasma lipoprotein levels, *JAMA* 247 (19), 2674, 1982.

15. Wood, P.D., Stefanick, M.L., Dreon, D.M., Frey-Hewitt, B., Garay, S.C., Williams, P.T., Superko, H.R., Fortmann, S.P., Albers, J.J., Vranizan, K.M. et al., Changes in plasma lipids and lipoproteins in overweight men during weight loss through dieting as compared with exercise, *N Engl J Med* 319 (18), 1173, 1988.

16. Williams, P.T., Krauss, R.M., Vranizan, K.M. and Wood, P.D., Changes in lipoprotein subfractions during diet-induced and exercise-induced weight loss in moderately overweight men, *Circulation* 81 (4), 1293, 1990.

17. Stefanick, M.L., Terry, R.B., Haskell, W.L. and Wood, P.D., Relationships of changes in postheparin hepatic and lipoprotein lipase to HDL-cholesterol changes following weight loss acheived by dieting versus exercise, in *Cardiovascular Disease: Molecular and Cellular Mechanisms, Prevention and Treatment*, Gallo, L., Ed., Plenum, Washington, D.C., 1987, pp. 61.

18. Stefanick, M.L., Mackey, S., Sheehan, M., Ellsworth, N., Haskell, W.L. and Wood, P.D., Effects of diet and exercise in men and postmenopausal women with low levels of HDL cholesterol and high levels of LDL cholesterol, *N Engl J Med* 339 (1), 12, 1998.

19. Blumenthal, J.A., Matthews, K., Fredrikson, M., Rifai, N., Schniebolk, S., German, D., Steege, J. and Rodin, J., Effects of exercise training on cardiovascular function and plasma lipid, lipoprotein and apolipoprotein concentrations in premenopausal and postmenopausal women, *Arterioscler Thromb* 11 (4), 912, 1991.

20. Grandjean, P.W., Crouse, S.F., O'Brien, B.C., Rohack, J.J. and Brown, J.A.,The effects of menopausal status and exercise training on serum lipids and the activities of intravascular enzymes related to lipid transport, *Metabolism* 47 (4), 377, 1998.

21. Halbert, J.A., Silagy, C.A., Finucane, P., Withers, R.T. and Hamdorf, P.A., Exercise training and blood lipids in hyperlipidemic and normolipidemic adults: a meta-analysis of randomized, controlled trials, *Eur J Clin Nutr* 53 (7), 514, 1999.

22. Thompson, P.D., Cullinane, E.M., Sady, S.P., Flynn, M.M., Bernier, D.N., Kantor, M.A., Saritelli, A.L. and Herbert, P.N.,Modest changes in high-density lipoprotein concentration and metabolism with prolonged exercise training, *Circulation* 78 (1), 25, 1988.

23. Simsolo, R.B., Ong, J.M. and Kern, P.A., The regulation of adipose tissue and muscle lipoprotein lipase in runners by detraining, *J Clin Invest* 92 (5), 2124, 1993.

24. Giada, F., Vigna, G.B., Vitale, E., Baldo-Enzi, G., Bertaglia, M., Crecca, R. and Fellin, R., Effect of age on the response of blood lipids, body composition and aerobic power to physical conditioning and deconditioning, *Metabolism* 44 (2), 161, 1995.

25. Cullinane, E., Siconolfi, S., Saritelli, A. and Thompson, P.D., Acute decrease in serum triglycerides with exercise: is there a threshold for an exercise effect?, *Metabolism* 31 (8), 844, 1982.

26. Klein, L., Miller, T.D., Radam, T.E., O'Brien, T., Nguyen, T.T. and Kottke, B.A., Acute physical exercise alters apolipoprotein E and C-III concentrations of apo E-rich very low density lipoprotein fraction, *Atherosclerosis* 97 (1), 37, 1992.

27. Crouse, S.F., O'Brien, B.C., Rohack, J.J., Lowe, R.C., Green, J.S., Tolson, H. and Reed, J.L., Changes in serum lipids and apolipoproteins after exercise in men with high cholesterol: influence of intensity, *J Appl Physiol* 79 (1), 279, 1995.

28. El-Sayed, M.S. and Rattu, A.J., Changes in lipid profile variables in response to submaximal and maximal exercise in trained cyclists, *Eur J Appl Occup Physiol* 73 (1-2), 88, 1996.

29. Ferguson, M.A., Alderson, N.L., Trost, S.G., Essig, D.A., Burke, J.R. and Durstine, J.L., Effects of four different single exercise sessions on lipids, lipoproteins and lipoprotein lipase, *J Appl Physiol* 85 (3), 1169, 1998.

30. Ginsburg, G.S., Agil, A., O'Toole, M., Rimm, E., Douglas, P.S. and Rifai, N., Effects of a single bout of ultraendurance exercise on lipid levels and susceptibility of lipids to peroxidation in triathletes, *JAMA* 276 (3), 221, 1996.

31. Skinner, E.R., Watt, C. and Maughan, R.J., The acute effect of marathon running on plasma lipoproteins in female subjects, *Eur J Appl Physiol Occup Physiol* 56 (4), 451, 1987.

32. Patsch, W., Brown, S.A., Gotto, A.M., Jr. and Young, R.L., The effect of triphasic oral contraceptives on plasma lipids and lipoproteins, *Am J Obstet Gynecol* 161 (5), 1396, 1989.

33. Tonolo, G., Ciccarese, M., Brizzi, P., Milia, S., Dessole, S., Puddu, L., Secchi, G. and Maioli, M., Cyclical variation of plasma lipids, apolipoproteins and lipoprotein(a) during menstrual cycle of normal women, *Am J Physiol* 269 (6 Pt 1), E1101, 1995.

34. Pronk, N.P., Crouse, S.F., O'Brien, B.C. and Rohack, J.J., Acute effects of walking on serum lipids and lipoproteins in women, *J Sports Med Phys Fitness* 35 (1), 50, 1995.

35. Imamura, H., Katagiri, S., Uchid, K., Miyamoto, N., Nakano, H. and Shirota, T., Acute effects of moderate exercise on serum lipids, lipoproteins and apolipoproteins in sedentary young women, *Clin Exp Pharmacol Physiol* 27 (12), 975, 2000.

36. Gordon, P.M., Visich, P.S., Goss, F.L., Fowler, S., Warty, V., Denys, B.J., Metz, K.F. and Robertson, J., Comparison of exercise and normal variability on HDL cholesterol concentrations and lipolytic activity, *Int J Sports Med* 17 (5), 332, 1996.

37. Grandjean, P.W., Crouse, S.F. and Rohack, J.J., Influence of cholesterol status on blood lipid and lipoprotein enzyme responses to aerobic exercise, *J Appl Physiol* 89 (2), 472, 2000.

38. Wild, S.H., Fortmann, S.P. and Marcovina, S.M., A prospective case-control study of lipoprotein(a) levels and apo(a) size and risk of coronary heart disease in Stanford Five-City Project participants, *Arterioscler Thromb Vasc Biol* 17 (2), 239, 1997.

39. Mackinnon, L.T., Hubinger, L. and Lepre, F., Effects of physical activity and diet on lipoprotein(a), *Med Sci Sports Exerc* 29 (11), 1429, 1997.

40. Mackinnon, L.T. and Hubinger, L.M., Effects of exercise on lipoprotein(a), *Sports Med* 28 (1), 11, 1999.

41. Ponjee, G.A., Janssen, E.M. and van Wersch, J.W., Long-term physical exercise and lipoprotein(a) levels in a previously sedentary male and female population, *Ann Clin Biochem* 32 (Pt 2), 181, 1995.

42. Holme, I., Urdal, P., Anderssen, S. and Hjermann, I., Exercise-induced increase in lipoprotein (a), *Atherosclerosis* 122 (1), 97, 1996.

43. Chance, B., Sies, H. and Boveris, A., Hydroperoxide metabolism in mammalian organs, *Physiol Rev* 59 (3), 527, 1979.

44. Sanchez-Quesada, J.L., Ortega, H., Payes-Romero, A., Serrat-Serrat, J., Gonzalez-Sastre, F., Lasuncion, M.A. and Ordonez-Llanos, J., LDL from aerobically-trained subjects shows higher resistance to oxidative modification than LDL from sedentary subjects, *Atherosclerosis* 132 (2), 207, 1997.

45. Vasankari, T., Lehtonen-Veromaa, M., Mottonen, T., Ahotupa, M., Irjala, K., Heinonen, O., Leino, A. and Viikari, J.,Reduced mildly oxidized LDL in young female athletes, *Atherosclerosis* 151 (2), 399, 2000.

46. Vasankari, T.J., Kujala, U.M., Vasankari, T.M. and Ahotupa, M., Reduced oxidized LDL levels after a 10-month exercise program, *Med Sci Sports Exerc* 30 (10), 1496, 1998.

47. Seip, R.L., Moulin, P., Cocke, T., Tall, A., Kohrt, W.M., Mankowitz, K., Semenkovich, C.F., Ostlund, R. and Schonfeld, G., Exercise training decreases plasma cholesteryl ester transfer protein, *Arterioscler Thromb* 13 (9), 1359, 1993.

48. Williams, P.T., Albers, J.J., Krauss, R.M. and Wood, P.D.,Associations of lecithin:cholesterol acyltransferase (LCAT) mass concentrations with exercise, weight loss and plasma lipoprotein subfraction concentrations in men, *Atherosclerosis* 82 (1-2), 53, 1990.

49. Frey, I., Baumstark, M.W., Berg, A. and Keul, J., Influence of acute maximal exercise on lecithin:cholesterol acyltransferase activity in healthy adults of differing aerobic performance, *Eur J Appl Physiol Occup Physiol* 62 (1), 31, 1991.

50. Schijf, C.P., van der Mooren, M.J., Doesburg, W.H., Thomas, C.M. and Rolland, R., Differences in serum lipids, lipoproteins, sex hormone binding globulin and testosterone between the follicular and the luteal phase of the menstrual cycle, *Acta Endocrinol (Copenh)* 129 (2), 130, 1993.

51. Poehlman, E.T., Toth, M.J., Ades, P.A. and Rosen, C.J., Menopause-associated changes in plasma lipids, insulin-like growth factor I and blood pressure: a longitudinal study, *Eur J Clin Invest* 27 (4), 322, 1997.

52. Stevenson, J.C., Crook, D. and Godsland, I.F., Influence of age and menopause on serum lipids and lipoproteins in healthy women, *Atherosclerosis* 98 (1), 83, 1993.

53. Munster, K., Helm, P. and Schmidt, L., Secondary amenorrhea: prevalence and medical contact — a cross-sectional study from a Danish county, *Br J Obstet Gynaecol* 99 (5), 430, 1992.

54. Tomten, S.E., Prevalence of menstrual dysfunction in Norwegian long-distance runners participating in the Oslo Marathon games, *Scand J Med Sci Sports* 6 (3), 164, 1996.

55. Kaiserauer, S., Snyder, A.C., Sleeper, M. and Zierath, J.,Nutritional, physiological and menstrual status of distance runners, *Med Sci Sports Exerc* 21 (2), 120, 1989.

56. Lamon-Fava, S., Fisher, E.C., Nelson, M.E., Evans, W.J., Millar, J.S., Ordovas, J.M. and Schaefer, E.J., Effect of exercise and menstrual cycle status on plasma lipids, low density lipoprotein particle size and apolipoproteins, *J Clin Endocrinol Metab* 68 (1), 17, 1989.

57. Friday, K.E., Drinkwater, B.L., Bruemmer, B., Chesnut, C., 3rd and Chait, A., Elevated plasma low-density lipoprotein and high-density lipoprotein cholesterol levels in amenorrheic athletes: effects of endogenous hormone status and nutrient intake, *J Clin Endocrinol Metab* 77 (6), 1605, 1993.

58. Perry, A.C., Crane, L.S., Applegate, B., Marquez-Sterling, S., Signorile, J.F. and Miller, P.C., Nutrient intake and psychological and physiological assessment in eumenorrheic and amenorrheic female athletes: a preliminary study, *Int J Sport Nutr* 6 (1), 3, 1996.

59. Connor, S.L., Connor, W.E., Sexton, G., Calvin, L. and Bacon, S., The effects of age, body weight and family relationships on plasma lipoproteins and lipids in men, women and children of randomly selected families, *Circulation* 65 (7), 1290, 1982.

60. Frohlich, J.J., Effects of alcohol on plasma lipoprotein metabolism, *Clin Chim Acta* 246 (1-2), 39, 1996.

61. Eagles, C.J. and Martin, U., Non-pharmacological modification of cardiac risk factors: part 3. Smoking cessation and alcohol consumption, *J Clin Pharm Ther* 23 (1), 1, 1998.

62. Labib, M. and Haddon, A., The adverse effects of anabolic steroids on serum lipids, *Ann Clin Biochem* 33 (Pt 3), 263, 1996.

63. Friedewald, W.T., Levy, R.I. and Fredrickson, D.S., Estimation of the concentration of low-density lipoprotein cholesterol in plasma, without use of the preparative ultracentrifuge, *Clin Chem* 18 (6), 499, 1972.

64. Anonymous, Executive summary of the third report of the National Cholesterol Education Program (NCEP) expert panel on detection, evaluation and treatment of high blood cholesterol in adults (Adult Treatment Panel III), *JAMA* 285 (19), 2486, 2001.

65. Grover, S.A., Palmer, C.S. and Coupal, L., Serum lipid screening to identify high-risk individuals for coronary death. The results of the Lipid Research Clinics prevalence cohort, *Arch Intern Med* 154 (6), 679, 1994.

66. Fodor, J.G., Frohlich, J.J., Genest, J.J., Jr. and McPherson, P.R., Recommendations for the management and treatment of dyslipidemia. Report of the Working Group on Hypercholesterolemia and Other Dyslipidemias, *CMAJ* 162 (10), 1441, 2000.

12

Assessment of Protein Status in Athletes

Stuart M. Phillips

CONTENTS

I. Introduction

During aerobic exercise, the main substrates oxidized are carbohydrate (CHO) and, to a lesser degree, fat. The oxidation of these fuels follows an inverse relationship, with the contribution of CHO to energy cost of exercise becoming greater at high exercise intensities and the contribution of fat greater at lower intensities.[1] The contribution of energy supplied by protein oxidation to the energy cost of exercise is, however, relatively small. Estimates of the contribution of protein oxidation to the energy cost of exercise have been made from urea excretion (sweat and urine) and direct measure-

0-8493-0927-1/02/$0.00+$1.50

ments of protein oxidation using amino acid tracers.[2-7] While there is some degree of variation in these estimates, the contribution of protein to endurance-type exercise energy is generally considered to be somewhere from less than 1% up to the highest estimates of ~5–6% of total exercising energy expenditure.[2,3]

Of concern to athletes is whether habitual exercise, either aerobic or resistance-based, increases the need for dietary protein. In theory, an increase in amino acid oxidation observed during endurance exercise[2-6] might be accompanied, perhaps, by an increased rate of protein breakdown. Taken together, increased rates of amino acid oxidation and an increased rate of protein degradation, either from muscle or other tissues (predominantly splanchnic), along with protein needed to repair the ultra-structural damage in muscle tissue occurring as a result of some eccentric component to the activity, could combine to increase an endurance athlete's requirement for dietary protein. Certain studies have corroborated the hypothesis that protein requirements are higher than established requirements in endurance-trained athletes.[3,5,7-9]

Resistance exercise is not characterized by high rates of substrate oxidation and, in fact, during resistance exercise, amino acid oxidation is unchanged from rest.[10] However, during the postexercise period, resistance exercise is characterized by a period of time lasting as long as 48 h,[11] during which rates of muscle protein synthesis are elevated above resting levels.[12-18] The observation that protein synthesis rates are elevated following acute bouts of resistance exercise along with observations of increases in lean body mass (LBM) and muscle hypertrophy following chronic resistance training.[19-22] Again the increased protein synthesis and greater net protein balance (synthesis minus breakdown), in addition to protein needed to repair any ultra-structural damage in muscle tissue occurring as a result of some eccentric component to the activity,[23,24] may lead to an increased requirement for dietary protein in athletes wishing to increase their lean body mass.[7,8] Studies have been conducted in which the protein requirements of resistance-trained athletes have been directly examined and the protein requirements of these persons have been determined to be greater than those of comparable sedentary persons.[3,5,7-9]

Despite the preceding proposed rationales for why an athlete *might* have an increased requirement for dietary protein, in addition to some experimental evidence,[3,5,7,9] there is also no consensus, at least in peer-reviewed scientific literature, as to whether habitual resistance exercise increases protein requirements.[25-27] That there is no general concurrence on the issue of an elevated dietary protein requirement for athletes likely arises from a number of confounding issues including variability in the intensity, duration and mode of exercise; variability in the period of adaptation to different (nonhabitual) protein and energy intakes; and differing methodology. Even at present it is less than clear what the best method is when it comes to estimating protein requirements.[28,29] Finally, it has been proposed that there are inherent problems that may be unsolvable in conducting studies of protein requirements in habitually active persons,[26] which have led to a flawed interpretation of data from studies in which the dietary protein requirements in athletes have been found to be elevated.[3,5,7-9]

The purpose of this chapter is to review the available data regarding protein and amino acid turnover and metabolism that occurs during and following endurance and resistance exercise in an attempt to determine whether athletes have elevated protein requirements relative to a sedentary population.

II. Protein Turnover

Proteins are constantly and simultaneously being synthesized and degraded (Figure 12.1). This constant synthesis and degradation provides a means for rapid response to a particular stimulus, due to the amplified response following a decrease or increase in either synthesis or breakdown. Protein synthesis is a complex process governed by a number of factors,[30,31] including gene expression, translational mechanisms, amino acid supply and hormonal milieu. In general, protein synthesis is stimulated by anabolic hormones (insulin, insulin-like growth factor-I, testosterone and growth hormone) and also by substrate supply (i.e., amino acids, in particular leucine). While at least one study has shown that provision of nonprotein substrates (i.e., glucose) can stimulate protein synthesis, particularly in the post-exercise period,[32] it is likely that this effect is due to insulin and not nonprotein calories per se. Another, more recent, study has confirmed that glucose and lipids do not stimulate protein synthesis.[33]

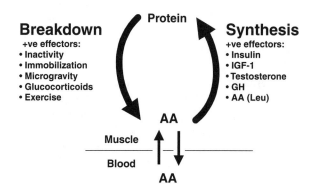

FIGURE 12.1
A schematic representation of protein turnover in muscle showing factors that stimulate both protein breakdown and protein synthesis. IGF-1 = insulin-like growth factor 1; GH = growth hormone; AA = amino acid; and Leu = leucine.

A. Protein Turnover and Endurance Exercise

Endurance exercise is fueled for the most part by fat and carbohydrate, but amino acids are also oxidized. While the contribution of amino acids to endurance-type activities are small, it is important to appreciate that, if exercise is of sufficient intensity and frequency, even a small amount of amino acid oxidation could, cumulatively, impact protein requirements. The interaction between skeletal muscle demand for oxidizable substrates and non-muscle sources of such substrates has been the subject of extensive investigation. Exchange of amino acids between muscle and non-muscle (primarily splanchnic) compartments is of particular relevance for amino acid metabolism. It is necessary to gain an understanding of the metabolism of amino acids, the inter-organ flow of amino acids and how these factors interact to determine protein requirements.

B. Skeletal Muscle Protein Metabolism and Protein Turnover

Muscle proteins form the greatest reservoir of protein within the body; however, their rate of turnover is relatively slow compared with splanchnic and blood-borne proteins. This slow turnover of muscle proteins means that, while exercise can induce an acute change in protein oxidation,[3,6] changes in protein breakdown in muscle are not thought to take place in response to exercise.[34-36] However, a suppression of protein synthesis during endurance exercise may mean that more amino acids are available for oxidation.[37,38]

Human muscle can oxidize at least seven amino acids (leucine, isoleucine, valine, glutamate, asparagine, aspartate and alanine).[39] Of these amino acids, however, oxidation of only the branched chain amino acids (BCAA) appears to be increased during catabolic states such as exercise.[39] Other amino acids that arise due to intramuscular proteolysis are simply exported from muscle during exercise.[40,41] The vast majority (> 60%) of amino acids exported from exercising muscle during exercise are in the form of alanine and glutamine,[42,43] a loss that is far greater than their abundance in skeletal muscle (generally 8–10% of muscle protein).[44] Of particular importance to amino acid flux during exercise is the fact that oxidation of the three BCAA (leucine, isoleucine and valine), in particular leucine, is accelerated relative to the oxidation of other amino acids.[36,45,46] The increased BCAA oxidation during exercise is due to the synergistic effects of a high abundance of BCAA in skeletal muscle protein (~ 20% of all muscle protein, by content) along with the fact that the activity of the enzymes responsible for the transamination (branched-chain aminotransferases, BCAAT) and subsequent oxidation (branched-chain keto-acid dehydrogenase, BCKAD) are also relatively high in muscle.[47,48]

The BCKAD enzyme is a mitochondrial-located multisubunit enzyme similar to pyruvate dehydrogenase in nature and in the mechanisms of its regulation.[47] Exercise stimulates activation of BCKAD, due possibly to a decrease in the ratio of ATP/ADP, or an increase in intramuscular acidity.[47,49]

In theory, however, because training induces an increase in the number of mitochondria,[50,51] the maximal activity of BCKAD should also increase. However, endurance training also results in the ability to better defend against changes in the ATP/ADP ratio;[52] hence, the proportion of the active form of BCKAD would be expected to decrease as a result of training. However, using leucine oxidation as a surrogate marker of BCKAD activity, the effect of training on this enzyme complex is entirely inconclusive with studies showing (1) increases in leucine oxidation following training, (2) no change and even (3) increases.[46,53-57] Recently, in a cross-sectional comparison in which leucine oxidation was compared at the same relative workload in trained and untrained athletes, it was concluded that training status did not affect leucine oxidation, when results were corrected for fat-free mass.[57] Using a longitudinal design, leucine oxidation and the abundance and activation state of the BCKAD enzyme were examined in humans by McKenzie and co-workers.[56] In this study, it was observed that, while training increased the maximal activity of the BCKAD enzyme, the percentage of active BCKAD during exercise was reduced, as was leucine oxidation, relative to the pretrained state, at the same absolute *and* relative workloads posttraining and that this result was unaffected by correcting for fat-free mass. McKenzie et al.[56] concluded that endurance training actually reduces the exercise-induced increase in leucine oxidation, due to a reduction in the activation of BCKAD.

Because it appears that muscle does not take up BCAA during exercise, at least not in appreciable quantities,[43,58-60] the increase in leucine oxidation observed during exercise should arise, for the most part, due to an increase in muscle protein breakdown within the muscle. An increase in muscle proteolysis during exercise would then supply leucine and other BCAA to the intramuscular free amino acid pool. In fact, MacLean et al. have shown that ingestion of BCAA reduces proteolysis, at least as measured by amino acid release across the exercising leg.[59] However, even the highest estimates of the rate of protein breakdown that might be occurring during endurance exercise cannot account for the nitrogen, in the form of amino acids, that leaves muscle during exercise.[61] A reasonable candidate amino acid, which might supply the source of nitrogen to account for the efflux from muscle, would be glutamine, given its large quantity in skeletal muscle. At present, however, no evidence in humans exists to support this idea.

In summary, while muscle has the capacity to oxidize a number of amino acids, oxidation of the BCAA, particularly leucine, is markedly increased during endurance exercise[2-6] and in direct proportion to exercise intensity.[62] Despite the acute exercise-induced rise in leucine oxidation, endurance training appears to decrease, or have no affect on, leucine oxidation at both absolute and relative workloads.[56,57] While leucine and possibly other BCAA oxidation is markedly increased during endurance exercise, it does not appear that this can account for the increase in amino nitrogen, carried as glutamine and alanine, that leaves muscle during exercise. It may be that muscle is able to take up sufficient quantities of glutamate, which may also act as a source of nitrogen for formation of alanine and glutamine in particular. Of particular interest is that the nitrogen arising from leucine transamination does not appear to result in increased ureagenesis.[63] The other possible fate of the nitrogen from BCAA transamination occurring in the muscle, because it is not incorporated into urea, may be incorporation back into proteins in the liver.[64]

C. Splanchnic Tissue Protein Turnover

In addition to skeletal muscle proteins, several other labile pools of protein also exist, namely splanchnic and blood-borne proteins. The breakdown of splanchnic proteins during exercise provides amino acids for other tissues, chiefly muscle.[65,66] However, the turnover of blood-bone proteins may also be stimulated by exercise.[64]

Alanine and glutamine that are released from skeletal muscle during exercise can serve as precursors for gluconeogenesis after the nitrogen is incorporated into urea.[42,44] Moreover, other amino acids (serine, proline and glycine) are also taken up in increasing quantities by the liver during prolonged exercise.[42] This occurs at the same time that there is a marked increase in the free concentration of amino acids in liver following exercise.[67] The significance of these findings is that liver not only increases the uptake of amino acids during exercise but that the rate of proteolysis in the liver is increased markedly by exercise, potentially to provide gluconeogenic carbon skeletons. The ~10–12% decrease in liver protein content following 2–3 h of exhaustive exercise that was observed by Kasperek[68] lends some support to the contention that the proteolysis within the liver is increased to potentially provide amino acids for gluconeogensis. What is bewildering, however, is how increase in hepatic protein breakdown[68] and increased amino acid uptake[42] during exercise can be reconciled with a lack of increase in urea production.[34,63,64]

Other investigations have also shown that exercise stimulates the gut[69] and liver[65] to release essential amino acids either as a result of an increase in proteolysis or a reduction in the synthetic rate of proteins, either of which would allow for more free amino acids to leave their respective tissues. The fate of the amino acids released from either gut or liver may be to provide gluconeogenic precursors to maintain glucose homeostasis[69] or to provide other tissues such as muscle with a source of fuel.[65] Recent measurements of gut mucosal protein synthetic rates in humans show that this tissue has a much higher (~50-fold) fractional protein synthetic rate than that of muscle.[70] Hence, even a small exercise-induced suppression in the protein synthetic rate of the gut would allow amino acids to be released. The idea that during exercise the gut could act as a labile pool of amino acids for other tissues, including liver and muscle, is an interesting one but also one that would appear difficult to study in humans.

As previously commented, a confusing observation with respect to protein turnover and of importance in a discussion of protein requirements, is the observation that increased uptake of amino acids by the liver and an apparent increased hepatic proteolysis does not result in appreciable urea formation.[34,63,64] This observation is particularly important when one considers the fact that nitrogen uptake by the liver during endurance exercise is almost complete (i.e., uptake matches delivery).[69] A possibility that could explain this phenomenon is that the amino acids could have been incorporated back into plasma proteins, as suggested by the results of Carraro et al.[64] Such a hypothesis, depending on the efficiency of this "recycling" of nitrogen, has obvious implications for protein requirements. It remains to be seen whether similar increases in the fractional turnover rates of other plasma proteins can be observed and what effect higher intensities of exercise might have on this protein cycling.

III. Protein Turnover and Resistance Exercise

Proteins are constantly and simultaneously being synthesized and degraded, This turnover of body proteins serves several functions:

- Replacement of damaged proteins[23,24]
- Degradation of proteins to supply amino acids for oxidation
- Remodeling of proteins due to external stimuli such as changes in hormone concentration or resistive contractile activity

Both repair of damaged proteins and remodeling of structural proteins appear to occur as a result of a resistive exercise stimulus.[71-73] However, in human muscle, the process of myofibrillar protein turnover, at least that induced by resistive exercise, appears to be a relatively slow one.[74-77] This slow turnover of muscle proteins means that resistive exercise, while it can induce changes in muscle fiber type and increase fiber diameter, requires a repeated exercise stimulus and a relatively prolonged period of time (at least 4 weeks) to see the outward change in phenotype (fiber type) and longer periods (at least 6–8 weeks) to observe hypertrophy.[21,74,77-79] Because resistance exercise does not induce an acute increase in protein turnover nor oxidation,[10] it is the postexercise period when changes in muscle protein turnover, more specifically an increase in muscle protein synthesis, occur; this assertion has been confirmed numerous times in both animals[80-82] and humans.[11-16]

Resistance exercise results in fundamentally different adaptations compared with those induced by endurance exercise, because the result is an increase in muscle fiber diameter.[83-85] To allow an increase in fiber diameter, there must be synthesis of new muscle proteins, ~60–70% of which are myofibrillar,[86] mostly actin and myosin,[87,88] in nature. During the period of fiber hypertrophy there also needs to be a net positive protein balance, that is, muscle protein synthesis must chronically exceed muscle protein breakdown. A variety of investigations have shown that resistance exercise stimulates mixed muscle protein synthesis[11,13,14,16] in trained and untrained subjects. The time course of protein synthesis following an isolated bout of resistance exercise appears to be somewhat different in untrained subjects, for whom changes in mixed muscle protein fractional synthetic rate (FSR) persist for up to 48 h post-exercise.[11] Mixed muscle protein FSR in trained persons is back to resting levels by 36 h postexercise, suggesting a diminished synthetic response in protein turnover in trained persons.[89] Results from cross-sectional comparisons also show that prolonged resistance training actually attenuates the acute immediate response of muscle protein synthesis to an isolated bout of resistance exercise,[12,82] which might be expected as a general adaptation response to training. Recently, we have confirmed these cross-sectional findings[12,82] using a longitudinal design (S.M. Phillips and M.A. Tarnopolsky, unpublished observations). The implications of these findings[12,82,89] are that trained persons would likely require less protein to support the maximal synthetic response to a given workout.

While resistance exercise stimulates an increase in the synthetic rate of muscle proteins,[11,13,14,16] there is also a concomitant increase in the rate of muscle protein breakdown.[11,12,16] The tight relationship between muscle protein synthesis and breakdown has been observed in a number of studies where the two variables have been simultaneously measured.[11,12,16,90] In fact, a hypothesis has been advanced that describes the link between muscle protein synthesis and breakdown, in combination with amino acid supply, as being critical in determining the degree of post-exercise muscle protein accretion or reduction.[91,92]

Using a surrogate marker of muscle myofibrillar protein degradation, urinary 3-methylhistidine (3-MH), others have observed increases[93-95] or no change[11,14,96] following resistance exercise. It is unclear why there is such disparity in the results from studies using 3-MH as an indicator of muscle proteolysis and results from studies in which muscle protein breakdown has been directly measured. The pitfalls of using 3-MH as an index of muscle protein degradation are well documented, however, and are related to the unknown contribution of splanchnic tissue proteolysis, which contains significant quantities of actin.[97] Given the observation that protein synthetic rates in intestinal tissue are almost 50 times higher than those of muscle,[70] it is not unreasonable that breakdown rates in intestinal tissue might be similarly elevated relative to those observed in skeletal muscle. If one also considers the observation that exercise induces a significant increase in splanchnic tissue protein degradation,[65] then the utility of 3-MH in measuring exercise-induced muscle myofibrillar protein breakdown is likely limited at best.

In studies where protein degradation has been directly measured following resistance exercise, it has consistently been shown that resistance exercise stimulates muscle protein degradation.[11,16,98] In every study that has measured muscle protein balance (synthesis minus breakdown) following resistive exercise, it has also been shown that, while synthesis is markedly elevated (in some cases > 150% above baseline levels) muscle balance is negative[11,12,16] until amino acids are provided either intravenously (to simulate postprandial concentrations) or orally.[17,99,100] This feeding-induced stimulation of muscle protein synthesis[17,99-102] has been shown to be independent of insulin[103] and is likely reflective of an increased delivery of amino acids to the intramuscular free pool.[92,104]

Increases in mixed muscle protein synthesis induced by resistance exercise can be relatively large (i.e., > 150% above resting).[11,13,14,16] Until the appearance of some recent studies,[87,88] the increase in *mixed* muscle protein synthesis seen after resistance exercise could not conclusively be established as the result of an increase in myofibrillar protein synthesis per se.[11,12,14] While a resistance exercise-induced increase in myofibrillar protein synthesis may seem intuitive, because resistance exercise eventually results in hypertrophy as a result of the accumulation of force-producing myofibrillar proteins,[83-85] recent studies have now established that this is the case.[87,88] These findings clearly establish that the increases in *mixed* muscle protein synthesis observed following exercise[11,13,14,16] are predominantly due to myofibrillar protein synthesis, most likely of myosin heavy chain and actin.[87,88] This conclusion gains further weight when one considers that myofibrillar proteins compose the majority of proteins in muscle.

Several studies have now been published in which the adaptations in muscle cross-sectional area and muscle fiber characteristics following resistance-training programs were reported for females.[74,76,84] These investigations have shown that, despite a markedly (~10-fold) lower serum testosterone concentration, women who follow a progressive resistive program will demonstrate skeletal muscle hypertrophy.[84] In addition, resistance exercise training in women results, quite rapidly, in changes in strength and muscle fiber characteristics similar to those that occur in males.[74] However, the results from Alway et al.,[84] examining highly trained resistance athletes of both sexes, show that highly trained males have greater muscle cross-sectional area (~76%) and muscle fiber diameters (~100%) than highly trained female bodybuilders. These findings indicate that longer-term training results in differences that favor greater muscle hypertrophy in male athletes. Despite the obvious differences in testosterone concentration, an intriguing question is whether there is a sexually dimorphic response that favors males in the exercise-induced expression of the muscle-derived autocrine form of insulin-like growth factor 1 (IGF-1, recently termed MGF for muscle growth factor),[107] which has recently been shown to have marked effects on muscle hypertrophy[105,106] (see reference 107 for review); this hypothesis remains to be tested, however.

Resistance exercise induces an increase in muscle fiber size provided a progressive stimulus of sufficient intensity is applied. The increased fiber size is due to a chronic period where protein synthesis has exceeded protein breakdown. During this period, new proteins are added to preexisting fibers; existing proteins are likely degraded at a higher rate as a result of the resistive stimulus. Which degradative pathway(s) are responsible for this increased proteolysis is unknown; however, recent evidence has shown that the ATP-dependent ubiquitin-proteasome pathway (AUPP) is upregulated in response to chronic muscle stimulation.[108] It seems reasonable to suggest that the AUPP, given the proportion of proteolysis accounted for by this pathway,[109] is also activated and active in the remodeling of muscle proteins seen during resistance exercise. It has recently been demonstrated that the exercise-induced increases in protein synthesis are due to increased synthesis of myofibrillar proteins, which would be predicted simply based on the protein composition of muscle. Whether the increases in protein synthesis that are induced by resistance exercise result in an increase in protein requirement, as is the popular impression, will be examined subsequently.

IV. Protein Requirements

Figure 12.1 shows the general scheme of protein turnover that occurs in all body tissues. A very high percentage of all amino acids that are released into the intracellular free amino acid pool are reincorporated back into protein, but not all amino acids are "recycled." Those amino acids that are lost from the amino acid pool are, for the most part, transported back to the liver, where they are metabolized and their nitrogen is released as urea. Because some amino acids cannot be synthesized in human tissue (i.e., essential amino acids) and intracellular reuse (i.e., reincorporation of amino acids arising from protein breakdown, see Figure 12.1) is not 100% efficient, we have a daily requirement for dietary protein.

A. Habitual Protein Intakes

Having established the fundamental processes by which protein requirements *might* be elevated in athletes, any discussion of how much dietary protein these persons do require must be preceded by an analysis of how much protein athletes and habitually exercising persons consume on a daily basis. Tables 12.1 and 12.2 show, respectively, the reported habitual dietary protein intakes of persons engaged in regular endurance activities (running, cycling and triathlon training) and resistive training.

As is plainly obvious from both tables, all athletes are reportedly consuming in excess of *all* current recommended levels of protein intake including the Recommended Nutrient Intake (RNI; Canada), Recommended Dietary Allowance (RDA; USA), the World Health Organization and even the most recent Dietary Reference Intakes (DRI; Canada and USA).[119-122] The only group of athletes that may be at risk for suboptimal protein intakes, if one accepts that athletes' reported dietary intakes are accurate with respect to the recommended intakes for protein, might be female endurance athletes (see Table 12.1). Such a supposition should be

TABLE 12.1

Habitual Reported Protein Intakes for Endurance-
Trained Athletes

Reference	N	Protein Intake g protein/kg^{-1}/d^{-1}
110	51 (female)[a]	1. 6 ± 0. 6
111	13 (female, EM)	1. 1 ± 0. 5
	14 (female, AM)	1. 2 ± 0. 5
112	6 (female, EM)	1. 3 ± 0. 4
	11 (female, AM)	1. 0 ± 0. 5
113	17 (female, EM)	1. 0 ± 0. 4
	11 (female, AM)	0. 7 ± 0. 4
3	6 (male)	1. 9 ± 0. 2
	6 (female, EM)	1. 0 ± 0. 1
114	5 (male)	2. 2 ± 0. 5
2	7 (male)	1. 8 ± 0. 4
	8 (female, EM)	1. 0 ± 0. 2
8	6 (male)	1. 5 ± 0. 3
115	8 (male)	1. 9 ± 1. 0
	8 (female, EM)	1. 2 ± 0. 3
Means	32 (male)	1.8 ± 0.4[b]
	109 (female, EM)	1.2 ± 0.3[c]
	36 (female, AM)	1.0 ± 0.4[d]

Values are means ± SD

EM – eumenorrheic

AM – amenorrheic

[a] menstrual status not stated (assumed to be EM, unless otherwise indicated)

[b] 14 ± 2% of total reported energy intake

[c] 13 ± 3% of total reported energy intake

[d] 15 ± 1% of total reported energy intake

cautionary, however, because it is documented that females — and athletic females in particular — habitually underreport their energy intakes;[123,124] hence, it is likely that females also underreport their protein intake. Another group of athletes, who fall into a separate category and deserve particular attention from a nutritional standpoint, are female athletes involved in sports that engender a regrettable preoccupation with the weight- and esthetically oriented facets of competition and performance (i.e., gymnasts, figure skaters and dancers). These athletes are well known for their "marginal" nutritional practices and should be appropriately instructed, in concert with their coaches and parents or guardians, as to how they should achieve optimal performance through their diet involving neither overly restrictive nor disordered patterns of eating.[125,126]

Despite an apparent adequate consumption of protein by most athletes, many have pointed out that the recommended protein intakes do not contain a necessary allowance for physical activity.[3,5,7-9] This apparent "oversight" in setting protein requirements could possibly be due to a number of reasons:

TABLE 12.2

Reported Habitual Protein Intakes in
Resistance-Trained Athletes and
Bodybuilders

Reference	N	Protein Intake g protein/kg^{-1}/d^{-1}
13	12 (BB)	1. 6 ± 0. 5
116	76 (BB)	2. 4 ± 0. 6
25	26 (BB)[a]	1. 9 ± 0. 5
117	12 (BB)	1. 4 ± 0. 2
32	10 (RA)	1. 6 ± 0. 2
118	30 (RA)	2. 5 ± 0. 8
	6 (BB)	2. 3 ± 0. 7
8	6 (BB)	2. 7 ± 0. 5
7	7 (RA)	1. 8 ± 0. 4
Mean	138 (BB)	2. 1±0. 5[b]
	47 (RA)	2. 0±0. 4[c]

Values are means ± SD

RA – resistance-trained athletes (includes football and rugby players)

BB – bodybuilders
[a] includes both males and females
[b] 19 ± 3% of total reported energy intake
[c] 18 ± 2% of total reported energy intake

In general, protein requirements are not elevated in any group of habitually exercising (be it endurance- or resistance-type activities) persons. Moreover, even if protein requirements were increased for athletes, the population requirements plus the built in safety margin inherent in all current recommendations[119-122] are more than adequate to compensate for any increase in requirement for dietary protein.

Those setting the protein requirements believe that because (see Tables 12.1 and 12.2) people who perform regular exercise, and the North American population in general, have above-requirement intakes of protein, it is not necessary to make any increased allowance.

The percentage of the general population who perform enough exercise to elevate their protein requirements is not sufficient to warrant inclusion of their increased requirements in current recommendations. It should, however, be noted that many have noted that habitual performance of physical activity does not increase protein requirements and may, in fact, increase the efficiency of protein use and hence actually decrease the need for protein.[25-27,127,128]

B. Protein Requirements for Endurance Trained Athletes

Numerous methods have been used to examine protein metabolism in athletes and sedentary persons alike, but requirements for dietary protein have always been and continue to be determined using nitrogen balance measurements. This is in spite of criticism suggesting inherent flaws in the nitrogen balance approach for determining protein requirements that can result in spurious results.[26,129-131] A suggested alternative approach to using only nitrogen balance, which has been implemented in both sedentary and exercising individuals, has been the inclusion of amino acid tracer methodologies.[129,130,132,133] Despite the criticisms of the nitrogen balance method, however, it is still the method used to establish protein requirements for sedentary individuals;[119-122] hence, a review of the dietary protein requirements for athletes should include only those studies that have used this methodology.

When male and training-matched females were fed the Canadian RNI for protein for a period of 10 days prior to a 3-day nitrogen balance experiment, it was observed that all athletes were in negative nitrogen balance.[3] In addition, by utilizing a stable-isotope-labeled infusion of leucine to examine protein turnover during a 90-minute (65% of peak oxygen uptake) run in both males and females, an attempt was made to determine a possible mechanism of the increased requirement for protein.[3] It was observed that 90 minutes of moderate-intensity exercise resulted in leucine oxidation during exercise that was 70% greater in trained male athletes than in their training-matched female counterparts.[4] Calculations revealed that ~ 90% of the negative nitrogen balance could be accounted for by the leucine oxidation that occurred during the 90-minute exercise bout, assuming an average value for tissue leucine content.[3] The sex-based difference in leucine oxidation was a main effect, however, and the increased leucine oxidation was evident at rest in the male athletes.[3] Subsequently, measurements of BCKAD activity have shown that, at rest, females had a lower activity than male.s[56] It is unclear, however, whether the results obtained[3] can be generalized to include conditions when adequate protein intakes are consumed, because the aforementioned subjects were in negative nitrogen balance.

Studying habitually exercising athletes, Friedman and Lemon[9] conducted experiments to determine nitrogen balance and dietary protein requirement when athletes were consuming two levels of protein intakes. On the low intake (~ 0.86 g protein·kg^{-1}·d^{-1}) the athletes were in negative nitrogen balance. Both of these studies[3,9] indicate that the Canadian RNI and the USA RDA for protein (0.86 g protein·kg^{-1}·d^{-1}) were inadequate for habitually exercising athletes. The mean protein intake to maintain zero nitrogen balance, in a group of middle-aged and young endurance athletes, was 0.94 g protein·kg^{-1}·d^{-1} (~ 109% of the protein RNI/RDA), which translated into an actual "safe" protein requirement (i.e., included an estimate to cover all individuals) of 1.26 g protein·kg^{-1}·d^{-1}.[5,120] A weakness of the previous studies, however, was the failure to include any sedentary controls.[3,5,9] When a sedentary control group was included, Tarnopolsky et al.[8] found that protein requirements of a group of endurance athletes were 1.67 times those of the control group; this finding resulted in a calculated daily protein requirement of 1.6 g protein·kg^{-1}·d^{-1}(~ 186% of the RNI for protein). A potential weakness of this study,[8] however, was that all of the protein intakes fed to the participants were above requirement, which may have biased the estimates toward higher dietary requirement estimates.[25] It should be pointed out that in all the studies mentioned above,[3,5,8,9] the adaptation periods to the protein intake(s) studied were at least 10 days in duration, which appears to be adequate for adaptation of specific urea cycle and other protein metabolic enzymes.[134]

A retrospective analysis of nitrogen balance data[3,5,8,9] collected in people performing reasonably intense aerobic-based exercise reveals that nitrogen balance is generally negative when these people consume protein at or near the RNI/RDA/DRI. In fact, Figure 12.2 shows a graph of reported nitrogen balances (46 data points) seen at various protein intakes in endurance-trained athletes.[3,5,8,9] A regression line drawn through these data shows that nitrogen balance is achieved at a protein intake almost 24% greater than the RDA/RNI/DRI (1.07g protein·kg^{-1}·d^{-1}; see Figure 12.2). Inclusion of a 95% confidence interval to the regression line to achieve zero balance to provide a margin of safe intake given the small numbers of athletes examined in the studies included in the analysis, yields a safe protein intake of 1.11 g protein·kg^{-1}·d^{-1}, which is almost 30% greater than the current RDA/RNI/DRI (see Figure 12.1). The evidence presented in Figure 12.2 would appear to be rather convincing, to most, that endurance-based exercise elevates the requirement for dietary protein. Other researchers who have examined the issue of protein requirements in exercising humans have concluded, however, that endurance exercise does not elevate the requirement for dietary protein.[27,128,135] In the latter studies, it was shown that exercise actually improves the economy of nitrogen (protein) utilization;[27,128,135] however, high quality egg protein was being ingested and all subjects were meticulously monitored to ensure they were in energy balance. A diet based entirely on egg protein differs from that used in previous studies in which protein was from mixed sources, which would likely be more reflective of what an athlete habitually ingests.[3,5,8,9] Further, in at least two of the previous studies, the athletes were checked to ensure that they were weight-stable,[3,8] meaning that energy balance must have been sufficient. However, in conflict with the finding that exercise training increases the requirements for dietary protein,[3,5,8,9] chronic aerobic exercise (training) results in a reduction, or at least no change, in the exercise-induced rise in leucine oxidation.[56,57] Other data, in which prolonged isotope infusions were utilized, have also shown that two exercise bouts (90 minutes, each at 50% of VO$_{2\,peak}$) resulted in neither negative leucine nor nitrogen balance while consuming 1 g protein·kg–1·d–1 (~ 100 mg leucine·kg^{-1}·d^{-1}).[35] In addition, estimates of protein turnover from leucine oxidation, which was only moderately increased (a minimal estimate of the increase in leucine oxidation was 27% above resting, whereas a maximal estimate was closer to 45%, depending on which bicarbonate retention factor was employed) during exercise, compared quite well with protein turnover data from urea nitrogen kinetics, which showed very little change throughout rest, exercise and recovery.[35] Hence, on a day-to-day basis, these researchers[35] concluded that despite a total of 3h of moderate exercise (one 1.5-h bout during the fed-state and one 1.5-h bout while fasted), could be supported by a protein intake of only 1 g protein·kg^{-1}·d^{-1}.

In extreme conditions of strenuous daily exercise, such as the Tour de France, lean body mass can be maintained when energy requirements are adequate.[114] These findings[114] are particularly impressive when one considers that the daily energy expenditures of these athletes were in the range of 27–38 MJ·d^{-1} and nitrogen balance was not significantly different from zero.[136,137] It should be made apparent, however, that protein intakes in these athletes were always > 1.4 g protein·kg^{-1}·d^{-1}.[136,137]

Several investigations, which have utilized nitrogen balance methodology, support the thesis that endurance exercise increases the requirement for dietary protein in endurance athletes.[3,5,8,9] It is important to mention that several studies have found that endurance exercise programs have actually reduced dietary protein requirements due to an improvement in the nitrogen retention.[27,128,135] The exercise-induced increase in nitrogen retention could, however, be a reflection of accommodative mechanisms, possibly due to a reduction in protein synthesis of a particular protein or muscle proteins in general, rather than an improved "economy of nitrogen utilization" as hypothesized by the authors.[27,128,135] Because no dynamic mechanisms can be determined from nitrogen balance data, neither an accommodative nor an improved economy hypothesis can be conclusively given for the findings.[27,128,135] This highlights one of the greatest shortcomings of the nitrogen balance method; that is, the "black box" approach to determining protein requirements; where protein *in* minus protein *out* equals requirement with no understanding of how or why these findings occurred.

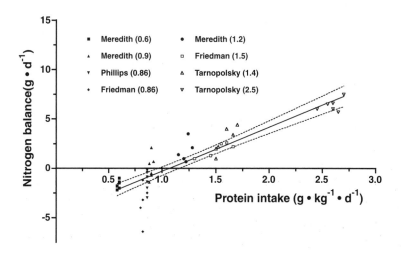

FIGURE 12.2
Nitrogen balance data from four studies that have reported nitrogen balance and protein requirement data for endurance-trained athletes. Data are taken from references 3, 5, 8 and 9. Numbers within brackets beside authors' names are approximate protein intakes in g protein·kg^{-1}·d^{-1}.

Some studies that have examined the "extremes" of endurance exercise tolerance have showed that maintenance of nitrogen balance can be achieved when energy balance is maintained.[114,136,137] Finally, it is difficult to reconcile a finding of increased protein requirements for endurance athletes (Figure 12.2) with the observation that exercise training results in a reduction in leucine (and hence protein) oxidation and BCKAD activation.[56] Obviously, the issue of protein requirements for endurance athletes is one that is difficult to settle absolutely. From a purely research-based perspective, however, it would appear (Figure 12.2) as if protein requirements are greater than those for sedentary persons. How much greater an athlete's requirements for dietary protein are would likely depend on training status, frequency and intensity of training and a host of other factors. Moreover, in longitudinal studies, as opposed to the mostly cross-sectional data presented in Figure 12.2, nitrogen balance actually adapts with exercise training to become more positive.[27] These findings[27] are consistent with data that has shown a training-induced *reduction* in the exercise-induced *activation* of the rate-limiting enzyme for BCAA oxidation, BCKAD.[56] Similar findings of an exercise-induced increase in efficiency of protein use have been reported when day-to-day nitrogen balance was examined in persons beginning an exercise program (Figure 12.3). Moreover, in an early study by Gontzea and others,[138] nitrogen balance became transiently negative at the onset of an exercise-training program, but the subjects were able to achieve zero nitrogen balance after 10–15 days of training consuming 1 g protein·kg^{-1}·d^{-1}. It is unknown whether what was reported[138] (see Figure 12.3) constitutes a transient increase in the oxidation and breakdown of protein, after which enzymes have adapted, or an accommodative mechanism[129,130] that has resulted in the suboptimal rate of incorporation of amino acids into protein (i.e., muscle protein). In addition, the impact that energy balance has on protein requirements is highlighted when one recognizes that the subjects that Gontzea et al.[138] studied were consuming energy intakes 10% greater than their calculated requirement, even when they began their daily exercise protocol. In fact, the energy balance of an athlete may be the most important factor, even more so than protein intake, in the determination of a requirement for dietary protein. Because, if energy balance can be achieved, then nitrogen balance can also be achieved, even at what would generally be considered low-to-marginal protein intakes.[27,128] Moreover, it has been known for some time that consumption of carbohydrate is protein sparing;[32,139] hence, the recommendation that endurance athletes consume a high-carbohydrate diet to enhance their performance[126] may also result in conservation of body protein. Therefore, from a practical perspective, any increase in dietary protein requirements (Figure 12.2) may be somewhat immaterial, provided athletes are consuming a *mixed* diet containing sufficient energy to cover their daily energy expenditure. If such is the case, they will almost certainly be getting enough protein to cover requirements, particularly if they are consuming a diet relatively high in carbohydrates (a usual recommendation is for a competitive athlete to consume > 6 g carbohydrate·kg^{-1}).[126] From a practical perspective therefore, it makes more sense and is more appropriate to recommend that likely more than 10%, no more than 15%, and at most 20% of dietary calories come from protein. This recommendation holds so long as athletes are consuming a mixed diet (one that follows current guidelines is more than sufficient)[140,141] with sufficient energy. At risk for developing a deficiency in terms of their protein intake are those athletes who consume marginal energy intakes.[126] These athletes, almost exclusively females,[125] should be monitored closely, not only for low protein intake, but also because they are likely at risk for developing other nutritional deficiencies.[126]

C. Protein Requirements for Resistance Trained Athletes

Tarnopolsky and co-workers[8] conducted a study using the nitrogen balance approach to examine the protein requirements of a group of resistance-trained athletes and a group of sedentary controls. As pointed out earlier, Tarnopolsky et al.[10] have demonstrated that an isolated bout of resistance exercise did not increase leucine oxidation or perturb whole body protein turnover, likely because of the periodic recovery that occurs during a resistance vs. an endurance workout. Hence, it would appear that any extra protein required by strength-trained individuals is likely directed toward muscular hypertrophy in the earlier phases of training, when muscle mass is still increasing. However, it should be stressed that, in highly trained powerlifters and bodybuilders, it is unlikely that dietary protein requirements are elevated much more than those of a sedentary person. In fact, any increase in protein requirements for such a highly trained group of individuals is likely only due to an increased rate of resting protein turnover. In support of the idea that training might induce an increase in resting muscle protein turnover, protein requirements of highly trained bodybuilders were found to be only 12% greater than those of sedentary controls, who had a protein requirement of 0.84 g protein·kg^{-1}·d^{-1}.[8] The results of this study[8] do highlight a puzzling result, however, that is evident in Figure 12.4. For example, on a protein intake (actually equivalent to the habitual protein requirement of bodybuilders) of ~2.8 g protein·kg^{-1}·d^{-1}, all bodybuilders were in highly positive nitrogen balance (~12-20 g N·d^{-1}). When extrapolated back to actual protein, this would have meant that the bodybuilders should have gained ~ 300–500g of lean mass/d^{-1} (assuming muscle is 75% water and assuming that no other pool of body protein significantly increased in size), which obviously did not occur.[8] The increasingly positive nitrogen balance, associated with higher protein intakes, that was observed in this[8] and other[7,117] studies is often incorrectly used to justify why high protein intakes are needed for resistance-trained athletes. Such shortcomings of nitrogen balance have long been recognized and have led to the recommendation of combining tracer and nitrogen balance approaches to determining protein requirements.[130,142]

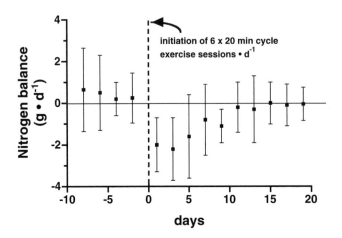

FIGURE 12.3
The time course of adaptation in nitrogen balance, following the initiation of endurance exercise training in novices (adapted from Gontzea et al.[138]). All subjects were consuming 1 g protein·kg⁻¹·d⁻¹throughout the experiment and energy 10% greater than their calculated requirement. Values are means ± SD.

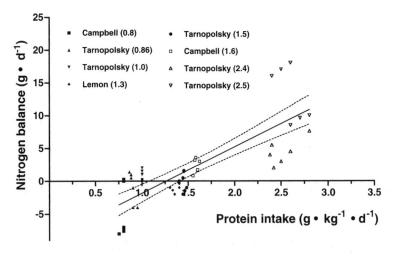

FIGURE 12.4
Nitrogen balance data from four studies that have reported nitrogen balance and protein requirement data for resistance-trained athletes and bodybuilders. Data are taken from references 7, 8, 117 and 143. Numbers within brackets beside authors' names are approximate protein intakes in g protein·kg⁻¹·d⁻¹.

Using a combination of nitrogen balance along with kinetic measurements of whole-body protein turnover, football and rugby players had protein requirements almost ~ 100% greater than those of a sedentary control group.[7] In fact, consumption of the low-protein diet (0.86 g protein·kg⁻¹·d⁻¹) by the strength trained group resulted in an accommodated state where whole body protein synthesis was reduced compared with the medium (1.4 g protein·kg^{-1}·d^{-1}) and high protein (2.4 g protein·kg^{-1}·d^{-1}) diets.

In contrast to the results of Tarnopolsky et al.,[7,8] nitrogen balance studies conducted in the elderly have shown that initiating a moderate program of strength training resulted in reduced protein requirements due to the anabolic stimulus of the resistance exercise.[143] However, even following 10 weeks of comparatively mild resistance training, there was no evidence of muscle hypertrophy in people consuming either 0.8 or 1.6 g protein·kg^{-1}·d^{-1}. The results of Campbell et al.[143] are remarkably similar to those reported by Torun et al.[127] showing that isometric exercise improved protein utilization. Hence, while resistance exercise did improve nitrogen balance,[143] the results of Campbell and co-workers and Torun et al.[127] may not be directly applicable to younger resistance training athletes who are trying to gain lean mass and stimulate hypertrophy. Nonetheless, support for the possibility that more intense resistance exercise can improve nitrogen economy can be seen in the results of Phillips et al.,[11] who showed that, in the fasted state, an isolated bout of resistance exercise resulted in increased muscle net protein balance, implying an improved intracellular reutilization of amino acids. Others have also observed that exercise per se vs. the creation of an energy deficit via diet, results in improved dietary protein retention.[27,127,128] That the athletes studied by Tarnopolsky et al.[7,8] were all highly trained at the time of study and were performing exercise that was more intense than that described in the studies that showed a reduction in protein requirements,[27,138,143] may be a reason for the discrepancy. It is of paramount importance to understand the concepts of adaptation and accommodation in regards to protein requirements,[129,130,142] particularly where athletes are concerned. This contention is highlighted by studies that have shown that protein balance can be achieved in exercising persons at very low to moderate protein intakes (i.e., ~ 1 g protein· kg–1·d^{-1}or less),[27,35,127,128,138,143] albeit at rather modest levels of exercise. It has been emphasized that obtaining nitrogen balance, particularly in long term studies, may be less reflective of requirement but rather of mechanisms that result in an accommodated state.[130] At issue is whether the accommodation, by athletes, to the lower protein intakes results in a reduced level of synthesis of some protein(s) that might eventually compromise performance; however, to substantiate such a proposition would be very difficult given the inherent problems in conducting long-term studies involving dietary control in athletes. Millward[25,26] has detailed some of the reasons questions of protein requirements are hard to determine in an exercising population.

A retrospective analysis of nitrogen balance data[7,8,117,143] from persons (50 data points) who were in a steady state of training and performing structured rigorous training involving resistance exercise is shown in Figure 12.4. A regression line drawn through these data show that nitrogen balance is achieved at a protein intake almost 46% greater than the RDA/RNI/DRI (1.26g protein·kg^{-1}·d^{-1}; see Figure 12.4). Inclusion of a 95% confidence interval in the regression line to achieve zero balance yields a safe protein intake of

1.35 g protein·kg–1·d⁻¹ (Figure 12.4) or almost 60% greater than the current RDA/RNI/DRI.

There is no doubt that the data presented in Figure 12.4 represent data from a variety of studies from athletes completing resistance exercise at a variety of intensities, with a variety of levels of experience. Assuredly, exercise intensity, duration, frequency and training status will impact on whether someone requires more protein. The data of Gontzea et al.,[138] shown in Figure 12.2, highlight the fact that unaccustomed exercise can induce a negative nitrogen balance, though transiently. Moreover, Lemon et al.[117] showed that novice weightlifters required more dietary protein (1.4-1.5 g protein·kg⁻¹·d⁻¹) than do more experienced weightlifters (1.05 g protein·kg⁻¹·d⁻¹) as reported in an earlier study.[8] In addition, when intense weightlifting is combined with training for sports with both power and aerobic bases (rugby and football) protein requirements have been reported to be as high as 1.76 g protein·kg⁻¹·d⁻¹.[7] As discussed earlier, the underlying reason for a training-induced reduction in dietary protein requirements[7,8,117] for strength-trained persons likely relates to the fact that it is early in a resistance training program when the largest gains in lean body mass and the greatest rates of muscle hypertrophy are seen.[84] Hence, after the introductory phase of beginning a strength training program and initial gains in lean mass are made, it is hard to reconcile that resistance "trained" athletes would have markedly elevated protein requirements. Instead, experienced weightlifters and bodybuilders not using anabolic steroids might require protein to support a slight elevation in basal (i.e., beyond 48 h after their last workout) protein turnover. Cross-sectional data from Phillips et al.[12] demonstrate support for the postulate that trained resistance athletes, whether male or female, have an elevated turnover of muscle proteins at rest (~ 24% elevation in FSR at rest in trained vs. untrained). These observations of a training-induced elevation in FSR[12] have recently been confirmed longitudinally following 8 weeks of training in previously untrained novices (S.M. Phillips, unpublished observations).

Can a general recommendation for the dietary protein requirement for weightlifters, bodybuilders, or any athlete desiring to gain lean mass, whether uninitiated or experienced, be made? First, a theoretical calculation *might* demonstrate to those who believe that, no matter what is recommended for dietary protein requirement for those desiring to gain lean mass, dietary protein must be greater than 2 g protein·kg⁻¹·d⁻¹ and that supplemental protein is necessary to gain muscle mass or strength.[8,116] Some data used in this calculation comes from the studies generated by animal scientists who have dedicated far more effort to determining the most cost-efficient (and hence protein content perspective) way of increasing lean mass gains in growing steers.[144,145]

If we take the theoretical example of a person who initially weighs 100 kg (220 lb) and in a given year gains 10 kg (22 lb) of muscle (it needs to be strongly emphasized that this gain is purely muscle and not just body mass), this represents a highly impressive gain of lean muscle mass and likely at the "outer limit" of possible gains in lean body mass, without anabolic steroids. The question is, how much extra protein (if any) would this individual have to consume?

1. 10kg muscle = 2.5kg protein (assuming 75% of muscle mass is water).

2. Then 2.5kg protein = 2500g in one year or 2500g/365d/100kg = 0.0685 g protein·kg^{-1}·d^{-1}that is gained.

3. Assuming that, based on some values calculated from growing steers,[144,145] eight times as much protein needs to be consumed to lay down the same amount of mass (note, this mass gain is not all muscle in steers and so application of this value to humans represents an overestimate): 0.0685 • 8 = 0.55 g protein·kg^{-1}·d^{-1}.

4. Assuming that the RNI/RDA/DRI is sufficient to cover all other protein needs, 0.86 g protein·kg^{-1}·d^{-1} + 0.55 g protein·kg^{-1}·d^{-1} = 1.41 g protein·kg^{-1}·d^{-1}.

What this calculation *does not* take into account is that resistance exercise actually increases the efficiency of protein and amino acid utilization (i.e., net muscle protein balance is less negative), which would actually reduce the amount of protein required to gain the 10 kg of muscle. An increased efficiency of protein utilization following intense resistance exercise has been shown acutely,[11] chronically,[12] and in nitrogen balance studies.[27,143] Campbell et al.[143] reported that 11 weeks of resistance training improved nitrogen balance by ~13mg N·kg^{-1}·d^{-1} or ~82 mg protein·kg^{-1}·d^{-1}, which would reduce the estimated dietary protein requirement of 1.41 g protein·kg^{-1}·d^{-1} to 1.33 g protein·kg^{-1}·d^{-1}. Put in practical terms, 1.33 g protein·kg^{-1}·d^{-1} for someone who weighs 110 kg (242 lb) would be equivalent to four glasses (~1000 ml) of low-fat milk, one can of tuna (~115g), a 6-oz skinless roast chicken breast (~170g), one cup of low fat yogurt (~245g) and four slices (184g) of whole-wheat bread. The same diet would provide only 6300 kJ, or ~1500 kcal and would provide 37% of one's energy from protein; however, it serves to illustrate how easy it is to obtain sufficient quantities of high quality protein from normal dietary sources. For an athlete in training, this sort of daily consumption is relatively easy to achieve without the use of protein supplements. Moreover, the training-induced improvement in nitrogen balance reported by Campbell et al.[143] occurred in a group of elderly persons who did not experience significant muscular hypertrophy, likely due to the moderate training stimulus they received despite 11 weeks of resistance training. Hence, it may be that, with more intense resistance exercise programs resulting eventually in significant fiber hypertrophy, the efficiency of nitrogen utilization may be even greater than that reported previously.[143]

While there is only weak evidence linking persistently high protein diets (Table 12.2) with adverse health consequences such as renal disease and poor bone health, Price et al.[146] have shown that high protein diets, once initiated, should be maintained to preserve lean mass. Essentially, what has been

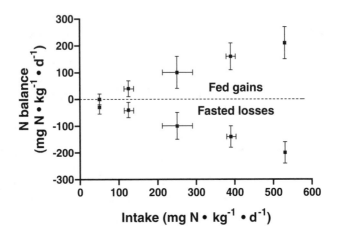

FIGURE 12.5
Fed and fasted cycling of protein turnover with increasing protein intakes (adapted from Price et al.[146]).

shown is that high protein diets, while they may result in high fed gains (i.e., stimulation of protein synthesis); there is a concomitant high fasting loss of protein (see Figure 12.5).[146,147] These findings[146,147] have implications for athletes who habitually consume high dietary protein intakes; they run the "risk" of losing lean body mass if they do not consistently follow this practice. The fasting loss of protein (i.e., lean body mass) arises due to the fact that urea cycle and amino acid oxidative enzymes adapt to higher protein intakes via an increase in activity;[143] hence, when one consumes high protein liver and potentially muscle, amino acid oxidative capacity is increased and hence with greater protein intake an increasingly larger proportion of dietary protein is directed toward oxidation. This assertion is supported as can be seen in Figure 12.5, which is adapted from the data of Price et al.[146] that shows greater fasting oxidative losses of amino acids concomitant with greater fed gains (protein synthesis) with increasing protein intakes. Accordingly, the pattern of consuming a large amount of dietary protein must be maintained because a significant time period must elapse before fasting losses are reduced (i.e., the time taken for urea cycle and amino acid oxidative enzymes to adapt), which would lead to significant lean body mass losses.[147]

It is apparent that, a *meaningful* recommendation for strength training athletes for a recommended dietary protein intake, based on the literature, is confounded by numerous factors including training status and combination of strength training with other modalities (sprint or aerobic exercise) and methodological considerations. What is certain, however, is that, even those athletes who have as their goal the gain of an impressive amount of lean mass, they do not require an enormous increase in protein intake. Consequently, as with my recommendation for the dietary protein intake for endurance athletes, I believe that even the most ardent strength-training athletes need not consume any more than 15% of their dietary calories in the form of protein. These same athletes should, however, be getting at least 10% of their dietary energy from protein, so long as they are consuming sufficient protein to cover their energy needs or surfeit energy required for optimal weight gain. It should be emphasized that, for even for larger athletes (100 kg and greater); a sufficient energy intake to cover caloric requirements for weight gain during intense training may be in excess of $18MJ/d^{-1}$ (~4300 kcal). Hence, protein intakes as high as 20% of such an energy intake would mean a daily protein intake of $215g/d^{-1}$, which would definitely be excessive by any standard (2.15 g $protein \cdot kg^{-1} \cdot d^{-1}$). Hence, protein needs of this group of athletes generally should be balanced against what is considered necessary.

V. Future Directions

Given the opposing points of view regarding protein requirements for athletes,[3,5,7-9.25-27,127,128] there is no doubt that future studies to examine protein requirements and even amino acid requirements during endurance exercise should to be conducted. Some definitive studies, if properly conducted and controlled, might serve to clear up much of the controversy[3,5,7-9.25-27,127,128] surrounding protein requirements in habitually active persons. The first study would be to have a group of highly trained endurance athletes having relatively high daily training volumes randomly consume protein at three different levels for prolonged periods of time (at least 3–4 weeks). As in a traditional nitrogen balance experiment, protein would be consumed at a sub-adequate (0.6 g $protein \cdot kg^{-1} \cdot d^{-1}$), adequate (1.0 g $protein \cdot kg^{-1} \cdot d^{-1}$) and more than adequate (2 g $protein \cdot kg^{-1} \cdot d^{-1}$) level. Each protein intake would have a period at the end of which measurements of protein kinetics, using appropriate stable isotope tracers, for muscle protein, plasma protein (albumin, fibrinogen, fibronectin), as well as whole-body protein turnover and nitrogen balance. In addition, and most importantly from an athlete's perspective, performance would be measured. This study has the following advantages:

1. Studying previously habitually trained athletes so the transient negative nitrogen balance seen at training onset[138] would not be a complicating factor

2. A prolonged period of adaptation to each diet to account for adaptations in enzymes involved in intramuscular protein metabolism and liver urea cycle enzymes

3. Measurement of protein kinetics for muscle, some blood proteins and at the whole body level, at each level of protein intake to account for adaptations in synthesis and turnover

4. Measurement of performance, which for athletes is the most important outcome

A second study would be similar to the one previously described, but obviously to include resistance trained athletes. This study would have the same advantages as outlined above, but would definitively show that high protein intakes are of no benefit in the maintenance of strength and lean mass for these athletes.

A third study would be to allow three comparatively large (N = 20 per group) groups of athletes who where inexperienced weightlifters to initiate a weightlifting program. Each group would have their diet manipulated so that they were consuming either 0.86 g protein$\cdot$ kg$^{-1}\cdot$d^{-1} (the current RNI/ RDA/DRI), 1.2 g protein$\cdot$ kg$^{-1}\cdot$d^{-1} (at or close to the average protein intake for a lacto-ovo, meat-eating North American male), or 2.2 g protein$\cdot$kg$^{-1}\cdot$d^{-1} (at or close to the habitual dietary protein intake for many strength-training athletes). Measures of muscle protein and whole-body protein kinetics, as well as nitrogen balance, should then be made at the beginning, in response to an acute bout of resistance exercise and at the end of their training programs, also in response to an acute bout of resistance exercise, which should last at least 12 weeks. The degree of muscle hypertrophy could be assessed both by biopsy techniques as well as by various imaging methods for all limb musculature and gains in lean mass could be measured using dual-energy x-ray absorptiometry. These measures should be made at 2-week intervals during the training program to assess the time course of changes in these parameters. This study would provide a reasonably definitive answer as to whether recommended protein intakes could support the same degree and rate of muscular hypertrophy and lean mass gain vs. higher protein intakes. Measurements of protein turnover in various body compartments, using isotopic tracers, would allow for the determination of the kinetic responses to each protein intake. A sufficient sample size (N = 20) would ensure that the inherent variability in measures of lean mass and fiber type and size would not mask a significant effect, should one be observed.

VI. Summary

No current recommendations for dietary protein intake include an allowance for physical activity. This is despite some evidence that regular aerobic-based exercise apparently results in an elevated requirement for dietary protein (see Figure 12.2). The basis for an elevated protein requirement in endurance athletes is the increased amino acid oxidation seen during exercise; however, whether amino acids other than leucine are oxidized to any appreciable extent during exercise appears unlikely. Despite the fact that endurance exercise results in an elevated amino acid oxidation, exercise training appears to lower, if not obliterate, the acute exercise-induced rise in amino acid oxidation, a finding that calls into question the thesis that endurance exercise elevates any requirement for dietary protein. In addition, in spite of reports showing that protein requirements are elevated in endurance-trained athletes, other reports show that habitual exercise lowers the requirements for dietary protein. Hence, it would appear that a conclusion that dynamic endurance-based exercise elevates proteins to any appreciable extent is impossible to make. In addition, the reported dietary protein intakes of endurance-trained athletes are far in excess of any current recommendation, due for the most part to their need to consume energy to balance their high daily expenditure. Hence, it is unlikely that endurance trained athletes require a highly specific recommendation for dietary protein intake. Instead, this author believes it is far more practical and applicable to give the recommendation that at least 10% and no more than 20% of dietary energy, provided the diet is varied and mixed and that energy is sufficient to cover energy expenditure, should come from protein for this group of athletes.

Strength-trained athletes habitually consume protein in excess of recommended intakes (Table 12.2). Some studies have reported that consumption of protein at levels greater than the RNI/RDA/DRI might be beneficial for strength trained athletes, because they appear to have protein requirements above those of sedentary persons (Figure 12.4). However, another body of literature indicates that strength training results in reduced protein requirements due to the anabolic nature of the activity. Support for such a supposition also comes from a consideration of a longitudinal examination of protein requirements in a group of elderly persons showing that 11 weeks of weightlifting resulted in increased retention of nitrogen.[143] Moreover, calculation of protein requirements for even the largest lean mass gains do not support the idea that supplementation with protein is necessary, provided that a mixed diet providing sufficient energy is consumed. Moreover, it is apparent that, while consumption of excessively high protein intakes leads to larger fed-state gains in lean body mass, it also results in greater fasted losses (see Figure 12.5). Are protein requirements for strength-training athletes truly elevated? Once again, it is almost impossible to clearly establish an exact protein intake for strength training individuals; however, a practical recommendation is, as with endurance athletes, that at least 10% and no more than 20% of dietary energy come from protein, in a mixed omnivorous diet that covers energy requirements.

Finally, it is this author's belief that a safe upper limit for dietary protein intakes should also be imposed with endurance- and strength-trained athletes of no more than 1.3–1.4 g protein·kg^{-1}·d^{-1}. Such a recommended intake may appear to be contraindicated, particularly in light of some of the recommended protein intakes to achieve nitrogen balance reported in individual studies.[5,7-9] However, in each study, no more than 6–8 participants were used and all relied on the short-term nitrogen balance methodology to establish requirement, an approach that has serious flaws.[130,132] Perhaps the most puzzling and troublesome flaw with the nitrogen balance methodology is the persistently positive nitrogen balance with increasing protein intakes (see

Figures 12.2 and 12.4). The highly positive nitrogen balance observed at high protein intakes would apparently result from an unbelievable expansion of body protein pools, namely an increase in lean body mass. Such an increase in lean body mass, as pointed out, cannot and does not occur. Until this problem with the nitrogen balance method is resolved, or unless the method is coupled with kinetic measures of amino acid turnover, a consensus cannot be reached when relying solely on this technique.

Undoubtedly, more research is required to answer some unresolved questions in the area of protein metabolism and requirements in athletes, whether they be endurance or strength-trained or beginning an exercise program. It is obvious to this author that future advances in methodology in amino acid metabolism, along with their successful and appropriate application, will allow for more definitive recommendations to be made to athletes. However, at this time, it appears that general recommendations for dietary protein (i.e., the current RNI/RDA/DRI) are adequate, provided a diet containing mixed food sources and sufficient energy is being consumed and there is no evidence that protein requirements are elevated to a degree that would call for supplemental protein to be consumed.

References

1. Romijn, J.A., Coyle, E.F., Sidossis, S., Gastaldelli, A., Horowitz, J.F., Endert, E. and Wolfe, R.R., Regulation of endogenous fat and carbohydrate metabolism in relation to exercise intensity and duration. *Am. J. Physiol.*, 265, E380-E391, 1993.
2. Tarnopolsky, M.A., Atkinson, S.A., Phillips, S.M. and MacDougall, J.D., Carbohydrate loading and metabolism during exercise in men and women. *J. Appl. Physiol.*, 78, 1360, 1995.
3. Phillips, S.M., Atkinson, S.A., Tarnopolsky, M.A. and MacDougall, J.D., Gender differences in leucine kinetics and nitrogen balance in endurance athletes. *J. Appl. Physiol.*, 75(5), 2134, 1994.
4. Tarnopolsky, L.J., MacDougall, J.D., Atkinson, S.A., Tarnopolsky, M.A. and Sutton, J.R., Gender differences in substrate for endurance exercise. *J. Appl. Physiol.*, 68, 302, 1990.
5. Meredith, C.N., Zackin, M.J., Frontera, W.R. and Evans, W.J., Dietary protein requirements and body protein metabolism in endurance-trained men. *J. Appl. Physiol.*, 66, 2850, 1989.
6. Knapik, J., Meredith, C.N., Jones, B., Fielding, R., Young, V. and Evans, W.J., Leucine metabolism during fasting and exercise. *J. Appl. Physiol.*, 70, 43, 1991.
7. Tarnopolsky, M.A., Atkinson, S.A., MacDougall, J.D., Chesley, A., Phillips, S. and Schwarcz, H.P., Evaluation of protein requirements for trained strength athletes. *J. Appl. Physiol.*, 73, 1986, 1992.
8. Tarnopolsky, M.A., MacDougall, J.D. and Atkinson, S.A., Influence of protein intake and training status on nitrogen balance and lean body mass. *J. Appl. Physiol.*, 64, 187, 1988.

9. Friedman, J.E. and Lemon, P.W., Effect of chronic endurance exercise on retention of dietary protein. *Int. J. Sports Med.,* 10, 118, 1989.

10. Tarnopolsky, M.A., Atkinson, S.A., MacDougall, J.D., Senor, B.B., Lemon, P.W.R. and Schwarcz, H., Whole body leucine metabolism during and after resistance exercise in fed humans. *Med. Sci. Sports Exerc.,* 23, 326, 1991.

11. Phillips, S.M., Tipton, K.D., Aarsland, A., Wolf, S.E. and Wolfe, R.R., Mixed muscle protein synthesis and breakdown following resistance exercise in humans. *Am. J. Physiol.,* 273, E99-E107, 1997.

12. Phillips, S.M., Tipton, K.D., Ferrando, A.A. and Wolfe, R.R., Resistance training reduces the acute exercise-induced increase in muscle protein turnover. *Am. J. Physiol.,* 276, E118-E124, 1999.

13. Chesley, A., MacDougall, J.D., Tarnopolsky, M.A., Atkinson, S.A. and Smith, K., Changes in human muscle protein synthesis after resistance exercise. *J. Appl. Physiol.,* 73, 1383, 1992.

14. Yarasheski, K.E., Zachwieja, J.F. and Bier, D.M., Acute effects of resistance exercise on muscle protein synthesis rate in young and elderly men and women. *Am. J. Physiol.,* 265, E210-E214, 1993.

15. Yarasheski, K.E., Pak-Loduca, J., Hasten, D.L., Obert, K.A., Brown, M.B. and Sinacore, D.R., Resistance exercise training increases mixed muscle protein synthesis rate in frail women and men > 76 years old. *Am. J. Physiol.,* 277, E118-E125, 1999.

16. Biolo, G., Maggi, S.P., Williams, B.D., Tipton, K.D. and Wolfe, R.R., Increased rates of muscle protein turnover and amino acid transport after resistance exercise in humans. *Am. J. Physiol.,* 268, E514-E520, 1995.

17. Biolo, G., Tipton, K.D., Klein, S. and Wolfe, R.R., An abundant supply of amino acids enhances the metabolic effect of exercise on muscle protein. *Am. J. Physiol.,* 273, E122-E129, 1997.

18. Biolo, G., Williams, B.D., Fleming, R.Y. and Wolfe, R.R., Insulin action on muscle protein kinetics and amino acid transport during recovery after resistance exercise (in process citation). *Diabetes,* 48(5), 949-957, 1999.

19. MacDougall, J.D., Ward, G.R., Sale, D.G. and Sutton, J.R., Biochemical adaptation of human skeletal muscle to heavy resistance training and immobilization. *J. Appl. Physiol.,* 43, 700, 1977.

20. Nelson, M.E., Fiatarone, M.A., Layne, J.E., Trice, I., Economos, C.D., Fielding, R.A., Ma, R., Pierson, R.N. and Evans, W.J., Analysis of body-composition techniques and models for detecting change in soft tissue with strength training. *Am. J. Clin. Nutr,* 63, 678, 1996.

21. McCall, G.E., Byrnes, W.C., Dickinson, A., Pattany, P.M. and Fleck, S.J., Muscle fiber hypertrophy, hyperplasia and capillary density in college men after resistance training. *J. Appl. Physiol.,* 81, 2004, 1996.

22. Hortobagyi, T., Hill, J.P., Houmard, J.A., Fraser, D.D., Lambert, N.J. and Israel, R.G., Adaptive responses to muscle lengthening and shortening in humans. *J. Appl. Physiol.,* 80, 765, 1996.

23. Gibala, M.J., MacDougall, J.D., Tarnopolsky, M.A., Stauber, W.T. and Elorriaga, A., Changes in human skeletal muscle ultrastructure and force production after acute resistance exercise. *J. Appl. Physiol.,* 78, 702, 1995.

24. Gibala, M.J., Interisano, S.A., Tarnopolsky, M.A., Roy, B.D., MacDonald, J.R., Yarasheski, K.E. and MacDougall, J.D., Myofibrillar disruption following acute concentric and eccentric resistance exercise in strength-trained men. *Can. J. Appl. Physiol.,* 78, 656, 2000.

25. Millward, D.J., Bowtell, J.L., Pacy, P. and Rennie, M.J., Physical activity, protein metabolism and protein requirements. *Proc. Nutr. Soc.*, 53, 223, 1994.
26. Millward, D.J. Inherent difficulties in defining amino acid requirements in *The Role of Protein and Amino Acids in Sustaining and Enhancing Performance.*, Natl. Acad. Press, Washington, D.C.,169-216, 1999.
27. Butterfield, G.E. and Calloway, D.H., Physical activity improves protein utilization in young men. *Brit. J. Nutr.*, 51, 171, 1984.
28. Bier, D.M., Intrinsically difficult problems: the kinetics of body proteins and amino acid in man. *Diabetes Metab. Rev.*, 5, 111, 1989.
29. Millward, D.J. The endocrine response to dietary protein: the anabolic drive on growth. in *Milk Proteins,* Barth, C.A. and Schlimme E., Eds., Steinkoppf Verlag, Darmstadt, 1989.
30. Goldspink, G., Selective gene expression during adaptation of muscle in response to different physiological demands. *Comp. Biochem. Physiol. B Biochem. Mol. Biol.*, 120, 5, 1998.
31. Kimball, S.R. and Jefferson, L.S., Regulation of protein synthesis by branched-chain amino acids. *Curr Opin. Clin. Nutr. Metab. Care*, 4, 39, 2001.
32. Roy, B.D., Tarnopolsky, M.A., MacDougall, J.D., Fowles, J. and Yarasheski, K.E., Effect of glucose supplement timing on protein metabolism after resistance training. *J. Appl. Physiol.*, 82, 1882, 1997.
33. Svanberg, E., Moller-Loswick, A.C., Matthews, D.E., Korner, U., Andersson, M. and Lundholm, K., The role of glucose, long-chain triglycerides and amino acids for promotion of amino acid balance across peripheral tissues in man. *Clin. Physiol.*, 19, 311, 1999.
34. Carraro, F., Kimbrough, T.D. and Wolfe, R.R., Urea kinetics in humans at two levels of exercise intensity. *J. Appl. Physiol.*, 75, 1180, 1993.
35. El-Khoury, A.E., Forslund, A., Olsson, R., Branth, S., Sjödin, A., Andersson, A., Atkinson, A., Selvaraj, A., Hambraeus, L. and Young, V.R., Moderate exercise at energy balance does not affect 24-h leucine oxidation or nitrogen rentention in healthy men. *Am. J. Physiol.*, 273, E394-E407, 1997.
36. Bowtell, J.L., Leese, G.P., Smith, K., Watt, P.W., Nevill, A., Rooyackers, O., Wagenmakers, A.M. and Rennie, M.J., Modulation of whole body protein metabolism, during and after exercise, by variation of dietary protein. *J Appl. Physiol.*, 85, 1744, 1998.
37. Dohm, G.L., Kasperek, G.J., Tapscott, E.B. and Barakat, H.A., Protein metabolism during endurance exercise. *Fed. Proc.*, 44, 348, 1985.
38. Carraro, F., Stuart, C.A., Hartl, W.H., Rosenblatt, J. and Wolfe, R.R., Effect of exercise and recovery on muscle protein synthesis in human subjects. *Am. J. Physiol.*, 259, E470-E476, 1990.
39. Goldberg, A.L. and Chang, T.W., Regulation and significance of amino acid metabolism in skeletal muscle. *Fed. Proc.*, 37, 2301, 1978.
40. Biolo, G., Gastaldelli, A., Zhang, X.-J. and Wolfe, R.R., Protein synthesis and breakdown in skin and muscle: a leg model of amino acid kinetics. *Am. J. Physiol.*, 267, E467-E474, 1996.
41. Biolo, G., Fleming, D., Maggi, S.P. and Wolfe, R.R., Transmembrane transport and intracellular kinetics of amino acids in human skeletal muscle. *Am. J. Physiol.*, 268, E75-E84, 1995.
42. Ahlborg, G., Felig, P., Hagenfeldt, L., Hendler, R. and Wahren, J., Substrate turnover during prolonged exercise in man. *J. Clin. Invest.*, 53, 1080, 1974.

43. Graham, T.E., Turcotte, L.P., Kiens, B. and Richter, E.A., Training and muscle ammonia and amino acid metabolism in humans during prolonged exercise. *J. Appl. Physiol.*, 78, 725, 1995.
44. Felig, P., Amino acid metabolism in man. *Ann. Rev. Biochem.*, 44, 933, 1975.
45. Wolfe, R.R., Goodenough, R.D., Wolfe, M.H., Royle, G.T. and Nadel, E.R., Isotopic analysis of leucine and urea metabolism in exercising humans. *J. Appl. Physiol.*, 52, 458, 1982.
46. Henderson, S.C., Black, A.L. and Brooks, G.A., Leucine turnover and oxidation in trained rats during exercise. *Am. J. Physiol.*, 249, E137-E144, 1985.
47. Boyer, B. and Odessey, R., Kinetic characterization of branched chain ketoacid dehydrogenase. *Arch. Biochem. Biophys.*, 285, 1, 1991.
48. Khatra, B.S., Chawla, R.K., Sewell, C.W. and Rudman, D., Distribution of branched-chain α-keto acid dehydrogenases in primate tissues. *J. Clin. Invest.*, 59, 558, 1977.
49. May, R.C., Hara, Y., Kelly, R.A., Block, K.P., Buse, M.G. and Mitch, W.E., Branched-chain amino acid metabolism in rat muscle: abnormal regulation in acidosis. *Am. J. Physiol.*, 252, E712-E718, 1987.
50. Holloszy, J.O., Biochemical adaptations in muscle. Effects of exercise on mitochondrial oxygen uptake and respiratory enzyme activity in skeletal muscle. *J Biol Chem*, 242, 2278, 1967.
51. Holloszy, J.O. and Coyle, E.F., Adaptations of skeletal muscle to endurance exercise and their metabolic consequences. *J. Appl. Physiol.*, 56, 831, 1984.
52. Phillips, S.M., Green, H.J., Tarnopolsky, M.A., Heigenhauser, G.J.F. and Grant, S.M., Progressive effect of endurance training on metabolic adaptations in working skeletal muscle. *Am. J. Physiol.*, 270, E265-E272, 1996.
53. Dohm, G.L., Hecker, A.L., Brown, W.E., Klain, G.J., Puente, F.R., Askew, E.W. and Beecher, G.R., Adaptation of protein metabolism to endurance training. Increased amino acid oxidation in response to training. *Biochem J*, 164, 705, 1977.
54. Lemon, P.W., Benevenga, N.J., Mullin, J.P. and Nagle, F.J., Effect of daily exercise and food intake on leucine oxidation. *Biochem Med*, 33, 67, 1985.
55. Hood, D.A. and Terjung, R.L., Effect of endurance training on leucine metabolism in perfused rat skeletal muscle. *Am. J. Physiol.*, 253, E648-E656, 1987.
56. McKenzie, S., Phillips, S.M., Carter, S.L., Lowther, S., Gibala, M.J. and Tarnopolsky, M.A., Endurance exercise training attenuates leucine oxidation and BCOAD activation during exercise in humans. *Am. J. Physiol. Endocrinol. Metab.*, 278, E580-E587, 2000.
57. Lamont, L.S., McCullough, A.J. and Kalhan, S.C., Comparison of leucine kinetics in endurance-trained and sedentary humans. *J. Appl. Physiol.*, 86, 320, 1999.
58. MacLean, D.A., Graham, T.E. and Saltin, B., Branched-chain amino acids augment ammonia metabolism while attenuating protein breakdown during exercise. *Am. J. Physiol.*, 276, E1010-E1022, 1994.
59. MacLean, D.A. and Graham, T.E., Branched-chain amino acid supplementation augments plasma ammonia responses during exercise in humans. *J. Appl. Physiol.*, 74, 2711, 1993.
60. Katz, A., Broberg, S., Sahlin, K. and Wahren, J., Muscle ammonia metabolism and amino acid metabolism during dynamic exercise in man. *Clin. Physiol.*, 6, 365, 1986.
61. Eriksson, L.S., Broberg, S., Björkman, O. and Wahren, J., Ammonia metabolism during exercise in man. *Clin. Physiol.*, 5, 325, 1985.

62. Lemon, P.W., Nagle, F.J., Mullin, J.P. and Benevenga, N.J., *In vivo* leucine oxidation at rest and during two intensities of exercise. *J. Appl. Physiol.*, 53, 947, 1982.

63. Wolfe, R.R., Wolfe, M.H., Nadel, E.R. and Shaw, J.H., Isotopic determination of amino acid-urea interactions in exercise in humans. *J. Appl. Physiol.*, 56, 221, 1984.

64. Carraro, F., Hartl, W.H., Stuart, C.A., Layman, D.K., Jahoor, F. and Wolfe, R.R., Whole body and plasma protein synthesis in exercise and recovery in human subjects. *Am. J. Physiol.*, 258, E821, 1990.

65. Williams, B.D., Wolfe, R.R., Bracy, D.P. and Wasserman, D.H., Gut proteolysis contributes essential amino acids during exercise. *Am. J. Physiol.*, 270, E85-E90, 1996.

66. Dohm, G.L., Tapscott, E.B. and Kasperek, G.J., Protein degradation during endurance exercise and recovery. *Med. Sci. Sports Exerc.*, 19, 64, 1987.

67. Dohm, G.L., Beecher, G.R., Warren, R.Q. and Williams, R.T., The influence of exercise on free amino acid concentrations in rat tissues. *J. Appl. Physiol.*, 50, 41, 1982.

68. Kasperek, G.J., Dohm, G.L., Barakat, H.A., Strausbauch, D.W., Barnes, D.W. and Snider, R.D., The role of lysosomes in exercise-induced hepatic protein loss. *Biochem. J.*, 202, 281, 1982.

69. Wasserman, D.H., Geer, R.J., Williams, P.E., Becker, T.A., Lacy, D.B. and Abumrad, N.N., Interaction of gut and liver on nitrogen metabolism during exercise. *Metabolism*, 40, 168, 1991.

70. Nakshabendi, I.M., McKee, R., Downie, S., Russell, R.I. and Rennie, M.J., Rates of small intestinal mucosal protein synthesis in human jejunum and ileum. *Am. J. Physiol.*, 277, E1028-E1031, 1999.

71. Sultan, K.R., Dittrich, B.T. and Pette, D., Calpain activity in fast, slow, transforming and regenerating skeletal muscles of rat. *Am. J. Physiol. Cell Physiol.*, 279, C639-C647, 2000.

72. Wong, T.S. and Booth, F.W., Protein metabolism in rat tibialis anterior muscle after stimulated chronic concentric exercise. *J. Appl. Physiol.*, 69, 1709, 1990.

73. Wong, T.S. and Booth, F.W., Protein metabolism in rat tibialis anterior muscle after stimulated chronic eccentric exercise. *J. Appl. Physiol.*, 69, 1718, 1990.

74. Staron, R.S., Karapondo, D.L., Kraemer, W.J., Fry, A.C., Gordon, S.E., Falkel, J.E., Hagerman, F.C. and Hikida, R.S., Skeletal muscle adaptations during early phase of heavy-resistance training in men and women. *J. Appl. Physiol.*, 76, 1247, 1994.

75. Staron, R.S. and Johnson, P., Myosin polymorphism and differential expression in adult human skeletal muscle. *Comp. Biochem. Physiol.*, 106, 463, 1993.

76. Staron, R.S., Leonardi, M.J., Karapondo, D.L., Malicky, E.S., Falkel, JE, Hagerman, F.C. and Hikida, R.S., Strength and skeletal muscle adaptations in heavy-resistance- trained women after detraining and retraining. *J. Appl. Physiol.*, 70, 631, 1991.

77. Hortobagyi, T., Dempsey, L., Fraser, D., Zheng, D., Hamilton, G., Lambert, J. and Dohm, L., Changes in muscle strength, muscle fiber size and myofibrillar gene expression after immobilization and retraining in humans. *J. Physiol.*, 524, 293, 2000.

78. Green, H., Goreham, C., Ouyang, J., Ball-Burnett, M. and Ranney, D., Regulation of fiber size, oxidative potential and capillarization in human muscle by resistance exercise. *Am J Physiol*, 276, R591, 1999.

79. Phillips, S.M., Short-term training: when do repeated bouts of resistance exercise become training? *Can. J. Appl. Physiol.,* 25, 185, 2000.

80. Farrell, P.A., Fedele, M.J., Vary, T.C., Kimball, S.R., Lang, C.H. and Jefferson, L.S., Regulation of protein synthesis after acute resistance exercise in diabetic rats. *Am. J. Physiol.,* 276, E721-E727, 1999.

81. Farrell, P.A., Fedele, M.J., Vary, T.C., Kimball, S.R. and Jefferson, L.S., Effects of intensity of acute-resistance exercise on rates of protein synthesis in moderately diabetic rats. *J. Appl. Physiol.,* 85, 2291, 1998.

82. Farrell, P.A., Fedele, M.J., Hernandez, J., Fluckey, J.D., Miller, J.L., III, Lang, C.H., Vary, T.C., Kimball, S.R. and Jefferson, L.S., Hypertrophy of skeletal muscle in diabetic rats in response to chronic resistance exercise. *J. Appl. Physiol.,* 87, 1075, 1999.

83. Roman, W.J., Fleckenstein, J., Stray-Gundersen, J., Alway, S.E., Peshock, R. and Gonyea, W.J., Adaptations in the elbow flexors of elderly males after heavy-resistance training. *J. Appl. Physiol.,* 74, 750, 1993.

84. Alway, S.E., Grumbt, W.H., Stray-Gundersen, J. and Gonyea, W.J., Effects of resistance training on elbow flexors of highly competitive bodybuilders. *J. Appl. Physiol.,* 72, 1512, 1992.

85. Housch, T.J., Housch, D.J., Weir, J.P. and Weir, L.L., Effects of eccentric-only resistance training and detraining. *Int. J. Sports Med.,* 17, 145, 1996.

86. Welle, S., Thornton, C., Jozefowicz, R. and Statt, M., Myofibrillar protein synthesis in young and old men. *Am. J. Physiol.,* 264, E693-E698, 1993.

87. Hasten, D.L., Morris, G.S., Ramanadham, S. and Yarasheski, K.E., Isolation of human skeletal muscle myosin heavy chain and actin for measurement of fractional synthesis rates. *Am. J. Physiol.,* 275, E1092-E1099, 1998.

88. Hasten, D.L., Pak-Loduca, J., Obert, K.A. and Yarasheski, K.E., Resistance exercise acutely increases MHC and mixed muscle protein synthesis rates in 78-84 and 23-32 yr olds. *Am. J. Physiol.,* 278, E620-E626, 2000.

89. MacDougall, J.D., Gibala, M.J., Tarnopolsky, M.A., MacDonald, J.R., Interisano, S.A. and Yarasheski, K.E., The time course for elevated muscle protein synthesis following heavy resistance exercise. *Can. J. Appl. Physiol.,* 20, 480, 1995.

90. Ferrando, A.A., Tipton, K.D., Doyle, D., Phillips, S.M., Cortiella, J. and Wolfe, R.R., Testosterone injection stimulates net protein synthesis but not tissue amino acid transport. *Am. J. Physiol.,* 275, E864-E871, 1998.

91. Wolfe, R.R., Protein supplements and exercise. *Am. J. Clin. Nutr,* 72, 551S, 2000.

92. Tipton, K.D. and Wolfe, R.R., Exercise-induced changes in protein metabolism. *Acta Physiol. Scand.,* 162, 377, 1998.

93. Dohm, G.L., Israel, R.G., Breedlove, R.L., Williams, R.T. and Askew, E.W., Biphasic changes in 3-methylhistidine excretion in humans after exercise. *Am. J. Physiol.,* 248, E588-E592, 1985.

94. Dohm, G.L., Williams, R.T., Kasperek, G.J. and van Rij, A.M., Increased excretion of urea and N^t-methylhistidine by rats and humans after a bout of exercise. *J. Appl. Physiol.,* 52, 27, 1982.

95. Pivarnick, J.M., Hickson, J.F. and Wolinsky, I., Urinary 3-methylhistidine excretion increases with repeated weight training exercise. *Med. Sci. Sports Exerc.,* 21, 283, 1989.

96. Hickson, J.F., Wolinsky, I., Rodriguez, G.P., Pivarnick, J.M., Kent, M.C. and Shier, N.W., Failure of weight training to affect urinary indices of protein metabolism in men. *Med. Sci. Sports Exerc.,* 18, 563, 1986.

97. Rennie, M.J. and Millward, D.J., 3-Methylhistidine excretion and the urinary 3-methylhistidine/creatinine ratio are poor indicators of skeletal muscle protein breakdown. *Clin. Sci.,* 65, 217, 1983.

98. Fu, A. and Nair, K.S., Age effect on fibrinogen and albumin synthesis in humans. *Am. J. Physiol.,* 275, E1023-E1030, 1998.

99. Rasmussen, B.B., Tipton, K.D., Miller, S.L., Wolf, S.E. and Wolfe, R.R., An oral essential amino acid-carbohydrate supplement enhances muscle protein anabolism after resistance exercise. *J. Appl. Physiol.,* 88, 386, 2000.

100. Tipton, K.D., Ferrando, A.A., Phillips, S.M., Doyle, D.J. and Wolfe, R.R., Postexercise net protein synthesis in human muscle from orally administered amino acids. *Am. J. Physiol.,* 276, E628-E634, 1999.

101. Svanberg, E., Möller-Loswick, A.-C., Matthews, D.E., Korner, U., Andersson, M. and Lundholm, K., Effects of amino acids on synthesis and degradation of skeletal muscle proteins in humans. *Am. J. Physiol.,* 271, E718-E724, 1996.

102. Svanberg, E., Ohlsson, C., Hyltander, A. and Lundholm, K.G., The role of diet components, gastrointestinal factors and muscle innervation on activation of protein synthesis in skeletal muscles following oral refeeding. *Nutrition,* 15, 257, 1999.

103. Svanberg, E., Jefferson, L.S., Lundholm, K. and Kimball, S.R., Postprandial stimulation of muscle protein synthesis is independent of changes in insulin. *Am. J. Physiol.,* 272, E841-E847, 1997.

104. Svanberg, E., Amino acids may be intrinsic regulators of protein synthesis in response to feeding. *Clin. Nutr.,* 17, 77, 1998.

105. Adams, G.R. and McCue, S.A., Localized infusion of IGF-I results in skeletal muscle hypertrophy in rats. *J. Appl. Physiol.,* 84, 1716, 1998.

106. Russell-Jones, D.L., Umpleby, A.M., Hennessy, T.R., Bowes, S.B., Shojaee-Moradie, F., Hopkins, K.D., Jackson, N.C., Kelly, J.M., Jones, R.H. and Sonksen, P.H., Use of a leucine clamp to demonstrate that IGF-I actively stimulates protein synthesis in normal humans. *Am. J. Physiol.,* 267, E591, 1994.

107. Goldspink, G., Changes in muscle mass and phenotype and the expression of autocrine and systemic growth factors by muscle in response to stretch and overload. *J. Anat.,* 194, 323, 1999.

108. Ordway, G.A., Neufer, P.D., Chin, E.R. and Demartino, G.N., Chronic contractile activity upregulates the proteasome system in rabbit skeletal muscle. *J. Appl. Physiol.,* 88, 1134, 2000.

109. Attaix, D., Aurousseau, E., Combaret, L., Kee, A., Larbaud, D., Ralliere, C., Souweine, B., Taillandier, D. and Tilignac, T., Ubiquitin-proteasome-dependent proteolysis in skeletal muscle. *Reprod. Nutr. Dev.,* 38, 153, 1998.

110. Deuster, P.A., Kyle, S.B., Moser, P.B., Vigersky, R.A., Singh, A. and Schoomaker, E.B., Nutritional survey of highly trained women runners. *Am. J. Clin. Nutr.,* 44, 954, 1986.

111. Drinkwater, B.L., Nilson, K., Chesnut, C.H., III, Bremner, W.J., Shainholtz, S. and Southworth, M.B., Bone mineral content of amenorrheic and eumenorrheic athletes. *New Engl. J. Med.,* 311, 277, 1984.

112. Marcus, R., Cann, C., Madvig, P., Minkoff, J., Goddard, M., Bayer, M., Martin, M., Gaudiani, L., Haskell, W. and Genant, H., Menstrual function and bone mass in elite women distance runners. Endocrine and metabolic features. *Ann. Intern. Med.,* 102, 158, 1985.

113. Nelson, M.E., Fisher, E.C., Catsos, P.D., Meredith, C.N., Turksoy, R.N. and Evans, W.J., Diet and bone status in amenorrheic runners. *Am. J. Clin. Nutr.*, 43, 910, 1986.

114. Saris, W.H., Erp-Baart, M.A., Brouns, F., Westerterp, K.R. and ten Hoor, F., Study on food intake and energy expenditure during extreme sustained exercise: the Tour de France. *Int. J. Sports Med.*, 10, S26-S31, 1989.

115. Tarnopolsky, M.A., Bosman, M., MacDonald, J.R., Vandeputte, D., Martin, J. and Roy, B.D., Postexercise protein-carbohydrate and carbohydrate supplements increase muscle glycogen in men and women. *J. Appl. Physiol.*, 83, 1877, 1997.

116. Faber, M. and Benade, A.J., Nutrient intake and dietary supplementation in bodybuilders. *S. Afr. Med. J.*, 72, 831, 1987.

117. Lemon, P.W., Tarnopolsky, M.A., MacDougall, J.D. and Atkinson, S.A., Protein requirements and muscle mass/strength changes during intensive training in novice bodybuilders. *J. Appl. Physiol.*, 73, 767, 1992.

118. Short, S.H. and Short, W.R., Four-year study of university athletes' dietary intake. *J. Am. Diet. Assoc.*, 82, 632, 1983.

119. Energy and Protein Requirements. Report of a Joint FAO/WHO/UNU Expert Consultation. (Tech. Rep. No. 724). Geneva,Switzerland, World Health Organization.

120. Nutrition recommendations: The Report of the Scientific Review Committee. Ottawa, Canada, Canadian Government Publishing Centre.

121. Institute of Medicine F.N.B. *Dietary Reference Intakes for Protein*. Washington, D.C., National Academy Press.

122. National Research Council. *Recommended Dietary Allowances*. 10th ed. Washington D.C., National Academy Press., 1995.

123. Schoeller, D.A., Limitations in the assessment of dietary energy intake by self-report. *Metabolism*, 44 (Suppl), 22, 1995.

124. Schoeller, D.A., How accurate is self-reported dietary energy intake? *Nutr. Rev.*, 48, 373, 1990.

125. Manore, M.M., Nutritional needs of the female athlete. *Clin. Sports. Med.*, 18, 549, 1999.

126. Joint Position Statement: nutrition and athletic performance. American College of Sports Medicine, American Dietetic Association and Dietitians of Canada. *Med. Sci. Sports Exerc.*, 32, 2130, 2000.

127. Torun, B., Scrimshaw, N.S. and Young, V.R., Effect of isometric exercises on body potassium and dietary protein requirements of young men. *Am. J. Clin. Nutr.*, 30, 1983, 1977.

128. Todd, K.S., Butterfield, G.E. and Calloway, D.H., Nitrogen balance in men with adequate and deficient energy intake at three levels of work. *J. Nutr.*, 114, 2107, 1984.

129. Young, V.R. and Marchini, J.S., Mechanisms and nutritional significance of metabolic responses to altered intakes or protein and amino acids with reference to nutritional adaptation in humans. *Am. J. Clin. Nutr.*, 51, 270, 1990.

130. Young, V.R., Nutritional balance studies: indicators of human requirements or adaptive mechanisms? *J. Nutr.*, 116, 70, 1985.

131. Millward, D.J., Human amino acid requirements. *J. Nutr.*, 127, 1842, 1997.

132. Young, V.R., 1987 McCollum award lecture. Kinetics of human amino acid metabolism: nutritional implications and some lessons. *Am. J. Clin. Nutr.*, 46, 709, 1987.

133. Young, V.R., Bier, D.M. and Pellett, P.L., A theoretical basis for increasing current estimates of the amino acid requirements in adult man, with experimental support. *Am. J. Clin. Nutr.*, 50, 80, 1989.

134. Das, T.K. and Waterlow, J.C., The rate of adaptation of urea cycle enzymes, amino transferases and glutamine dehydrogenases to changes in dietary protein intake. *Brit. J. Nutr.*, 32, 353, 1974.

135. Butterfield, G.E., Whole-body protein utilization in humans. *Med. Sci. Sports Exerc.*, 19, S167-S165, 1987.

136. Brouns, F., Saris, W.H., Stroecken, J., Beckers, E., Thijssen, R., Rehrer, N.J. and ten Hoor, F., Eating, drinking and cycling. A controlled Tour de France simulation study, Part II. Effect of diet manipulation. *Int. J. Sports Med.*, 10, S41-S48, 1989.

137. Brouns, F., Saris, W.H., Stroecken, J., Beckers, E., Thijssen, R., Rehrer, N.J. and ten Hoor, F., Eating, drinking and cycling. A controlled Tour de France simulation study, Part I. *Int. J. Sports Med.*, 10, S32-S40, 1989.

138. Gontzea, I., Sutzescu, P. and Dumitrache, S., The influence of adaptation to physical effort on nitrogen balance in man. *Nutr. Rep. Int.*, 22, 231, 1975.

139. Richardson, D.P., Wayler, A.H., Scrimshaw, N.S. and Young, V.R., Quantitative effect of an isoenergetic exchange of fat for carbohydrate on dietary protein utilization in healthy young men. *Am. J. Clin. Nutr.*, 32, 2217, 1979.

140. Canada's Food Guide to Healthy Eating. Ottawa, Canada, Minister of Supply and Services Canada, 1992.

141. Food Guide Pyramid: A Guide to Daily Food Choices. Home and Garden Bulletin No. 252. Washington, D.C., US Dept. of Agriculture, Human Nutrition Information Service, 1992.

142. Young, V.R., Gucalp, C., Rand, W.M., Matthews, D.E. and Bier, D.M., Leucine kinetics during three weeks at submaintenance-to-maintenance intakes of leucine in men: adaptation and accommodation. *Hum. Nutr. Clin. Nutr.*, 41C, 1, 1987.

143. Campbell, W.W., Crim, M.C., Young, V.R., Joseph, L.J. and Evans, W.J., Effects of resistance training and dietary protein intake on protein metabolism in older adults. *Am. J. Physiol.*, 268, E1143-E1153, 1995.

144. Veira, D.M., Butler, G., Proulx, J.G. and Poste, L.M., Utilization of grass silage by cattle: effect of supplementation with different sources and amounts of protein. *J. Anim. Sci.*, 72, 1403, 1994.

145. Rumsey, T.S., McLeod, K., Elsasser, T.H., Kahl, S. and Baldwin, R.L., Performance and carcass merit of growing beef steers with chlortetracycline-modified sensitivity to pituitary releasing hormones and fed two dietary protein levels. *J. Anim. Sci.*, 78, 2765, 2000.

146. Price, G.M., Halliday, D., Pacy, P.J., Quevedo, M.R. and Millward, D.J., Nitrogen homeostasis in man: influence of protein intake on the amplitude of diurnal cycling of body nitrogen. *Clin. Sci.*, 86, 91, 1994.

147. Quevedo, M.R., Price, G.M., Halliday, D., Pacy, P.J. and Millward, D.J., Nitrogen homoeostasis in man: diurnal changes in nitrogen excretion, leucine oxidation and whole body leucine kinetics during a reduction from a high to a moderate protein intake. *Clin. Sci.*, 86, 185, 1994.

13

Assessment of Vitamin Status in Athletes

Helena B. Löest and Mark D. Haub

CONTENTS

I. Introduction

Vitamins are organic compounds required in small amounts not only for survival, but also for athletic competitions. In general, vitamins cannot be synthesized in large enough quantities endogenously to meet metabolic requirements for efficient daily functioning and therefore, must be consumed.[1,2] To function physiologically, some vitamins must be converted to an active form or be incorporated into coenzymes, while some are capable of functioning without any modifications.[2]

The vitamin status of athletes is often assumed based on outcomes of estimates of dietary intake (e.g., diet recall and diet records). Given the metabolic demands of athletes, especially athletes training and performing in events that rely heavily on bioenergetic pathways, it may be an unfortunate speculation to base nutritional recommendations on guidelines geared toward the general population. Conversely, those same athletes will not likely experience vitamin deficiencies if consuming a balanced and varied diet to meet energy demands. For detailed insight into vitamin functions,

0-8493-0927-1/02/$0.00+$1.50
© 2002 by CRC Press LLC

adequate intake values and food sources, other resources are available.[2] Also, the assumption of vitamin status from diet records or recall does not always account for differences in vitamin bioavailability or activity. The efficiency of vitamin absorption needs to be considered, as well as the interaction of the vitamin with other nutrients or compounds that might render them less available.

However, given the temporal and financial costs associated with many biochemical assessments, not to mention the means of collecting tissue samples from athletes, the vitamin status of and requirements for athletes are not fully known. With increasing interest in nutritional supplements and functional foods, the area of micronutrient analysis will likely expand to better determine their mechanisms of action. Therefore, the purpose of this chapter is to convey vitamin assessment strategies for those wanting to better determine vitamin status in athletes or research volunteers performing exercise interventions. Suggestions for the appropriate biological sample type (i.e., blood, tissue or urine) will be discussed for those vitamins that have been demonstrated to potentially yield differences in concluding vitamin status. It must be noted that few studies have examined the influence of acute or chronic exercise on values of specific vitamins using human subjects. Therefore, caution and an open mind must be used when applying the following information.

In general, two critical issues to bear in mind when analyzing samples for vitamin content are: 1) to utilize an acceptable vitamin extraction procedure and, 2) to ensure that appropriate measures or precautions are made to minimize the deactivation of the vitamin(s) being measured. For example, when assessing biochemical vitamin status, many factors may influence the analysis (e.g., vitamin stability, see Table 13.1). If these influencing factors are not accounted for or controlled, the results will be of lesser value.

II. Analytical Considerations

A. Stability of Vitamins

One problem that occurs with the analysis of vitamins is their instability under certain conditions (exposure to light, oxygen, metals, etc.; see Table 13.1). This instability leads to changes in the structure (inactive form) and may ultimately yield spurious results. Therefore, it is critical to account for as many potential sample contaminants as possible.[3] For example, when vitamin D is exposed to light it will convert to isotachysterol and the 5,6-*trans*-isomer. As noted in Table 13.2 and in the summary of assessments, most individual and multi-analyte vitamin assessments require specific preparations and procedures; therefore, *post hoc* vitamin assessments are generally difficult to perform adequately.

TABLE 13.1

Factors Responsible for Degrading or Inactivating Fat-Soluble and Some Water-Soluble Vitamins (Free Forms In Solution) that Can Influence Analysis Results

Vitamins	A	D	E	K	B_1	B_2	B_6	B_{12}	C	Niacin	Biotin	Folate#	Pantothenic Acid	Prevention
Influencing Factors														
Air (O_2)§	✓	✓	✓					✓	✓			✓		Exclude oxygen or air by replacement of inert gas.
Heat	✓	✓	✓		✓	✓	✓		✓		✓	✓	✓	Work at lowest temperatures possible, store below –20°C (preferably –70°C).
Light, UV	✓	✓	✓	✓	✓	✓	✓	✓	✓		✓	✓		Avoid sunlight (UV), and use dim lights.
Metals/Minerals	✓	✓	✓	✓				✓	✓			✓		Avoid adding metals.
Acid	✓	✓		✓	✓	✓	✓	✓				✓	✓	Use acid free solvents.
Alkali		✓		✓				✓			✓	✓	✓	
Water		✓			✓	✓	✓					✓	✓	
Reducing Agents				✓	✓									
Oxidizing Agents	✓	✓						✓						
Antioxidant	*	*	*	*								*		
Other		Iodine		Sulfite								Sulphurous acid, nitrite		
References	11,32,33	11,32-34	11,32,33	11,32,33	1,11,20,33,34	1,11,33	1,11,33,34	1,11,15,33,34	1,6,11	11	1,33,34	1,11,15,33	1,33	

* Add an antioxidant like butylated hydroxytoluene (BHT), α–tocopherol, Vitamin C, propylgallate to samples prior to analysis to protect from oxidation[11]

Folate exists in various forms and each form is sensitive to different factors.

§ Try to avoid exposure to air or oxygen during sampling or analysis; the vitamins may be more stable in the absence of oxygen, and this may minimize the sensitivity to these other factors.[11]

Exposure of some vitamins to more than one of these factors can have an additive effect; more losses occur when exposed to more than one factor.[11]

TABLE 13.2

Biochemical Indices to Assess Vitamin Status

Vitamin	Component	Biochemical Tests for Status Assessment
Vitamin A (retinoids)		Colorimetry, spectrophotometry, fluorometry, capillary electrophoresis[11]; high pressure liquid chromatography (HPLC), thin-layer chromatography (TLC)[11,33]; gas chromatography (GC)[7]; and , immunological, or molecular biological techniques[9]
	Blood	Serum β carotene levels[2] Plasma retinal levels (only reduced if liver stores are depleted)[2] Relative dose response (RDR) & Modified relative dose response (MRDR)[9] (Most representative of current status, and determine liver stores in a non-invasive way[5,9,40]) Retinol binding proteins (RBP)[5,9] Plasma retinol (generally accepted[9]) and carotenoid analysis[5,41,42] (plasma retinol need not be adjusted for lipoprotein concentration)[18]
	Liver	Liver retinol levels[43] (not practical)[9]
	Tear fluid	Conjunctival impression cytology (CIC)[9] (Least representative of current status[5,9]) Tear analysis[5]
	Other	Dark adaptation test or night blindness determination[5,8]
Vitamin D		HPLC, TLC, colorimetry, radioimmunoassay, gas chromatography-mass spectrometry (GC-MS)[33], ligand-binding[11]
	Blood	Plasma/serum vitamin D levels[2,10] (need not be adjusted for lipoprotein lipid content)[18] Serum 25-OH-vitamin D levels is the sum of diet intake and production from sun exposure[10] - the most valuable determinant of vitamin D status[10,11] Specific competitive protein binding assay for determination of 25-OH-vitamin D and 1-25(OH)$_2$ vitamin D (of little value)[10,11] Radio receptor assay, using ^{3}H metabolites is a specific way to determine 1-25(OH)$_2$ vitamin D[11] (also of little value)[10] Plasma alkaline phosphatase activity[2,11]
	Tissue	Blood and tissue vitamin D metabolites are acceptable status indicators, but are non-specific[11]
	Other	Indirect determination: serum calcium levels[2] Clinical trial of supplementation[5]

TABLE 13.2 (CONTINUED)

Biochemical Indices to Assess Vitamin Status

Vitamin	Component	Biochemical Tests for Status Assessment
Vitamin E (αTP)		Colorimetry, spectrophotometry, spectrofluorometry, TLC, HPLC, and GC[11,14]
	Blood	Serum αTP[14] in relation to serum triglyceride levels[5]
		Platelet αTP levels in relation to serum triglyceride levels[5]
		Plasma αTP is not a good indicator for toxic levels, because it reaches a plateau[17]
		Erythrocyte α TP levels[14]
	Adipose	Adipose αTP levels in relation to serum triglyceride levels[5]
		Adipose α P levels increase linearly with dietary intake of vitamin E[15]. Assess long term vitamin E status[17]
	Muscle	Muscle αTP levels,[14] in close metabolic equilibrium with plasma α TP[44]
	Urine	Urinary excretion of vitamin E may indicate excessive vitamin E intakes[16]
		Urinary excretion of vitamin E metabolite α CEHC is not used to assess vitamin E status[16]
	Other	Erythrocyte hemolysis by peroxide[2,5] is inversely related to plasma αTP concentrations[16]
		Breath ethane[16] and pentane[13], levels are lipid peroxidation markers, high levels show depleted stores[17]
		Functional tests: vitamin E status can be assessed by oxidative changes in lipids:
		(1) Erythrocyte malondialdehyde test (in vitro) by H_2O_2 exposure[13]
		(2) Erythrocyte malondialdehyde test with thiobarbituric acid[13]
	Recommendation	Evaluate vitamin E levels in conjunction with blood lipid levels because vitamin E is carried on lipid-protein complexes called lipoproteins. Evaluating blood vitamin E levels alone when assessing vitamin E status, is misleading[16]
		It is more useful to use more than one biochemical test to assess vitamin E status[13]
Vitamin K (phyloquinone)		HPLC, TLC, colorimetry, GC-MS[33,45]
	Blood	Plasma prothrombin concentrations[2,45]
		Plasma phylloquinone[13] reflects phylloquinone intakes[45], but does not correlate well with vitamin K status[45]

TABLE 13.2 (CONTINUED)

Biochemical Indices to Assess Vitamin Status

Vitamin	Component	Biochemical Tests for Status Assessment
		Plasma or serum des-γ-carboxyprothrombin (DCP) -most sensitive indicator of vitamin K status[5,18,21,45]
		DCP: Prothrombin ratios[13]
		Direct chromatographic vitamin K assays[46]
	Urine	Urinary γ-carboxyglutamic acid[13]
	Other	Hydroxyapatite binding capacity of osteocalcin[13]
		Ratio of prothrombin activity to the total immunochemical equivalents of prothrombin[45]
		Ratio of Simplastin thromboplastin activated prothrombin time to activated by *Echis carnatus* venom (S:E ratio)[45]
		Bleeding and clotting time[5]
		Prothrombin time[5] (still used, but is insensitive and non-specific as primary method to determine vitamin K status[36])
		Measurements of uncarboxylated osteocalcin[45]
	Recommendation	Use both the plasma prothrombin measurements and DCP[13]
		Plasma or serum des-γ-carboxyprothrombin (DCP) and osteocalcin -most sensitive indicator of vitamin K status[5,18,21,45]
Thiamin (B₁)		HPLC,[5,19,33] TLC,[33] ion exchange chromatography,[47] colorimetry,[5] enzymatic[5,19,21] and microbiological assays[5,33]
	Blood	ETKAC (erythrocyte transketolase activity)[5,19,21] (highly reliable method to determine status)[11]
		Serum thiamin levels,[5,19,20] -insensitive status indicator[11]
		Thiamin pyrophosphate (TPPE) test of erythrocytes[19-21]
		Blood pyruvate, lactate, and α ketoglutarate levels[20]
		Whole blood (*Lactobacillus viridescens* assay),[48] -insensitive status indicator[11]
		Erythrocyte thiamin levels, -insensitive status indicator[11]
	Urine	Urinary excretions of thiamin (reflect thiamin status of the previous 24 h)[2,5]
		Urinary excretions of thiamin metabolites[20]
	Body fluids	Microbiological assays[5,33]
	Other	*Ex vivo* lymphocyte growth response[5]
		Cerebrospinal fluid (CSF) thiamin levels[20]
	Recommendation	Use ETKAC and TPPE together to assess thiamin status for most reliable results[20]

TABLE 13.2 (CONTINUED)

Biochemical Indices to Assess Vitamin Status

Vitamin	Component	Biochemical Tests for Status Assessment
		Use more than one method or test to assess thiamin status[48]
Riboflavin (B[2])		HPLC,[5,22,33] TLC,[33,49] fluorometry,[5,22] enzymatic[2,5,23] and microbiological assays[5,33]
	Blood	Erythrocyte glutathione reductase activity coefficient (EGRAC)[2,22,23] is the most common and most sensitive to tissue stores[22,23] Blood riboflavin levels[22] is an insensitive indicator of riboflavin status[23] Erythrocyte riboflavin levels[22] is an insensitive indicator of riboflavin status[23]
	Urine	24 h collection of urinary excretions of riboflavin reflects dietary intake,[22] and is not a sensitive indicator for tissue stores[22] Urinary excretions collected 1) at random, 2) after fasting, 3) a 24 h specimen, and 4) after load return test[22] Ratio of urinary riboflavin levels to creatinine levels[21]
	Body fluids	Microbiological assays[5,33]
	Other	*Ex vivo* lymphocyte growth response[5]
	Recommendation	EGRAC together with urinary excretion test[11,23]
Niacin		HPLC,[33] chromatography,[24] colorimetry,[50] fluorometry,[24] enzymatic[24] and microbiological assays[2,5,33]
	Blood	Serum niacin level determination is not a sensitive test,[21] it reflects dietary intake, not tissue stores[11] Erythrocyte NAD levels[5] Erythrocyte NAD:NADP ratio[5] is used to evaluate niacin status[24]
	Blood and tissue	Lowry method measures NAD and NADP by using specific dehydrogenase enzymes[24]
	Urine	Excretion of N'-methylnicotinamide (NMN) and 2-pyridone[5] after a tryptophan dose[2]-widely used method[21] Ratio of 2-pyridone to NMN is a recommended method[23]
	Body fluids	Microbiological assays[5,50] (*Lactobacillus plantarum*)[3]
	Other	*Ex vivo* lymphocyte growth response[5] NMN excretion expressed as mmol / mol creatinine is not an accurate method[21]

TABLE 13.2 (CONTINUED)

Biochemical Indices to Assess Vitamin Status

Vitamin	Component	Biochemical Tests for Status Assessment
		Dowley-1-formate chromatography is used to separate the puridine nucleotides (NAD/H and NADP/H) and NMN[24]
		NMN assessment done after 4-5 hr after a 50 mg load of nicotinamide[23]
Vitamin B$_6$		HPLC,[33] TLC,[33] GC,[51] enzymatic[5,25] and microbiological assays[5,33]
	Blood	Plasma pyridoxal phosphate (PLP) concentrations[25,52] most often used, and correlates with tissue stores[11]
		Plasma total vitamin B$_6$ levels or plasma PL levels[25]
		*Plasma homocysteine levels[5] after a methionine load[15,21,25] reflect hepatic vitamin B$_6$ status[25]
		Serum 4-PA levels[5]
		Erythrocyte PLP levels are useful as an additional index[25]
		*Erythrocyte ALT and AST activation coefficients[5,15,21,25,53] reflect long term vitamin B$_6$ status because of the lifetime of the erythrocyte[25]
		Erythrocyte α-EGOT measurements[54]
	Urine	Urinary 4-PA excretion,[2,15,25] which is a short term indicator[25] that reflects dietary intake[21]
		Urinary total vitamin B$_6$[25]
		Urinary pyridoxal lactone[15]
		*Urinary metabolite (xanthurenic and kynurenic acid) excretion[5] after a tryptophan load[11,15,21,25] reflect hepatic vitamin B$_6$ status[25]
		*Urinary homocysteine levels[5] after a methionine load[15,21,25] reflect hepatic vitamin B$_6$ status[25]
		Urinary PL expressed as mg per g creatinine[11]
	Body fluids	Microbiological assays[5,33,54]
	Other	*Oxalate excretion[25] less common method
		*EEG pattern[25] less common method
		Ex vivo lymphocyte growth response[5]
		Plasma or urine amino acid levels and ratios[5]
	Recommendation	Use at least two biochemical indices; one must be the PLP test.
		Plasma PLP and tryptophan load test together is an excellent biochemical confirmation of vitamin B$_6$ status[11]
		(*) These are indirect methods that does not necessarily reflect total vitamin B$_6$ in tissue or serum, they indirectly reflect PLP in certain tissue[21,25]

TABLE 13.2 (CONTINUED)

Biochemical Indices to Assess Vitamin Status

Vitamin	Component	Biochemical Tests for Status Assessment
Cobalamin (B$_{12}$)		Radioimmunoassay;[26,33] microbiological assays, dual isotope methods[5]
	Blood	Serum cobalamin assay is a standard method[5,26] Erythrocyte vitamin B$_{12}$ measurement is a common biochemical test[11] Holo TC-II (vitamin B$_{12}$ transporter) measurements detect early vitamin B$_{12}$ deficiency[11,26] Plasma total vitamin B$_{12}$ levels[21]
	Plasma and urine	Measurement of substrates, methylmalonic acid (MMA) and homocysteine, of two vitamin B$_{12}$ dependent enzymes is a new and more accurate way of assessing intracellular deficiencies[5,26] Plasma MMA measurements are better than plasma homocysteine measurements[26]
	Urine	Urinary total vitamin B$_{12}$ levels[21]
	Biological fluids	Microbiological assays[5,33]
	Other	Vitamin B$_{12}$ deficiency is reflected by high levels of 2-methylcitrate, N,N-dimethylglycine, N-methylglycine and cystathionine *Ex vivo* lymphocyte growth response[5] Shillings test or dual isotope variations for vitamin B$_{12}$ absorption[5]
Folate		HPLC,[33] radioimmunoassy,[33] radiometry,[27] fluorometry,[27,55] TLC,[27] enzymatic assay[27]
	Blood	Serum folic acid levels[2,5,21]; should not be used by itself[11,56] Erythrocyte folic acid levels[2,5,21] Serum or erythrocyte THF by radio isotope assay[27] Serum or erythrocyte 5-methyl THF[27] Serum folate activity[27] Erythrocyte folate status is a reliable indicator for long term of folate status,[21] and tissue stores[11,28,56] Serum homocysteine concentration is an ancillary indicator of folate adequacy[28]
	Urine	Urinary folate levels[2] Urinary N-formimino glutamic acid indicates comprised folate stores[15] indirectly, but is not sensitive enough and not used frequently[11]
	Biological fluids	Microbiological assays[5,33] (*Lactobacillus rhamnosus*)[3]
	Other	*Ex vivo* lymphocyte growth response[5] Neutrophil hypersegmentation[5,56]

TABLE 13.2 (CONTINUED)

Biochemical Indices to Assess Vitamin Status

Vitamin	Component	Biochemical Tests for Status Assessment
		Dihydrofolate reductase (DHFR) inhibition assay[55]
Biotin		HPLC,[29,33] fluorescent assay,[29] TLC,[33] microbiological assay,[2,5,33] colorimetry[5]
	Blood	Whole blood biotin levels (not a sensitive indicator)[11,29] Avidin-binding assay[29,57,58] Derivatives of biotin[29]
	Urine	Urinary biotin levels[2,5,15] Urinary excretion of 3-hydroxyisovaleric acid (inversely related to biotin status),[30] is a sensitive, early detector of biotin deficiencies[11,30]
	Biological fluids	Microbiological assays[5,33]
	Other	*Ex vivo* lymphocyte growth response[5] Propionyl-CoA carboxylase and pyruvate carboxylase (biotin dependent enzymes) activity in hair roots[59]
	Recommendation	Chromatographic separation of biotin analogues together with avidin-binding assay[29]
Pantothenic acid		HPLC,[33] colorimetry,[5] microbiological assay[5,33]
	Blood	Whole blood pantothenic acid levels (not very sensitive)[5,11] Serum pantothenic acid (not very sensitive)[11]
	Urine	Urinary pantothenic acid levels (not very sensitive)[5,11]
	Biological fluids	Microbiological assays,[5,33] using yeast and lactobacillus for blood and urine pantothenic acid measurements[2,31]
	Other	*Ex vivo* lymphocyte growth response[5]
Vitamin C		HPLC,[5,60] TLC[33,60] GC;[60] spectrophotometry, fluorometry, chromatography, electrochemical techniques[6]
	Blood	Serum ascorbate levels[60]-easy to perform, and most often used, also reliable[2,6] Leukocyte ascorbate levels-most reliable[6] (reflect tissue and blood ascorbate content and correlates with liver ascorbate[6,11,16]) Platelet ascorbate level[6]
	Urine	Urinary ascorbate level measurement is not a good indicator of vitamin C status, because vitamin C is reabsorbed by the kidneys[6], but is a good indicator for current status[11]

TABLE 13.2 (CONTINUED)

Biochemical Indices to Assess Vitamin Status

Vitamin	Component	Biochemical Tests for Status Assessment
	Saliva	Salivary ascorbate level measurement is not a good indicator of vitamin C status[6]
	Other	Oral loading test[5]
		Recently the automated and microtiter plate spectrophotometric method has been used for measurement of plasma and leukocyte ascorbate, it is fast and has high sensitivity[6]
		Whole blood and red blood cell ascorbate measurements are less sensitive[6]

B. Vitamin Bioavailability, Active Forms and Storage

Basing vitamin status solely on nutrient intake values may yield inaccurate estimations of vitamin status, which may in turn lead to either a vitamin deficiency or toxicity. This results from interactions of micronutrients and other dietary consumables on the absorption and availability of other nutrients. The assessment of an athlete's menu may generate a different picture of vitamin status from what is derived from the analysis of biochemical samples. This conflict may go unnoticed if vitamin intake alone is assessed. This may be common in some instances, as the availability of computer-assisted nutrient analysis programs has increased, whereas the access to biochemical assessment equipment may be limited to some (if not many) coaches or athletes. Table 13.3 displays the tissues or sample sites that can be used for assessment, as well as the compound and analytical method used to verify vitamin status.

This oversight may occur with the assessment of vitamin B_6. Two sources of dietary vitamin B_6 are pyrodoxine (PN) and pyrodoxine-5'-β-D-glucoside (PN-glucoside). Both PN and PN-glucoside are converted to vitamin B_6; however, the conversion of PN-glucoside is less than that of PN, and PN-glucoside slightly inhibits the conversion of PN.[4] Therefore, if athletes ingest foods that contain higher levels of PN-glucoside, then their actual vitamin B_6 levels may not adequately reflect vitamin B_6 intake, unless the nutrient assessment procedure accounts for the influence of PN-glucoside.

Another complication may arise when measuring serum or plasma levels of particular vitamins. The concentrations of vitamins in circulation may reflect only the current vitamin status, whereas, if the storage forms (if applicable) of the vitamin were assessed, a deficiency might be evident. That is, the individual has limited stored vitamin levels available for continued normal functioning, even when the circulating levels are quite normal.

TABLE 13.3

The Active Forms and Storage Sites for Vitamins

Vitamin	Active Form(s)	
A	(all-trans) Retinol[2,9]	Liver (retinol) [2,9,32]
		Adipose tissue (carotenosis)[8]
	(all-trans) Retinal[2,9]	
	Retinoic acid[2,9]	
	β-cartotene	
D	1,25(OH)$_2$D[2, 35]	Skin (7-dehydrocholesterol)[36]
	24,25(OH)$_2$D[2]	
E	d-α-tocopherol (most active)[2,12]	Adipose (adipocytes)[2,15,17]
	β- tocopherol[2]	Lipid fractions of membranes[2]
	γ- tocopherol[2]	Adrenals, liver, and muscles[2,15]
	δ- tocopherol[2]	
	Trienols[2]	
K	Hydroquinone[37]	Adrenal glands, lungs, bone marrow, kidneys, and lymph nodes[13]
Thiamin (B$_1$)	Thiamin pyrophosphate (TPP)[2,15]	Skeletal muscle, liver, heart, kidneys, and brain[2,20]
Riboflavin (B$_2$)	FMN, FAD[2,33]	Liver, heart, and kidneys[2,15]
Niacin	NAD, NADP[2]	
Pyridoxine (B$_6$)	Pyridoxal phosphate (PP)[2]	Muscle,[2,25] liver[2]
(Cyano)cobalamin (B$_{12}$)	Methylcobalamin[2], adenosylcobalamin[2]	Liver[26], brain, kidney, spleen, and muscle[15]
Vitamin C	Reduced ascorbic acid (DHAA),[2] ascorbic acid (AA)[6,38]	Pituitary and adrenal glands,[6,15] leukocytes,[6] eye tissue,[16] less in saliva and plasma[6,16]
Biotin	Biocytin[2]	Muscle, brain, and liver[15]
Folate	Tetrahydrofolic acid (THF)[2]	Small amounts in liver, cerebrospinal fluid, bone marrow, spleen, and kidney[2]
Pantothenic acid	Portion of coenzyme A[2,39]	

C. Biochemical Indices to Assess Vitamin Status

Determining vitamin status is dependent on the source of sample used for quantification. For some vitamins, it may be more beneficial to measure stored levels vs. amounts in circulation, as the concentrations in circulation will not reflect a deficiency until the stored levels have been sufficiently diminished. On the other hand, assessing certain samples may not be justifiable. For example, liver samples provide an accurate measurement of vitamin A (retinol) levels, but the necessary biopsy would be excessive, as similar results can be obtained by measuring plasma retinol levels. Some have reported the assessment techniques using tear[5] or saliva samples[6] to assess vitamin status, but those minimally invasive techniques are generally less representative of the individual's vitamin status than results obtained from blood or tissue samples. Therefore, when assessing vitamin status, it is imperative to carefully select the sample source, preparatory methods and analytical techniques. Otherwise, the time and money spent for this assessment may not yield optimum results. In other words, the assessment would not have performed up to its potential.

III.   Assessment Guidelines and Considerations

The following information was compiled to aid in deciding which indices or techniques to choose to assess the status of a particular vitamin. These guidelines are not all-encompassing, as many of these procedures have not been used in conjunction with athletes. Additionally, other modifications or adjustments not mentioned here may need to be made given differences in analytical equipment and skill of personnel.

A. Vitamin A (Retinoids)

Several techniques and laboratory equipment can be used to assess vitamin A status (Table 13.2). Different forms of vitamin A (β-carotene, retinol, or retinal) can be determined from blood, liver or tear fluid. Carotenoid concentrations in blood and tissue samples usually reflect dietary intakes.[7] Vitamin A status can also be determined indirectly by conducting a night blindness test.[5,8] The relative dose response and modified relative dose response method, where liver stores are assessed by giving the person an oral vitamin A dose, is most representative and noninvasive.[9] The conjunctival impression cytology test is the analysis of vitamin A levels of cells taken from a person's eye, but is less representative of current vitamin A status.[9]

B. Vitamin D (Calciferol)

Different forms of vitamin D exist in blood and tissue, such as 25-OH vitamin D and 1,25 $(OH)_2$ vitamin D (Table 13.2). In assessing vitamin D status of the body, it is most valuable to assess 25-OH vitamin D levels in blood. The reason for this is that 25-OH vitamin D is converted to 1,25 $(OH)_2$ vitamin D (active form, Table 13.3). In the blood, 25-OH vitamin D is generally present in much higher concentrations than 1,25 $(OH)_2$ vitamin D,[10] so it will always be converted to the active form, even though the active form appears in low, normal or high concentrations. Other methods, such as assessing the proteins that carry vitamin A in the blood (retinol-binding proteins), enzymatic tests and receptor binding tests are also used, but are not as efficient as the method discussed earlier.[11]

C. Vitamin E (Tocopherols and Tocotrienols)

Alpha tocopherol (αTP) is the most active form of vitamin E in the body, and this form is assessed when determining vitamin E status.[2,12] Table 13.2 lists the different techniques to assess vitamin E status, such as the use of colorimetry, TLC, HPLC; the value of different methods are also mentioned. According to Groff and Gropper,[13] there is no single method that is very accurate in determining vitamin E status, therefore, it is recommended to use more than one biochemical test. Blood, erythrocyte, adipose, muscle and urine αTP levels have been used to determine vitamin E status.[14-16] Vitamin E protects lipids in the body against oxidative damage (peroxidation). By exposing samples to oxidation, vitamin E status can be determined by the time it takes for these samples to be damaged. High vitamin E levels in the samples will extend or delay the damage. Status can also be determined by measuring lipid peroxidation markers like breath ethane and pentane.[13,16,17] In the latter test, high levels of peroxidation markers show depleted vitamin E levels. Vitamin E is carried in the blood on lipid-protein complexes called lipoproteins and, when assessing vitamin E, the lipids in these lipoproteins must be taken into account, because assessment of blood vitamin E levels alone are misleading in determining vitamin E status.[18]

D. Vitamin K (Phylloquinone, Menaquinone and Menadione)

By measuring blood prothrombin, phylloquinone, or des-γ-carboxyprothrombin (DCP) levels (Table 13.2), vitamin K status can be assessed. Of these three, determining DCP by utilizing antibodies is the most valuable indicator. Other samples, such as urine, can also be used to determine vitamin K status. The recommendation, however, is to use DCP as well as blood prothrombin determinations.[13] Bleeding and clotting time of blood is also useful to determine vitamin K status.[5]

E.   Vitamin B$_1$ (Thiamin)

Erythrocyte (red blood cell) transketolase is an enzyme that needs thiamin to function and, when thiamin is depleted, this enzyme's activity decreases. Therefore, by measuring the enzyme activity, vitamin B$_1$ status can be determined.[19] Thiamin is needed in the form of thiamin pyrophosphate (TPP).[20] Erythrocyte transketolases activity can be measured by adding TPP to the reactions. After TPP is added, increased activity would indicate thiamin deficiency. This suggests there was not enough thiamin for the enzyme to function before the addition of TPP.[21] Other methods, such as serum thiamin, microbiological assays and erythrocyte thiamin levels are insensitive indicators of vitamin B_1 status (Table 13.2).

F. Vitamin B_2 (Riboflavin)

Erythrocyte glutathione reductase activity coefficient is a test utilizing the activity of the enzyme erythrocyte glutathione reductase to determine vitamin B_2 status[22] (Table 13.2) The activity of the enzyme is measured before and after addition of flavin-adenine dinucleotide (FAD), a coenzyme needed for the enzyme to function.[22,23] If the activity of the enzyme was low before and higher after the addition of FAD, that would suggest a vitamin deficiency. If there were no deficiency, the levels before and after FAD addition would be the same. Other methods, such as blood, red blood cell and urinary riboflavin levels are also used to assess vitamin B_2 levels, but are not very sensitive indicators.[22]

G. Niacin (Nicotinamide and Nicotinic Acid)

Niacin is a precursor for nicotinamide adenine dinucleotide (NAD), which is very important for biological functions.[24] Erythrocyte NAD levels as well as the ratio of erythrocyte NAD: NADP can be used to determine niacin status in blood.[24] The Lowry method uses specific dehydrogenase enzymes to measure NAD and NADP levels in blood and tissue.[24] Urinary excretions of niacin metabolites, such as N'-methylnicotinamide (NMN) and 2-pyridone, are also widely used methods in assessing niacin status (Table 13.3).[23]

H. Vitamin B_6

Table 13.2 displays methods by which vitamin B_6 can be assessed. Vitamin B_6 levels and vitamin B_6 metabolites in blood and urine samples are generally used for assessing this vitamin's status.[5,25] Pyridoxyl phosphate (PLP or PP) is the active form of vitamin B_6 and its levels in blood reflect tissue stores.[2,11] Enzymatic tests such as erythrocyte alanine transaminase (ALT) and erythrocyte aspartate transaminase (AST) indirectly reflect vitamin B_6 status.[5] A short-term indicator for vitamin B_6 status is urinary 4-pyridoxic acid (4-PA), a metabolite, representing 40% to 60% of the daily intake of vitamin B_6.[25] Urinary total vitamin B_6 levels represents 8% to 10% of the daily intake.[25]

I. Vitamin B_{12} (Cobalamin)

Vitamin B_{12} status is generally assessed using blood samples,[21] where total vitamin B_{12} levels are assessed (Table 13.2). Enzymatic tests are also used where substrates, such as methylmalonic acid and homocysteine, are measured. Vitamin B_{12}-dependent enzymes utilize these substrates. High substrate levels in blood or urine indicate that there is not enough vitamin B_{12} for the enzymes to function, so they cannot use the substrates. Therefore, high substrate levels indicate deficiency.[5,26]

J.   Vitamin C (Ascorbic and Hydroascorbic Acids)

Leukocyte (white blood cell) vitamin C (ascorbic acid) concentration, the most reliable determinant of vitamin C status, is not affected by recent fluctuations in the diet (Table 13.2).[6,11] It is representative of tissue and blood vitamin C status and is correlated with liver vitamin C stores.[6,11,16] Serum and platelet vitamin C levels can also be used to assess vitamin C status.[6] Urinary levels are not a good indicator because the kidney reabsorbs vitamin C.[6] Blood and urinary vitamin C levels also reflect recent dietary intake.[11]

K.   Folate (and Folacin)

Folate (folic acid) is present in the body in the form of tetrahydrofolate, which is very important for many biological pathways in the body.[27] By measuring metabolites of these pathways, folate status can be determined (Table 13.2). An example is urinary N-formiminoglutamic acid. This metabolite is involved in the breakdown of histidine to glutamic acid and requires the cofactor tetrahydrofolate. Without tetrahydrofolate, levels of N-formiminoglutamic acid in the blood will increase and lead to excretion in the urine.[15] Assessment of serum folic acid levels by itself should not be used for folate status determination.[11] Red blood cell folate levels represent tissue store, thus this measurement is a more reliable long-term indicator.[21,28]

L.   Biotin

A reduced biotin level in urine is a determinant of biotin deficiency.[29] Also, the metabolite 3-hydroxyisovaleric acid, which is excreted in urine, is inversely related to biotin status.[30] It is also a sensitive and early indicator of biotin deficiency.[11,30] Blood biotin levels are not sensitive indicators for biotin status, even if the avidin-binding assay or bioassays was used (Table 13.2).[29]

M.   Pantothenic Acid

Pantothenic acid is present in the body as part of acetyl coenzyme A (CoA), which plays a critical role in energy metabolism. After blood samples are obtained, certain enzymes, called hydrolytic enzymes, are needed to cleave pantothenic acid from CoA in order to be analyzed in the laboratory.[31] This cleavage is not needed for determining pantothenate levels in the urine, because hydrolytic enzymes present in the body have already cleaved pantothenate from CoA.[31] Other means of determining blood, tissue and urine pantothenate is by microbiological assays using yeast and lactobacillus[2] (Table 13.2).

IV. Assessment Methods

Absorption spectrophotometry is limited to vitamins with a strong chromaphore. Light spectrophotometry utilizes either ultraviolet or visible wavelengths to measure the sample. As the selected wavelength of light passes through the sample, the absorption of light will vary according to the sample. Based on a standard curve or derived regression equation, the absorption is proportional to the vitamin content of the sample.

Capillary electrophoresis is a high-performance analytical technique that can be used to separate a variety of charged and neutral components. When voltage is applied through the run buffer, the particles present will migrate through a tube at a velocity determined by their respective size and electric charge. This separation technique is synonymous with other forms of electrophoresis.

Chromatography (gas, thin-layer and paper) is a separation procedure similar to HPLC. It is capable of separating the desired compound, but cannot quantify the amount or concentration of the sample. For example, following gas chromatography, the sample is further assessed using mass spectroscopy to quantify the amount of the desired compound.

Electrochemical techniques are used following chromatography to quantify vitamin content. The procedure is based on the electrochemical qualities of each vitamin or vitamer.

Enzymatic and microbiological assays utilize chemical reagents to convert the vitamin or vitamer to a compound that is generally measurable by fluorometry or various types of spectrophotometry. Specific to microbiological assays, the sample is exposed to an organism that will grow only in the presence of the specific vitamin.

Fluorometry is similar to spectroscopy. The exception is that the fluorometer detects the fluorescence of compounds at different wavelengths. Therefore, if the assay reagent does not yield fluorescent compounds, the fluorometer will not be of value.

Gas chromatography-mass spectrometry (GC-MS). The gas chromatograph separates the compound of interest from other potentially interfering compounds and the mass spectrometer analyzes the purified sample over a time interval.

High pressure liquid chromatography (HPLC), can be used as a purification method and quantitative technique. Injecting the sample onto the column separates compounds. The various components in the sample pass through the column at different rates due to partitioning differences between the mobile liquid and stationary phases. HPLC also provides greater chromatographic selectivity than gas chromatography. Fluorescent detection is frequently used for quantifying several lipid- and water-soluble vitamins.

Ion exchange chromatography is commonly used in the purification of biological materials. Charged molecules in the liquid phase pass through the column until a binding site in the stationary phase appears. The molecule will not elute from the column until a solution of varying pH or ionic strength is passed through it. Separation by this method is highly selective.

Radioimmunoassay utilizes a labeled isotope to quantify a given compound. The radio-labeled isotope binds to the compound. The sample is analyzed in a scintillation counter. The greater the radioactive count, the greater amount of bound isotope.

V.   Summary of Vitamin Assessments

The intent of this chapter was to provide sport scientists with information regarding the assessment techniques to biochemically determine vitamin status. The assessment of vitamin status tends to require more analytical steps and stability-maintaining procedures than assessments of other nutrients (e.g., glucose, non-esterified fatty acids, etc.). If greater detail is desired, several texts can fully explain and discuss the chemical properties and analytical methods to assess each vitamin or vitamer.[1,11,32] Given the complex interactions among micronutrients, such as vitamins and other ingested compounds, it will be beneficial for scientists to assess vitamin status in athletes to justify or better explain biochemical occurrences affecting their training, competition, or recovery.

When initiating the process of assessing vitamin status, refer to texts or articles that not only explain the methods, but discuss the confounding analytical factors that lead to the conversion of inactive isomers or instability of the vitamin(s) being measured. These factors, in conjunction with the fact that few studies have demonstrated vitamin malnutrition in athletes, seem to minimize the interest in vitamin research in exercise science. However, the assessment of vitamin status may prove beneficial in better understanding performance outcomes of athletes with eating disorders, those who ingest megadoses of vitamins and other supplements or those performing high training volumes. Therefore, future research in vitamin assessment should investigate how nutrient or training status (for example, malnutrition or high training volume) alter the circulating and stored levels of vitamins and the subsequent effect on performance.

References

1. Ball, G.F.M. *Water-Soluble Vitamin Assays in Human Nutrition.* Chapman & Hall, London, 1994.
2. Driskell, J.A. *Sports Nutrition.* CRC, Boca Raton, FL, 2000.
3. Eittenmiller, R.R., Landen, W. O., Jr. and Augustin, J. Vitamin Analysis in *Food Analysis.* 2nd ed. Nielsen, S.S., Ed., Aspen, Gaithersburg, MD, 1998, 281.
4. Nakano H. and McMahon L.G., Gregory J.F. III., Pyridoxine-5'-beta-D-glucoside exhibits incomplete bioavailability as a source of vitamin B-6 and partially inhibits the utilization of co-ingested pyridoxine in humans. *J Nutr*;127(8):1508-13, 1997.
5. Bucci, L.R. Introduction in *Sports Nutrition: Vitamins and Trace Elements.* Wolinsky, I. and Driskell, J.A., Eds. CRC, Boca Raton, FL, 1997.
6. Jacob, R.A. Vitamin C in *Modern Nutrition in Health and Disease.* 9th ed. Shils, M.E. et al., Eds. Williams and Wilkins, Baltimore, MD, 1999, 467.
7. Lambert, W.E., Nelis, H.J., De Ruyter, M.G.M. andDe Leenheer, A.P. Vitamin A: Retinol, Carotenoids and Related Compounds in *Modern Chromatographic Analysis of the Vitamins.* De Leenheer A.P., Lambert, W E. and De Ruyter, M.G.M. Eds. Marcel Dekker. 1985, 1.
8. Stacewicz-Sapuntzakis, M. Vitamin A and Carotenoids in *Sports Nutrition: Vitamins and Trace Elements.* Wolinsky, I. and Driskell, J.A., Eds. CRC, Boca Raton, FL, 1997, 101.
9. Ross, A.C. Vitamin A and Retinoids in *Modern Nutrition in Health and Disease.* 9th Ed Shils, M.E., Olson, J.A., Shike, M. and Ross, A.C., Eds. Williams and Wilkins, Baltimore, MD, 1999, 305.
10. Holick, M.F. Vitamin D in *Modern Nutrition in Health and Disease.* 9th ed. Shils, M.E., Olson, J.A., Shike, M. and Ross, A.C., Eds. Williams and Wilkins, Baltimore, MD, 1999, 329.
11. Eitenmiller, R.R. and Landen, W.O., Jr., *Vitamin Analysis for the Health and Food Sciences.* CRC, Boca Raton, FL, 1999.
12. Kanter, M.M. Nutritional Antioxidants and Physical Activity in *Nutrition in Exercise and Sport.* 3rd ed. Wolinsky, I., Ed. CRC, Boca Raton, FL, 1998, 245.
13. Groff, J.L. and Gropper, S.S., *Advanced Nutrition and Human Metabolism.* 3rd ed. Wadsworth/Thomas Learning, Belmont, CA, 2000.
14. Nelis, H.J., De Bevere, V.O.R.C. and De Leenheer, A.P. Vitamin E: Tocopherols and Tocotrienols in *Modern Chromatographic Analysis of the Vitamins.* De Leenheer A.P., Lambert, W.E. and De Ruyter, M.G.M. Eds. Marcel Dekker, New York, 1985, 129.
15. Wildman, R.E.C. and Medeiros, D.M. *Advanced Human Nutrition.* CRC, Boca Raton, FL, 2000.
16. Institute of Medicine. *Dietary Reference Intakes for Vitamin C, Vitamin E, Selenium and Carotenoids: a Report of the Panel on Dietary Antioxidants and Related Compounds,* Subcommittees on Upper Reference Levels of Nutrients and of Interpretation and use of Dietary Reference Intakes and the Standing Committee on the Scientific Evaluation of Dietary Reference Intakes, Food and Nutrition Board, Institute of Medicine. National Academy Press, Washington, D.C., 2000.

17. Traber, M.G. Vitamin E in *Modern Nutrition in Health and Disease*. 9th ed. Shils, M.E. et al., Eds. Williams and Wilkins, Baltimore, MD, 1999, 347.
18. Traber, M.G. and Jialal, I. Measurement of lipid-soluble vitamins-further adjustment needed? *Lancet*, 335(9220): 2013, 2000.
19. Peifer, J.J. Thiamin in *Sports Nutrition: Vitamins and Trace Elements*. Wolinsky, I., Driskell, J.A., Eds. CRC, Boca Raton, FL, 1997, 47.
20. Tanphaichitr, V. Thiamin in *Modern Nutrition in Health and Disease*. 9th ed., Shils, M.E. et al., Eds. Williams and Wilkins, Baltimore, MD, 1999, 381.
21. Clarkson, P.M. Exercise and the B Vitamins in *Nutrition in Exercise and Sport*. 3rd ed. Wolinsky, I., Ed. CRC, Boca Raton, FL, 1998, 179.
22. McCormick, D.B. Riboflavin in *Modern Nutrition in Health and Disease*. 9th ed., Shils, M.E. et al., Eds. Williams and Wilkins, Baltimore, MD, 1999, 391.
23. Lewis, R.D. Riboflavin and Niacin in *Sports Nutrition: Vitamins and Trace Elements*. Wolinsky, I. and Driskell, J.A., Eds. CRC, Boca Raton, FL, 1997, 57.
24. Cervantes-Laurean, D., McElvaney, N.G. and Moss, J. Niacin in *Modern Nutrition in Health and Disease*. 9th ed. Shils, M.E. et al., Eds. Williams and Wilkins, Baltimore, MD, 1999, 401.
25. Leklem, J.E. Vitamin B_6 in *Modern Nutrition in Health and Disease*. 9th ed. Shils, M.E. et al., Eds. Williams and Wilkins, Baltimore, MD, 1999, 413.
26. Weir, D.G. and Scott, J.M. Vitamin B_{12} "Cobalamin" in *Modern Nutrition in Health and Disease*. 9th ed. Shils, M.E. et al., Eds. Williams and Wilkins, Baltimore, MD. 1999, 447.
27. Herbert, V. Folic Acid in *Modern Nutrition in Health and Disease*. 9th ed., Shils, M.E. et al., Eds. Williams and Wilkins, Baltimore, MD, 1999, 433.
28. Bailey, L.B. and Gregory, J.F III., Folate Metabolism and Requirements. *J Nutr*, 129:779, 1999.
29. Mock, D.M. Biotin in *Modern Nutrition in Health and Disease*. 9th ed., Shils, M.E. et al., Eds. Williams and Wilkins, Baltimore, MD, 1999, 459.
30. Mock, N.I., Malik, M.I., Stumph, P.J., Bishop, W.P. and Mock D.M. Increased urinary excretion of 3-hydroxyisovaleric acid and decreased excretion of biotin are sensitive early indicators of decreased biotin status in experimental biotin deficiencies. *Am J Clin Nutr*, 65(4): 951, 1997.
31. Plesofsky-Vig, N. Pantothenic Acid in *Modern Nutrition in Health and Disease*. 9th ed., Shils, M.E. et al., Eds. Williams and Wilkins, Baltimore, MD, 1999, 423.
32. Ball, G.F.M. *Fat-soluble Vitamin Assays in Food Analysis— A Comprehensive Review*. Elsevier, London, 1988.
33. Combs, G.F. *The Vitamins*, Academic, San Diego, CA, 1992.
34. Gregory, J.F., III, *Vitamins in Food Chemistry*. 3rd ed., Fennema, O.R., Ed. Marcel Dekker, New York, 1996, 531.
35. Jones, D., Seamark, D.A., Trafford, D.J.H. and Makin, H.L.J. Vitamin D: Cholecalciferol, Ergosterol and Hydroxylated metabolites in *Modern Chromatographic Analysis of the Vitamins*. De Leenheer A.P., Lambert, W.E. and De Ruyter, M.G.M. Eds. Marcel Dekker, 1985, 73.
36. Lewis, N.M. and Frederick, A.M. Vitamins D and K in *Sports Nutrition: Vitamins and Trace Elements*. Wolinsky, I. and Driskell, J.A., Eds. CRC, Boca Raton, FL, 1997, 111.
37. Voet, D. and Voet, J.G. *Biochemistry*, 2nd ed. John Wiley & Sons, NY. 1995, 1202.
38. Keith, R.E. Ascorbic Acid in *Sports Nutrition: Vitamins and Trace Elements*. Wolinsky, I. and Driskell, J.A., Eds. CRC, Boca Raton, FL, 1997, 29.

39. Thomas, E.A. Pantothenic Acid and Biotin in *Sports Nutrition: Vitamins and Trace Elements.* Wolinsky, I. and Driskell, J.A., Eds. CRC, Boca Raton, FL. 1997, 97.

40. Underwood, B.A. and Olson, J.A. A brief guide to current methods of assessing vitamin A status, International Vitamin A Consultative Group, ILSI-NF, Washington, D.C., 1993.

41. Barua, A.B. and Olson, J.A. Retinoyl ß-glucuronide: an endogenous compound of human blood. *Am. J. Clin. Nutr.* 43, 481, 1986.

42. Bieri, J.G., Brown, E.D. and Smith, J.C. Jr. Determination of individual carotenoids in human plasma by high performance liquid chromatography. *J Liq Chromatogr,* 8, 473,1985.

43. Got, L., Gousson, T. and Delacoux, E. Simultaneous determination of retinyl esters and retinol in human livers by reverse-phase high-performance liquid chromatography, *J Chromatogr B Biomed Appl*; 668(2):233, 1995.

44. Meydani, M., Fielding, R.A. and Fotouhi, N. Vitamin E in *Sports Nutrition: Vitamins and Trace Elements.* Wolinsky, I. and Driskell, J.A., Eds. CRC, Boca Raton, FL, 1997, 119.

45. Olson, R.E. Vitamin K in *Modern Nutrition in Health and Disease.* 9th ed. Shils, M.E. et al., Eds. Williams and Wilkins, Baltimore, MD, 1999, 363.

46. Lefevere, M.F.L., Clayeys, A.E. and De Leenheer, A.P. Vitamin K: Phylloquinone and menaquinones in *Modern Chromatographic Analysis of the Vitamins.* De Leenheer A.P., Lambert, W.E. and De Ruyter, M.G.M. Eds. Marcel Dekker, 1985, 201.

47. Kawasaki, T. and Sanemari, H. Vitamin B_1: Thiamins in *Modern Chromatographic Analysis of the Vitamins.* De Leenheer A.P., Lambert, W.E. and De Ruyter, M.G.M. Eds. Marcel Dekker, New York, 1985, 385.

48. Rokitzki, L., Sagredos, A., Logemann, E., Sauer, B., Buechner, M. and Keul, J. Vitamin B_1 status in athletes of various types of sports. *Med. Exer. Nutr. Health.* Cambridge, MA, 3(5): 240, 1994.

49. Marletta, M.A. and Light, D.R. Flavins in *Modern Chromatographic Analysis of the Vitamins.* De Leenheer A.P., Lambert, W.E. and De Ruyter, M.G.M. Eds. Marcel Dekker, New York, 1985, 413.

50. Hengen, N. and De Vries, J.X. Nicotinic Acid and Nicotinamide in *Modern Chromatographic Analysis of the Vitamins.* De Leenheer A.P., Lambert, W.E. and De Ruyter, M.G.M. Eds. Marcel Dekker, New York, 1985, 341.

51. Vanderslice, J.T., Brownlee, S.G., Cortissoz, M.E. and Maire, C.E. Vitamin B6 Analysis: Sample Preparation, Extraction Procedures and Chromatographic Separations in *Modern Chromatographic Analysis of the Vitamins.* De Leenheer A.P., Lambert, W.E. and De Ruyter, M.G.M. Eds. Marcel Dekker, New York, 1985, 435.

52. Guilland, J.C., Penaranda, T., Gallet, C., Boggio, V., Fuchs, F. and Klepping, J. Vitamin status of young athletes including the effects of supplementation. *Med Sci Sports Exerc,* 21(4):441, 1989.

53. Sampson, D.A. Vitamin B_6 in *Sports Nutrition: Vitamins and Trace Elements.* Wolinsky, I. and Driskell, J.A., Eds. CRC, Boca Raton, FL, 1997, 75.

54. Rokitzki, L., Sagredos, A.,Reuss, F., Buechner, M. and Keul, J. Acute changes in vitamin B_6 status in endurance athletes before and after a marathon. *Int J Sport Nutr,* 4(2): 154, 1994.

55. McCormack, J.J. and Newman, R.A. Chromatographic Studies on Folic Acid and Related Compounds in *Modern Chromatographic Analysis of the Vitamins.* De Leenheer A.P., Lambert, W.E. and De Ruyter, M.G.M. Eds. Marcel Dekker, New York, 1985, 303.

56. McMartin K. Folate and Vitamin B$_{12}$ in *Sports Nutrition: Vitamins and Trace Elements*. Wolinsky, I. and Driskell, J.A., Eds. CRC, Boca Raton, FL, 1997, 85.

57. Frappier, F. and Gaudry, M. Biotin in *Modern Chromatographic Analysis of the Vitamins*. De Leenheer A.P., Lambert, W.E. and De Ruyter, M.G.M. Eds. Marcel Dekker, New York, 1985, 477.

58. Mock, D.M., Stadler, D.D., Stratton, S.L. and Mock, N.I. Biotin status assessed longitudinally in pregnant women. *J Nutr*, 127(5): 710, 1997.

59. Wolf, B. and Raetz, H. The measurement of propionylcoA carboxylase and pyruvate carboxylase activity in hair roots: its use in the diagnosis of inherited biotin-dependent enzyme deficiencies. *Clin Chim Acta*, 130(1):25, 1983.

60. Bui-Nguyen, M.H. Ascorbic Acid and Related Compounds in *Modern Chromatographic Analysis of the Vitamins*. De Leenheer A.P., Lambert, W.E. and De Ruyter, M.G.M. Eds. Marcel Dekker, New York, 1985, 267.

14

Assessment of Mineral Status of Athletes

Henry C. Lukaski[a,b]

CONTENTS

[a] Mention of a trademark or proprietary product does not constitute a guarantee of warranty of the product by the United States Department of Agriculture and does not imply its approval to the exclusion of other products that may also be suitable.

[b] U.S. Department of Agriculture, Agricultural Research Service, Northern Plains Area is an equal opportunity/affirmative action employer and all agency services are available without discrimination.

I. Introduction

As knowledge of the biological roles that mineral elements play in the development and maintenance of physical fitness and performance grows, there is burgeoning need for tools to assess the adequacy of mineral element nutritional status of physically active persons. Pursuit of the appropriate assessment tool is complicated by theoretical and practical limitations. The ideal method is specific and sensitive; it distinguishes adequate from deficient nutritional status and discriminates graded degrees of nutritional deficiency. The method also is practical, convenient and noninvasive, reflects cellular mineral element content and adequacy of function and responds proportionally to changes in dietary intake. Unfortunately, no single method achieves all of these criteria. Thus, a compromise among available approaches is needed to accommodate the requirements of a valid and practical method to routinely assess human mineral nutritional status.[1]

This chapter details some basic approaches for assessment of mineral nutritional status with an emphasis on biochemical methods and indicators. The focus is mineral elements that are either acknowledged to have key roles in promoting physical performance or are used as performance-enhancing supplements; they include calcium, chromium, copper, iron, magnesium, phosphorus and zinc. This review supplements a previous publication of laboratory methods for nutritional status assessment.[2] It presents reference intervals of biochemical measures for assessment of mineral element status, features typical blood biochemical markers found in diverse groups of physically active persons and identifies physiological impairments or adaptations associated with altered mineral nutritional status.

A. Dietary Intake

The estimated daily intake of nutrients is a common indicator of nutritional status. The use of a self-reported dietary history or diet recall in conjunction with the availability of computerized programs and mineral nutrient data bases permits calculation of individual nutrient intakes from commonly consumed foods. Evaluation of adequacy of intake requires the comparison of self-reported intake with established national recommendations.[3,4] This approach relies on accurate recording or recall of amounts of specific foods, reporting of intake on days of the week that are representative of usual food consumption and nutrient databases that accurately reflect nutrient contents of the food consumed. Interpretation of adequacy of intake relies on the threshold of 70% of recommended intake. The tendency of individuals to report less food than they actually consume limits the accuracy of this approach.[5,6]

B. Blood Biochemical Measures

Blood biochemical analyses offer an unbiased alternative to self-reported food intakes. The concentrations of minerals in serum or plasma, mineral concentration in the cellular components of the blood, and the activities of mineral-containing enzymes or metalloenzymes in the circulation are routine assessment measures. The basis for these determinations is the assumption that these variables are proportional to their intracellular contents and thus reflect tissue or organ content and function. Some factors complicate the validity of these measures to index nutritional status. Circulating mineral element concentrations may be affected by factors unrelated to diet or whole-body mineral status (e.g., hormones, stress, inflammation, etc.). Importantly for physically active persons, alterations in the extracellular fluid volume may artificially increase concentration values, which may be corrected for decreases in plasma volume.[7,8]

1. Sample Collection

Accurate determination of mineral elements in biological specimens requires special precautions and presents specific analytical problems.[9] Use of consistent sampling procedures is mandatory because mineral element distributions in the same tissue are variable. Analysis of seemingly homogenous specimens such as blood may be markedly affected by sampling and processing procedures. Hemolysis or microhemolysis of a whole-blood sample can yield erroneously high plasma or serum concentrations of iron or zinc because erythrocyte concentrations of these and other minerals are more than 10 times greater than those in plasma.[10] Also, concentrations of zinc are 5 to 15% greater in serum than plasma because of release of zinc from platelets and erythrocytes during clotting. Selection of an anticoagulant also is important because of the potential expansion of plasma volume associated with intracellular fluid shifts.

2. Sample Contamination

The critical problem affecting the validity of mineral element analyses is sample contamination from external sources. In experimental and laboratory environments, mineral elements exist in nanogram (ng) and milligram (mg) amounts. Thus, a significant portion of an analytical value may be the result of contamination unless appropriate precautions are followed. Contamination, therefore, contributes to the wide variation of reported reference values, specifically in the mineral elements reported in the part per billion range (e.g., ng/g).

Many sources of contamination in the laboratory include dust, rubber, paper products, wood, metal surfaces, skin, dandruff and hair. Plastic and borosilicate glass are best suited for trace element analysis. Specifically, fluorocarbon, polyethylene and polypropylene plastics are recommended. Surfaces in contact with samples for analysis should be cleaned of adherent mineral elements by soaking with dilute nitric acid or commercial, metal-binding solutions. Water should meet or exceed American Chemical Society standards of 14 MΩ/cm^2 for elemental contamination or resistivity.[9] Reagents and anticoagulants should be free of mineral elements. Disposable syringes and stainless steel needles should be used for blood collection. Importantly, stainless steel needles are not acceptable for phlebotomy for chromium, nickel and other ultratrace elements unless they are siliconized; stainless steel contains high chromium and nickel contents. Commercially available evacuated blood collection tubes may be problematic if specimens contact the stopper. Mineral elements may leach from the stopper into the blood and thus contaminate the specimen.

3. Analytical Methods

Measurement of mineral elements in biological specimens requires analytical sensitivity, specificity, precision, accuracy and expedience. Analytical sensitivity is paramount because concentrations of trace and ultratrace elements occur in the microgram (mg) to ng/g range.

Although a variety of analytical techniques are available, atomic absorption spectrophotometry (AAS), emission spectroscopy including inductively coupled plasma emission spectroscopy (ICPES) and inductively coupled mass spectroscopy (ICPMS) are commonly used in clinical settings. The AAS method is the routine assessment tool of single mineral element analysis. Samples may be diluted and aspirated directly into the flame. Electrothermal or flameless AAS methods are available for micro samples and very low concentrations (< 50 ng/g). Background correction using Zeeman or deuterium arc techniques is often necessary with electrothermal AAS to overcome matrix or background interferences. The ICPES is a multi-elemental method that is replacing AAS for many mineral element applications. It enables simultaneous multi-elemental measurements over a wide analytical range.

4. Quality Control

Effective quality assurance procedures must be included in mineral element analysis plans because methods for mineral analysis generally are not standardized and are prone to interferences from biological matrices and external contamination. An effective quality control program for trace and ultratrace mineral analyses necessitates the following components. In each batch of samples, there should be reagent blanks, replicate analyses to estimate precision, and reference materials with known or certified concentrations of mineral elements prepared similarly to the unknown samples to enable assessment of accuracy and batch-to-batch precision. Importantly, the reference material should possess the same matrix and approximately the same amounts of analytes as the unknown samples. A variety of reference or control materials are available commercially.

II. Calcium

Calcium is a major mineral in the body; it serves to provide body structure, with more than 99% of body calcium stored in bone. The remainder of body calcium exists in tissues and extracellular fluid and acts to regulate a wide variety of body functions including muscle contraction, blood coagulation, enzyme activation, nerve transmission, signal transduction in hormone actions and membrane transport. Calcium in the plasma exists in different physiological forms. Approximately 50% of calcium is free or ionized; it is available for incorporation into intracellular compartments. Forty percent is bound to plasma proteins, mainly albumin; this binding is highly dependent on pH. About 20% of the protein-bound calcium is bound to globulins. The remaining 10% of plasma calcium is associated with diffusable anions including bicarbonate, lactate, citrate and phosphate. Factors such as diet, stress and illness alter the distribution of calcium among these three metabolic pools and thus affect the amounts of total and ionized calcium in the circulation.

A. Methods for Assessing Calcium Status

Assessment of calcium status relies on determination of either total or ionized calcium. Ionized calcium, also termed free calcium, is generally considered to be the physiological form of calcium because it is biologically active and is highly controlled by calcium-regulating hormones. Because approximately 60% of circulating calcium is bound to proteins, total calcium concentrations are markedly influenced by protein concentrations, principally albumin.

1. Total Serum Calcium

Three methods currently used to determine total calcium in biological fluids include photometric analysis, titration of a fluorescent calcium complex with EDTA or ethylene glycol tetraacetic acid (EGTA), and AAS. The approved reference method for measuring serum concentrations of calcium is AAS;[11] it provides improved accuracy and precision compared with the spectrophotometric methods. Detailed procedures for the determination of calcium in serum are available.[12]

2. Serum Ionized Calcium

Serum ionized calcium, which represents the majority of calcium in the circulation, is the physiologically active form of calcium. In contrast to total serum calcium, which may be normal in conditions characterized by neuromuscular irritability such as vitamin D-deficient rickets and hypoparathyroidism, serum ionized calcium concentration is reduced.

Physiological and measurement conditions, including changes in the specimen pH, the use of EDTA or heparin and high concentrations of magnesium and sodium, affect serum ionized calcium concentrations.[13] Because most anticoagulants bind calcium, serum is the preferred specimen for measuring ionized or free calcium. Common biologically active anions, including citrate, phosphate, oxalate and sulfate, form complexes with free calcium and thus may reduce its apparent concentration. The binding of free calcium by protein and relatively small anions is affected by pH both *in vivo* and *in vitro*. Biological specimens should be analyzed at the pH of the blood because of the inverse relationship between pH and ionized or free calcium. Anaerobic conditions should be maintained because specimens lose carbon dioxide and become more alkaline when exposed to air. Also, specimens should be handled with care to minimize metabolism of erythrocyte and leukocytes, which produce acids and decrease pH.

3. Calcium Reference Intervals and Data from Interventions in Physical Activity

In healthy adults, serum calcium concentrations range from 8.6 to 10.2 mg/dL or 2.15 to 2.55 mmol/L.[12] Concentrations decrease with age in men; females have slightly lower concentrations than males. Serum ionized calcium concentrations range from 4.64 to 5.28 mg/dL or 1.16 to 1.32 mmol/L in healthy adults.

Supplemental calcium in conjunction with a program of weight-bearing activity has been used to prevent and treat age-related bone loss in non-osteoporotic women.[14] However, when both treatments have been applied, no additive effects were found in elderly women.[15]

Calcium supplementation apparently does not influence the risk of developing bone stress injuries. Supplementation of healthy military recruits with 500 mg of calcium, as compared with placebo, had no effect on the frequency of overuse injuries during 9 weeks of physical training.[16] Because total daily calcium intake was at least 800 mg/d, the authors concluded that this amount of calcium was adequate to protect against overuse bone injuries.

Although the importance of measuring blood biochemical indicators of calcium status is well established in the evaluation of endocrine control of bone metabolism, measurements of calcium status in physically active persons are not common. Assessment of bone status relies on determinations of bone mass and quality with dual x-ray absorptiometry and determinations of circulating hormones involved in maintenance of bone accretion and turnover.

III. Chromium

Chromium is an ultratrace element; it facilitates the biological action of insulin in carbohydrate, protein and lipid metabolism.[17] Chromium, which binds to an intracellular, low-molecular weight chromium-binding protein, potentiates the auto-amplification of insulin signaling by stimulating the insulin receptor kinase activity in insulin-sensitive cells.[18] Insulin resistance may be a consequence of chromium deficiency because insulin apparently is inefficient as a regulator of glucose uptake and utilization without chromium. Because of analytical problems with measurements of very small concentrations of chromium in foods, beverages and biological samples as well as interferences with chromium contamination, human metabolic studies of chromium are very limited. Thus, inference of human chromium deficiency relies on improvement in glucose tolerance after supplementation.[17]

A. Method for Assessment of Chromium Status

Analytical limitations because of trace concentrations of chromium in human tissues and fluids have limited the identification of a reliable measure of body chromium status.[17] Early reports of serum and urinary chromium concentration were erroneous because of contaminations and other analytical problems. With improved method sensitivity and capability of identification and elimination of external chromium contamination, substantially decreased estimates of chromium concentration in biological and food samples appeared.

The preferred method for determination of chromium in biological samples is AAS with a graphite furnace and Zeeman correction.[19] Caution is advised to avoid any contact of a sample with any metal surface, including the use of stainless steel needles unless they are siliconized.

1. Reference Intervals and Data from Physically Active Persons

The current adult reference range for serum chromium concentration is < 0.05 to 0.5 µg/L or 1 to 10 nmol/L. Urinary chromium excretion is referenced at 100 to 200 ng/24h. Consumption of chromium supplements will increase daily urinary chromium output depending on the dose and duration of the supplement usage.

Data describing serum chromium concentrations and urinary chromium excretion are limited. Anderson and co-workers[20] reported significantly increased serum chromium concentrations in nine men after they ran 6 miles (10 km). Basal values were 0.12 ± 0.06 (mean $\pm$ SD) µg/L, increased to 0.17 ± 0.09 µg/L immediately after running, then to 0.19 ± 0.09 µg/L 2 h after exercise. Urinary chromium output also increased significantly from non-exercise values of 0.20 ± 0.12 to 0.37 ± 0.24 µg/d on the day of running. Among young men consuming self-selected diets and participating in an 8-wk resistance training program, serum chromium concentrations increased from 13 ± 4 to 14.5 ± 4 nmol/L.[21] With chromium supplementation (~ 180 µg/d as chromium picolinate), serum chromium increased from 13 ± 4 to 16 ± 3 nmol/L. Concomitantly, urinary chromium excretion increased only with chromium supplementation. Thus, both exercise and chromium supplementation affect serum and urinary chromium.

IV. Copper

The biochemical role for copper is primarily catalytic, with many copper metalloenzymes acting as oxidases to achieve the reduction of molecular oxygen. In these oxidation-reduction reactions, copper serves as the reactive center in the copper metalloenzymes. Some examples include ceruloplasmin, superoxide dismutase, dopamine-β-hydroxylase, lysyl oxidase, cytochrome c oxidase and tyrosinase.[22] Thus, copper plays a key role in supporting increased energy expenditure during physical activity.

Copper deficiency decreases the activity of copper metalloenzymes and results in marked biological impairments.[22] Defective connective tissue cross-links in heart, muscle and bone may be attributed to decreased lysyl oxidase activity. Hypopigmentation has been associated with depressed tyrosinase activity required for melanin synthesis. Oxidative damage in various organs, tissues and organelles has been shown to be the result of decreased superoxide dismutase activity. Altered catecholamine concentrations and hypothermia have been attributed to decreased dopamine-β-hydroxylase activity in brown adipose tissue.[23]

A. Methods for Copper Assessment

Biochemical indicators of copper nutritional status continue to undergo evaluation and validation. Despite the lack of an unequivocal marker of human copper nutritional status, a number of indices are useful in the diagnosis of human copper deficiency.

1. Serum or Plasma Copper Concentration

A common measure of copper status is serum or plasma copper concentration; low copper concentration in plasma or serum is an indicator of depleted body copper stores. Yet plasma copper concentrations are unreliable indicators of short-term marginal copper status in humans. Homeostatic mechanisms regulate plasma copper concentrations within a narrow range. Thus, plasma copper concentrations decrease only after significant depletion of body copper stores.[24] Factors independent of copper intake affect circulating copper concentrations. Women generally have higher plasma or serum copper concentrations than men; estrogen increases plasma copper concentrations in women taking oral contraceptive agents and postmenopausal women receiving estrogen therapy.[25] Plasma copper concentrations are increased in pregnancy, inflammation, infection and rheumatoid arthritis.[26] In contrast, general stress and glucocorticoid hormones increase plasma copper concentrations.[26] Thus, conditions that elevate serum copper may belie decreased serum copper even during copper deprivation. Also, circumstances that reduce serum copper should be eliminated before a valid assessment of copper nutritional status can be undertaken.

The method of choice for determination of plasma or serum copper is AAS after dilution of the specimen with deionized water. Hemolysis is not a major concern for copper determinations because concentrations of copper in erythrocytes and plasma are similar.

2. Ceruloplasmin

More than 80% of the copper in plasma is associated with the protein ceruloplasmin; changes in plasma copper are reflected in changes in the amount of this protein in the circulation. Both the enzymatic activity of ceruloplasmin and the immunoreactive protein ceruloplasmin respond similarly to age, sex and hormone use; they increase in pregnancy and in response to inflammation. Enzymatic activity of ceruloplasmin has been shown to be an indicator of copper status in animals and humans deprived of copper.[24]

Serum ceruloplasmin can be measured immunochemically or by its oxidase activity. The copper-depleted apo-ceruloplasmin is likely present in normal and copper-deficient serum.[24] Thus, chemical assays of its oxidase activity are preferred as an index of copper status. The specific activity of ceruloplasmin, defined as the ratio of enzymatic activity to the immunoreactive protein, may be a sensitive marker of copper status because it was inversely related to blood pressure response to hand-grip work.[27] This ratio is not affected by age, sex or hormone use.[24]

3. Superoxide Dismutase Activity

There are two distinct forms of copper, each of which utilizes copper in its reactive center. *Zinc superoxide dismutase (SOD)*: these isozymes are characterized by their cellular location and distribution among various tissues. The *erythrocyte isoform (SOD1)* is localized in the nucleus and cytoplasm and found principally in erythrocytes and liver cells.[28] However, the extracellular isoform (SOD3) is concentrated in the extracellular matrix of tissues, specifically lung and kidney and is the dominant extracellular antioxidant enzyme found in the serum.[29]

a.   Erythrocyte Superoxide Dismutase

Erythrocyte superoxide dismutase activity decreases during copper deficiency in humans and some animal species. It also is sensitive to changes in copper status, as shown in several studies of experimental copper deprivation.[24] Compared with other biochemical markers of copper status such as plasma copper and ceruloplasmin, erythrocyte superoxide dismutase activity is independent of age, sex and hormone use.[30]

b.   Extracellular Superoxide Dismutase

The extracellular superoxide dismutase is a secretory protein present in relatively reduced amounts in the circulation relative to its tissue source.[29] It is responsive to changes in copper[31] and zinc[32,33] intake in animal models. Some controversy exists regarding the specificity of the activity of extracellular superoxide dismutase as a functional indicator of copper or zinc status, as both conditions have been shown to reduce its activity.[34,35]

Biochemical assays for superoxide dismutase are based on the indirect measurement of activity that consists of a superoxide generating system and a superoxide indicator that is measured spectrophotometrically.[36] Addition of copper, zinc superoxide dismutase, specifically SOD1, inhibits the absorption change. The use of the autoxidation of pyrogallol is the method of choice for determination of erythrocyte superoxide dismutase activity.[37] In contrast, the autoxidation of xanthine by xanthine oxidase is the recommended method for determination of extracellular superoxide dismutase.[38]

A practical problem arises from the use of superoxide dismutase activities to assess copper status; there are no uniform reference ranges available. To facilitate the use of superoxide dismutase, it is suggested that reference ranges be developed in each laboratory and conditions used for analysis be maintained.

4.   Cytochrome C Oxidase Activity

Decreased tissue cytochrome c oxidase activity is an early and consistent trait of copper deficiency in animals. Reductions of 50% of normal cytochrome c oxidase activity are associated with impaired neurological, cardiac and muscle functions.[39] Studies in humans report that cytochrome c oxidase activities in platelets are decreased when dietary copper is restricted.[24,40] Cytochrome c oxidase activity in platelets and leukocytes paralleled copper status in animals;[41] the cytochrome c oxidase activity correlated directly with liver copper concentration, an established index of copper status in animals.

Available methods for determination of cytochrome c oxidase activity in blood cells and tissues utilize the spectrophotometric analysis of the oxidation of ferricytochrome c. A microassay has been described that uses a coupled reaction between cytochrome c and 3-3'-diaminobenzidine tetrachloride in microwell plates.[42]

Age apparently affects cytochrome c oxidase activity.[24,40] Platelet and leukocyte cytochrome c oxidase activity are higher in older than in young adults, but are not affected by sex or hormone use. Other factors that may limit the use of this marker include considerable between-individual variability, the labile nature of this enzyme and its sensitivity to minor variations in technique.

5.   Copper Reference Intervals and Data from Athletes

Serum copper concentrations are higher in women of child-bearing age, 80 to 190 µg/dL or 12.6 to 24.4 µmol/L, than in men, 70 to 140 µg/dL or 11 to

22 µmol/L. Serum copper is highest in pregnant women, 118 to 302 µg/dL or 18.5 to 47.4 µmol/L. The range of normal values for children 6 to 12 yrs of age is 80 to 90 µg/dL or 12.6 to 29.9 µmol/L.[11]

There is a paucity of data describing the copper status of athletes. Among nine healthy, middle-aged runners, serum copper was 93 ± 15 µg/dL.[20] In a sample of 44 male university athletes, plasma copper was 90 ± 14 µg/dL with hypocupremia (< 70 µg/dL) present in four of the men.[43] Plasma copper (95 ± 11 and 94 ± 10 µg/dL) and enzymatic ceruloplasmin (419 ± 37 and 397 ± 38 mg/L) were unchanged from preseason to end of the competitive season in 12 elite female university swimmers.[44] Similarly, plasma copper and enzymatic ceruloplasmin were within the range of normal values for male and female swimmers before and during a competitive season.[45] Interestingly, SOD1 activity increased significantly in response to swim training, despite reduced copper intake.[45] Apparently the increased activity of this enzyme was an adaptation to increased oxidative stress associated with aerobic training.

Copper status of runners has also been assessed. Anderson et al.[20] reported serum copper of 93 ± 5 µg/dL for nine trained runners. In contrast, Singh et al.[46] found increased plasma copper (18.8 ± 3.5 vs. 16.1 ± 3.1 µg/dL), decreased erythrocyte copper (1.06 ± 0.21 vs. 1.26 ± 0.15 µg/g) and similar enzymatic ceruloplasmin (287 ± 49 vs. 281 ± 50 mg/L) in 45 female runners compared with 27 nonrunners. Thus, exercise apparently induced a redistribution of copper in the women.

It is useful to acknowledge that the use of more than one biochemical measure of copper status will increase the probability of reliably identifying an individual as copper deficient or adequate. Thus, the use of multiple indicators, such as serum copper and platelet cytochrome c oxidase and superoxide dismutase, will enhance success of a valid assessment of copper nutritional status in physically active persons.

V. Iron

Iron serves as a component of a number of proteins, including enzymes and hemoglobin, that are required for metabolic energy production. More than 60% of iron in the body is found in hemoglobin in circulating erythrocytes. A readily mobilizable iron store accounts for another 25% of body iron. The remaining 15% is in myoglobin of muscle and a variety of iron-containing enzymes, such as the cytochromes, required for oxidative metabolism and other cellular functions. Thus, iron functions in delivery of oxygen to tissues and facilitates the use of oxygen at the cellular level.

Iron deficiency is one of the most prevalent micronutrient deficiencies in both industrialized and developing countries.[47] It is most common among children and women during their reproductive years; it may be seen among men as the result of chronic blood loss associated with parasitic load. Severe iron deficiency is manifest as anemia with adverse consequences such as impaired immune function, decreased work capacity, cold intolerance and compromised learning ability. In contrast, iron overload, which may be caused by progressive accumulation of iron in tissues (idiopathic hemochromatosis), may contribute to ischemic heart disease and cancer. It also may be the result of excessive use of iron supplements, injections of therapeutic iron or blood transfusions

A. Methods for Iron Assessment

Because the iron status of humans ranges from deficiency states to iron overload, a variety of biochemical indices are available. Some common measurements include hemoglobin, hematocrit, various erythrocyte indices, ferritin, serum iron, total iron-binding capacity, transferrin, transferrin saturation, free erythrocyte protoporphyrin, zinc protoporphyrin and transferrin receptors. These status indicators vary in their sensitivity and specificity.

1. Hemoglobin and Hematocrit

Measurement of hemoglobin concentration in whole blood is perhaps the most widely used assessment tool for iron deficiency anemia. As an indicator of iron deficiency, it is relatively insensitive and exhibits low specificity. Hemoglobin concentrations decrease only during the late stages of iron deficiency after tissue iron stores have been greatly reduced. Moreover, hemoglobin concentration may be affected by other nutritional perturbations such as folic acid, copper and vitamin B_{12} deficiency, and other conditions including pregnancy, tobacco smoking, infection and inflammation, as well as dehydration.[48] A common method for measurement of hemoglobin in blood includes spectrophotometry after anticoagulation with heparin or EDTA and conversion to cyanomethemoglobin.

Hematocrit or packed erythrocyte volume decreases after erythrocyte production has been reduced. Thus, it also is relatively insensitive and nonspecific because hematocrit is influenced by the same factors that affect hemoglobin concentrations, mainly changes in plasma volume.

2. Ferritin

Serum ferritin concentration is in equilibrium with body stores ,and variations in the quantity of iron in the storage compartment are reflected in serum ferritin concentration.[49] Serum ferritin concentration declines very early in the development of iron deficiency, well in advance of any reductions in hemoglobin or serum iron concentration. Thus, serum ferritin may serve as a useful indicator of iron deficiency. However, certain chronic conditions increase serum ferritin concentrations independently of iron intake. These conditions include chronic infections, inflammatory diseases, some malignancies and liver damage. Among healthy women depleted of iron by diet and phlebotomy, then repleted with iron, serum ferritin was the most sensitive measure of changes in iron status and stores.[50] Serum ferritin concentrations are currently determined by using immunological techniques. Commercial radioimmunoassay (RIA) and enzyme-linked immunosorbent assay (ELISA) kits are available.

3. Serum Iron, Total Iron-Binding Capacity, Transferrin and Transferrin Saturation

Measurement of iron and iron bound to transport proteins in the circulation provides another approach to assess iron nutritional status. Serum iron and total iron-binding capacity reflect the transit of iron from the reticuloendothelial system to the bone marrow. Transferrin, or the serum transport protein for iron, generally is only one third saturated with iron in normal circumstances. Transferrin may be measured immunologically, but practically, it is determined as total iron-binding capacity. The most useful measure of iron transport is transferrin saturation, the ratio of serum iron to total iron-binding capacity, because serum iron and iron-binding capacity respond in reciprocal manner to iron deficiency and overload. A transferrin saturation less than 16% indicates an inadequate iron intake; in contrast, iron saturation exceeding 55% reflects iron overload and possibly hemochromatosis.

Serum or plasma iron is measured by using chromogens, such as banthophenanthroline sulphonate and ferrozine and spectrophotometry. The use of AAS to measure serum or plasma iron is not recommended because AAS will determine the heme iron released during hemolysis; the colorimetric procedure does not detect heme iron. Total iron-binding capacity is determined by initially saturating the serum with excess iron, then adding magnesium carbonate to adsorb and remove excess iron not bound to transferrin.

4. Transferrin Receptor

The cell membranes of the developing erythrocyte precursors in bone marrow are very rich in transferrin receptors to which iron-transferrin complex binds before it is internalized and the iron is released from transferrin in the cytosol. The number of transferrin receptors increases during iron deficiency and decreases during iron excess. Studies in humans indicate that serum transferrin receptors decline as iron stores are depleted,[51] thus confirming the diagnostic value of serum transferrin receptor concentration as a measure of anemia. Circulating serum transferrin receptor concentrations increased only after iron stores were replenished but in advance of other markers of iron deficiency. The ratio of serum transferrin receptor to ferritin concentration shows an inverse relationship to iron status from usual iron stores to iron overload.[52] Thus, this ratio may be a practical and useful indicator of iron deficiency without anemia. Importantly, transferrin receptor concentration is not markedly affected by inflammation or liver disease, as is ferritin.[53] Transferrin receptor concentrations can be determined by using commercially available ELISA; care is required to minimize between-batch variability.

5.   Free Erythrocyte Protoporphyrin and Zinc Protoporphyrin

The concentrations of these proteins have been found to be sensitive indicators of iron-deficient erythrocyte production. In iron deficiency, these porphyrins accumulate in erythrocytes because a lack of iron decreases the rate of heme synthesis.[54] Changes in free erythrocyte protoporphyrin or zinc protoporphyrin are relatively insensitive to acute changes in iron status because iron stores must be depleted before heme synthesis is affected and because of the slow turnover rate of erythrocytes — 90 to 120 days. Free erythrocyte protoporphyrin and zinc protoporphyrin concentrations are measured spectrophotometrically.

6.   Iron Reference Intervals and Data from Athletes and Physically Active Persons

Serum iron concentrations range from 65 to 165 µg/dL or 11.6 to 31.3 µmol/L in men and 50 to 170 µg/dL or 9.0 to 30.4 µmol/L in women.[11] Total serum iron-binding capacity in healthy adults ranges from 250 to 425 µg/dL or 44.8 to 76.1 µmol/L. Serum ferritin concentrations range from 20 to 250 µg/L in men and 10 to 120 µg/L in women. Ferritin concentrations less than 10 µg/L indicate depleted iron stores, whereas concentrations greater than 300 µg/L suggest iron overload.

Iron status in athletes and physically active persons has been summarized in several reviews.[1,55] Iron-deficiency anemia, defined as hemoglobin concentrations less than 110 and 120 g/L in women and men, respectively, has been reported in physically active persons (Table 14.1). This severe iron deficiency is associated with reduced aerobic capacity in athletes and decreased work productivity in agricultural laborers. In some studies, the anemia is present in all of the subjects.[56] Generally, anemia is present in some but not all volunteers examined.[57-60] Perhaps more common is mild iron deficiency, characterized by decreased iron stores and increased iron-binding capacity. Since the initial finding that depleted body iron stores adversely affect submaximal work metabolism,[61] there has been increased awareness that iron deficiency without anemia is associated with impaired work ability. Studies of adolescents, particularly girls, show significant decreases in serum ferritin with normal hemoglobin concentrations and impaired training or endurance.[62,63] Among adults, iron-deficiency without anemia is manifest with alterations in endurance and performance and increased reliance on glycolytic metabolism.[64-66] Thus, surveys of athletes should include determinations of hemoglobin as well as measurements of body iron stores and transport iron.

VI.   Magnesium

Magnesium is an intracellular cation, second in concentration only to potassium. It is required in a wide variety of fundamental cellular processes that

TABLE 14.1

Selected Summary of Blood Biochemical Measures of Iron Status in Physically Active Individuals (Mean ± SD)

Source	Activity	Indicator*	Female	n	Male	n
Viteri and Torun[56]	Laboring	Hb			91 ± 11	78
Magnusson et al.[57]	Running	Hb			140 ± 5	5
		SF			31.0 ± 29.3	
		SFe			17.4 ± 8.3	
		TIBC			61.0 ± 2.1	
		TS			28.4 ± 13.8	
Celsing et al.[58]	Running	Hb			110 ± 7	9
Magazanik et al.[59]	Running	Hb	126 ± 9	11	148 ± 7	18
		SF	7.8 ± 8.8		28.8 ± 15.2	
		SFe	9.6 ± 2.6		13.6 ± 3.3	
		TIBC	72.8 ± 4.1		66.2 ± 4.6	
Rowland et al.[62]	Running	Hb	129 ± 5	14		
		SF	8.7 ± 3.5			
Rowland et al.[63]	Swimming	Hb	133 ± 8	15		
		SF	20.2 ± 13.7			
Newhouse et al.[60]	Running	Hb			130 ± 6	19
		SF			12.2 ± 4.3	
Lukaski et al.[64]	Cycling	Hb	120 ± 7	11		
		SF	6.0 ± 4.1			
Zhu and Haas[65]	Running	Hb	137 ± 8	17		
		SF	12.2 ± 8.1			
		STfR	6.0 ± 3.5			
		TIBC	60.7 ± 16.1			
		TS	19.0 ± 12.9			
Hinton et al.[66]	Running	Hb	133 ± 4	20		
		SF	8.1 ± 0.8			
		STfR	7.9 ± 0.7			
		SFe	13.4 ± 1.6			
		TIBC	65.0 ± 2.5			
		TS	20.9 ± 2.0			

* Hb = hemoglobin (g/L); SF = serum ferritin (µg/L); STFR = serum transferrin receptors (mg/L); SFE = serum iron (µmol/L); TIBC = total iron-binding capacity (µmol/L); TS = transferrin saturation (%).

support diverse physiological functions.[67] Magnesium is involved in more than 300 enzymatic reactions in which food is metabolized and new products are formed. Some of these reactions are involved in glycolysis, fat and protein metabolism, hydrolysis of adenosine triphosphate (ATP) and second messenger system and signal transduction. Magnesium also regulates membrane stability and neuromuscular, cardiovascular, immune and hormonal functions. Thus, magnesium status may be a limiting factor in physical performance.

A. Methods for Magnesium Assessment

Evaluation of human magnesium status is challenging; there is no simple, rapid and accurate laboratory test to indicate magnesium status.[67] A number of approaches have been used to assess magnesium status including determination of circulating magnesium, measurement of cellular magnesium content and indirect assessment of body magnesium stores.

1. Serum or Plasma Magnesium Concentration

Serum magnesium is the most commonly used indicator of magnesium status. Although a practical tool, serum or plasma magnesium is only an index of the presence or absence of magnesium deficiency. Low magnesium concentration or hypomagnesemia reliably indicates magnesium deficiency; however, its absence does not exclude significant magnesium depletion. The concentration of magnesium in serum has not been shown to be correlated with the concentration of magnesium in any other tissue pools except interstitial fluid, a component of the extracellular fluid.[68]

Serum, rather than plasma, is preferred because anticoagulants may be contaminated with magnesium or affect the assay procedure. It is critical to avoid hemolysis because the magnesium concentration of erythrocytes is three times as great as in serum. Magnesium concentration in serum is determined directly by flame AAS after diluting 50-fold with a lanthanum chloride or oxide diluent.

2. Ionized Magnesium Concentration

Magnesium in serum exists in several forms at physiological pH; protein-bound (19–34% of total), free magnesium ion (61–67% of the total) and complexed to certain anions (5–14% of the total).[69] The free or ionized magnesium is considered to be the metabolically active form.[70] Technology for measuring ionized magnesium in serum with ion-specific electrodes has only recently been available. Alternatively, the use of magnetic resonance spectroscopy provides the unique opportunity to measure intracellular magnesium in tissues *in vivo* at rest and during exercise.[71] This novel technology is restricted to a few research laboratories.

3. Magnesium Concentration in Muscle

More than 26% of the magnesium in the body is localized in muscle. Knowledge of the fundamental biological roles of magnesium in metabolism suggests that muscle is an appropriate tissue to sample in both healthy and ill persons to assess magnesium nutriture. Percutaneous skeletal muscle biopsy has been used to assess magnesium status in humans.[72] Factors such as being an invasive procedure and requiring special skills and equipment limit its general use.

4. Magnesium Content of Blood Cells

The mononucleated white cell has been proposed as a possible indicator of cellular magnesium status. In humans, magnesium concentrations of the mononucleated white cells do not correlate with serum or erythrocyte magnesium concentrations. However, several studies have shown a significant correlation between the magnesium concentration of the mononucleated cells and skeletal muscle magnesium.[70,71]

Another candidate measure of human magnesium status is erythrocyte magnesium. As with serum magnesium, erythrocyte magnesium has not been a significant predictor of tissue magnesium concentration. Although the clinical usefulness of determining erythrocyte magnesium is unclear, some studies have found that changes in erythrocyte magnesium reflect hypertension, chronic fatigue syndrome and premenstrual syndrome.[70]

5. Magnesium Retention after Acute Administration

Oral and intravenous magnesium loading tests have been described and perhaps are more widely used as a diagnostic tool than a measure of intracellular magnesium.[67] Persons with adequate magnesium in body pools generally excrete the vast majority (75 to 100%) of the administered dose with 24 to 48 hr compared with persons with depleted magnesium pools who retain a significant proportion of the dose. Sensitivity of the response as well as the need for normal kidney function and the lack of any disturbances in myocardial conductivity hamper the application of this test.

6. Magnesium Reference Intervals and Data from Athletes and Physically Active Persons

Total magnesium concentrations, as determined by AAS, range from 1.6 to 2.6 mg/dL or 0.66 to 1.07 mmol/L.[11] There is no apparent diurnal variation in total serum magnesium concentration.

Impetus for the measurement of magnesium status of physically active persons began with a report of hypomagnesemia (plasma magnesium = 0.60 mmol/L) associated with muscle spasms in a competitive tennis player.[73] Magnesium status of athletes has been reported (Table 14.2). Surveys of adult athletes participating in a variety of sports indicate values of plasma or serum magnesium in the range of normal values.[43,74–79] Similarly, children participating in swim training had normal values for plasma magnesium concentrations.[80] Intense anaerobic training transiently decreases plasma magnesium concentration with a parallel increase in urinary magnesium excretion.[81,82] Routine assessment of magnesium status is recommended because of the adverse effect of magnesium depletion on muscle function.

TABLE 14.2

Blood Biochemical Measurements of Magnesium Status in Athletes (Mean ± SD)

Source	Activity	Indicator*	Female	n	Male	n
Lukaski et al.[43]	Football, basketball, hockey, track & field	P			0.82 ± 0.09	44
Stendig-Lindberg et al.[74]	Hiking	S			0.83 ± 0.14	20
Deuster et al.[81]	Running	P			0.78 ± 0.03	13
Conn et al.[80]	Swimming	P	0.88 ± 0.04	13	0.82 ± 0.06	9
Fogelholm et al.[75]	Running	S			0.83 ± 0.02	114
Fogelholm et al.[76]	Variable†	S			0.85 ± 0.01	278
Cordova et al.[77]	Soccer	S			0.82 ± 0.04	18
		UF			0.47 ± 0.04	
	Volleyball	S			0.85 ± 0.04	12
		UF			0.50 ± 0.03	
Manore et al.[82]	Aerobic	P			0.95 ± 0.07	19
	Anaerobic	P			0.95 ± 0.07	18
Lukaski et al.[78]	Swimming	P	0.82 ± 0.04	10	0.87 ± 0.03	7
Lukaski et al.[79]	Swimming	P	0.85 ± 0.05	5	0.88 ± 0.05	5

* P = plasma (mmol/L); S = serum (mmol/L); UF = ultra filterable magnesium (mmol/L)

† Running, soccer, skiing, wrestling, track & field, weightlifting

VII. Phosphorus

Phosphorus in the form of inorganic or organic phosphate is the second most abundant mineral in the body. More than 85% of the phosphorus in the adult is present in the skeleton as either hydroxyapatite or as calcium phosphate. The remainder in cells of the soft tissues and the extracellular fluid is present as inorganic phosphate or in nucleic acids, phosphoproteins, phospholipids and high energy compounds including phosphocreatine (CP) and adenosine mono-, di- and triphosphates (AMP, ADP and ATP). Phosphorous is an essential factor in most energy-producing reactions of cells.

Phosphorus depletion results in low intracellular concentrations of phosphoglycerate, ATP and CP that adversely affect muscle function, work capacity and overall cardiorespiratory function. Impaired phosphorus status is associated with long-term total parenteral nutrition, metabolic perturbations associated with ketoacidosis, excessive use of antacids containing aluminum hydroxide or aluminum carbonate because aluminum complexes with phosphate.

A. Methods for Assessing Phosphorus Status

Serum phosphorus, measured as phosphate, is used most frequently to assess phosphorus status. Phosphate in serum exists both as the monovalent and divalent anion. The ratio of $H_2PO_4^{-1}$ to HPO_4^{-2} varies from 1:1 in acidosis to 1:4 at physiological pH and 1:9 in alkalosis. Approximately 55% of the phosphate in serum is free, 35% is complexed with sodium, calcium and magnesium and 10% is bound to protein.

Serum phosphorus concentrations are generally measured colorimetrically.[83] It is critical to separate blood cells from the serum as soon as possible because high concentrations of organic phosphate esters in cells may be hydrolyzed to inorganic phosphate during storage.

1. Phosphorus Reference Intervals and Data from Phosphate Supplementation Trials

Age affects the range of normal values for phosphorus. Values are higher in infancy, then decline throughout childhood until adulthood concentrations are reached. Serum phosphate, expressed as phosphorus, ranges from 4.0 to 7.0 mg/dL or 1.29 to 2.26 mmol/L in children and from 2.5 to 4.5 mg/dL or 0.81 to 1.45 mmol/L in healthy adults. Serum phosphate concentrations also are dependent on meals and variation in the secretion of hormones such as parathyroid hormone.

Determinations of serum phosphate have been used to evaluate the effects of phosphate supplements on physical performance rather than to assess phosphorus nutritional status.[84] As compared with placebo, ingestion of 1 gram of tribasic sodium phosphate for 4 days significantly increased basal serum phosphate concentration from 0.95 ± 0.17 to 1.11 ± 0.32 mmol/L in six male endurance athletes.[85] However, at peak exercise, there was no difference in serum phosphate concentrations (1.50 ± 0.19 vs 1.48 ± 0.21 mmol/L). Interestingly, most studies report greater increases in serum phosphate after a bout of acute exercise than after ingestion of phosphate-containing supplements.[84]

VIII. Zinc

The metabolic importance of zinc is emphasized by its vital role for growth and well-being of animals and plants. Zinc also exerts a key impact by its presence in more than 300 metalloenzymes participating in essentially all aspects of metabolism. Some important zinc-containing enzymes include RNA and DNA polymerase, carboxypeptidase, carbonic anhydrase and alcohol dehydrogenase.[86] Zinc also plays a regulatory role in gene expression by affecting gene structure and enzymatic activity.[86]

Zinc deficiency occurs in various stages in humans. In mild deficiency, general symptoms such as weight loss occur. Moderate deficiency is characterized by growth retardation in children and adolescents, mild dermatitis, impaired cognition, poor appetite, impaired immune function and abnormal adaptation to darkness. Characteristics of severe zinc deficiency include alopecia, weight loss, behavioral and neurophysiological disorders and ultimately death, if untreated.

A. Methods for Zinc Assessment

Two general approaches for laboratory assessment of zinc status include measurement of zinc in a body fluid and determination of activity of a specific zinc-dependent enzyme. Useful tests in the first category are determination of the zinc concentration of plasma or serum. Functional assessments of zinc-containing enzymes include determinations of enzymatic activity in blood and responses to controlled stressors such as exercise and ethanol administration. Although many of the tests have elicited diagnosis of zinc deficiency, no single test has been proven to be a definitive indicator of zinc status.

1. Plasma or Serum Zinc

Although the zinc concentration in plasma or serum often has been interpreted to indicate human zinc deficiency, it does not reflect whole-body zinc status universally. Concurrent conditions that decrease plasma zinc concentration without causing zinc depletion including nonfasting conditions, infection, inflammation, steroid use, pregnancy, low serum albumin associated with liver disease and malnutrition.

The most practical and reliable analytical method to determine plasma or serum zinc is AAS. The recommended approach is to use a five-fold dilution of plasma or serum and standards with 5% glycerol matrix with AAS.[87] Hemolysis must be avoided during sample acquisition and preparation because erythrocytes contain more than 10 times more zinc than plasma.

2. Zinc-Containing Enzyme Activities

Several zinc-containing enzymes, such as alkaline phosphatase, carbonic anhydrase, nucleoside phosphorylase and ribonuclease, are useful indicators of zinc deficiency. Decreased alkaline phosphatase activity in either serum or neutrophils has been shown in a number of human zinc-deficient conditions. Zinc-deficient patients supplemented with zinc responded with increases in alkaline phosphatase activity that paralleled the magnitude of zinc repletion. Similarly, carbonic anhydrase and nucleoside phosphorylase activities increased in sickle anemia patients treated with zinc. Enzyme assays that require reagents that contain zinc generally are unsuitable tests for assessing zinc status.

3. Zinc Reference Intervals and Data from Athletes

The accepted reference interval for zinc in plasma is 70 to 150 μg/dL or 10.7 to 22.9 μmol/L. Serum zinc concentrations are generally 5 to 15% higher than plasma values because of osmotic shifts of fluid into the extracellular fluid when various anticoagulants are used. Because of diurnal variation and significant effects of recent food ingestion, a fasting morning blood sample is recommended for routine assessment of human zinc status.

Because of the potential of zinc deficiency to adversely affect all aspects of metabolism, there has been an effort to assess zinc status in many groups of athletes (Table 14.3). Dressendorfer and Sockolov[88] found that 25% of 76 experienced marathon runners had serum zinc concentration less than 11.5 μmol/L. In a survey of elite German athletes, 25% of the men and women were identified as hypozincemic as defined by serum zinc concentrations less than 12.0 μmol/L.[89] Among male participants in a 500-km road race, pre-race serum concentrations were markedly depressed, with the majority of the values less than 11 μmol/L.[90] A similar pattern of low plasma zinc concentrations was found in elite female endurance runners by Deuster et al.[91] Other studies did not identify low zinc concentrations in runners,[20,46,76,93] swimmers,[46,79] skiers[92] or volleyball players.[94] However, some longitudinal studies of athletes showed small, nonsignificant decreases in serum zinc during periods of intensive training.[93,94]

Low serum zinc concentrations have been associated with decreased muscle strength and diminished exercise capacity. Adolescent gymnasts, screened for delayed pubertal maturation and growth, had serum zinc concentrations significantly less than age-matched nontraining adolescents (9.2 ± 0.4 vs. 12.4 ± 0.2 μmol/L).[95] Among the 21 gymnasts, the 12 girls had lower serum zinc than the nine boys (8.5 ± 0.3 vs. 10.1 ± 0.6 μmol/L). Serum zinc concentrations were significantly correlated ($r = 0.465$) with isometric adductor strength. Similarly, a screening of 21 male soccer players revealed that nine had low serum zinc concentrations (8.3 ± 0.2 μmol/L) and 12 had normal serum zinc (11.3 ± 0.2 μmol/L).[96] The hypozincemic men had significantly decreased peak power output and a lower lactate threshold. Thus, serum or plasma zinc concentration, specifically hypozincemia, may be a specific indicator of impaired physiological function.

IX. Other Minerals

Two additional minerals, manganese and selenium, are potentially important in the development of peak performance. Currently, these minerals have not been intensively studied in the interaction between intake and physical activity.

TABLE 14.3

Plasma Zinc Concentrations (μmol/L) of Athletes (Mean ± SD)

Source	Activity	Indicator	Female	n	Male	n
Dressendorfer and Sockolov[88]	Running	S			11.6 ± 2.0	77
Dressendorfer et al.[90]	Running	S			9.1 ± 1.3	12
Lukaski et al.[43]	Football, basketball, hockey, track & field	P			13.3 ± 1.1	44
Anderson et al.[20]	Running	S			12.4 ± 0.6	9
Deuster et al.[91]	Running	P	10.1 ± 0.4	13		
Lukaski et al.[45]	Swimming	P	12.6 ± 0.5	16	14.3 ± 0.5	13
Singh et al.[46]	Running	P	12.7 ± 0.3	45		
Couzy et al.[93]	Running	S			14.2 ± 0.8	6
Fogelholm et al.[75]	Running	S			13.6 ± 0.3	114
Fogelholm et al.[92]	Skiing	S	12.7 ± 0.3	19	14.1 ± 0.4	19
Lukaski et al.[78]	Swimming	P	12.7 ± 0.4	5	14.6 ± 0.4	5
Cordova and Navas[94]	Volleyball	S			14.6 ± 0.2	12

A. Manganese

Manganese is an essential nutrient involved in the formation of bone and connective tissue, in amino acid, cholesterol and carbohydrate metabolism and in the protection against oxidative damage. Manganese also acts as an enzyme activator either by binding to a substrate (e.g., ATP) or directly to the protein causing a conformation change. Manganese metalloenzymes include arginase, glutamine synthetase, phosphoenolpyruvate decarboxylase and manganese superoxide dismutase (SOD2) in mitochondria.[97] Although manganese deficiency has not been demonstrated in humans consuming natural diets, some maladies have been connected to possible disturbances in manganese metabolism. Seizure disorders in children without head injury have been associated with low blood and tissue manganese concentrations. Manganese deficiency was suggested as an etiological factor in the development of hip abnormalities and some joint diseases.[98]

1. Methods for Manganese Assessment

Laboratory tests for reliable assessment of manganese status have not been established. Measurement of manganese concentration in whole blood or serum is the most common approach to estimate changes in manganese metabolism or status. It is assumed that whole-blood manganese and manganese in blood cells reflect body manganese stores in tissues. An advantage of whole blood compared with plasma or serum manganese concentration is that hemolysis of erythrocytes markedly affects plasma or serum manganese concentration. However, the wide variability in whole-blood manganese concentration may preclude its widespread use as a reliable manganese status indicator.[99] The large variation in reported manganese concentrations may be attributed partially to sample contamination during collection and processing and the use of relatively insensitive and nonspecific analytical methods. Recent evidence indicates that the manganese concentration and manganese superoxide dismutase activity in lymphocytes are sensitive to manganese status.[100] Factors, such as ethanol intake[101] and dietary polyunsaturated fatty acids,[102] independent of manganese intake may affect SOD2 activity.

Because of the low concentrations of manganese in blood and urine, AAS with Zeeman background correction is the method of choice.[103] Determination of SOD2 uses the pyrogallol method for superoxide dismutase activity after inactivation of SOD1 and SOD3 with cyanide or azide.[37]

2. Manganese Reference Intervals

Current reference intervals for blood manganese are 0.4 to 1.1 µg/L or 7.0 to 20.0 nmol/L for serum or plasma and 7.7 to 12.1 µg/L or 140 to 220 nmol/L for whole blood.[103]

B. Selenium

Selenium is a trace element that is essential, yet toxic when consumed in excessive amounts. Selenium exerts biological actions largely through association with proteins, termed selenoproteins,[104] including glutathione peroxidases and iodothyronine deiodinases that protect against oxidative stress and activation of triiodothyronine from thyroxine, respectively. Other selenium-containing proteins include selenoprotein P, which facilitates selenium transport between tissues and extracellular antioxidant defense and selenoprotein W, which protects against pathological muscle degeneration. Each of these selenium-containing enzymes and proteins are significantly decreased in dietary selenium deficiency.

1. Methods for Selenium Assessment

Determinations of urinary and blood selenium are practical and useful measures of human selenium status. Plasma or serum concentrations may be a more sensitive indicator of selenium status than whole-blood concentrations. Determination of erythrocyte glutathione peroxidase activity has been shown to correlate with blood selenium; it represents a functional test of selenium status. Assay of selenoprotein P, the major selenium-containing protein in the plasma, also is a useful and sensitive measure of selenium status.

The recommended methods for determining selenium in biological specimens are flameless AAS with Zeeman background correction and spectrofluorometry. The characteristic of selenium to form covalent organic compounds impacts its analytical determinations in two distinct practices. The organo-selenium forms are likely to be volatile and, therefore, may be lost in certain preparatory steps, such as high-temperature ashing. Also, the simple reduction of sample selenium to the volatile hydride form allows the determination of selenium by the AAS hydride generation technique.

2. Selenium Reference Intervals

Reported selenium concentrations from healthy adults range from 58 to 234 µg/L in whole blood, 75 to 240 µg/L in erythrocytes, 46 to 143 µg/L in serum or plasma and 7 to 160 µg/L excretion in urine. Blood and tissue selenium contents vary with selenium status of the specific geographic area.

Studies examining the effects of dietary selenium on exercise metabolism and performance are very limited. Studies of rats fed low-selenium diets consistently report lower tissue glutathione peroxidase activity compared with values from animals fed an adequate selenium diet.[105] There are no data available describing the interaction of dietary selenium and exercise in humans.

X. Summary and Conclusions

There is increasing evidence that many of the mineral elements play important biological roles in the development and maintenance of human physical work capacity and performance. One factor limiting research on the interaction of mineral intake and physiological function during work has been the lack of awareness of the need for appropriate procedures for collection of blood and methods of analysis of specimens for valid determinations of mineral elements. Although caution is needed to eliminate contamination of plasma, serum and blood cells during phlebotomy and processing, appropriate guidelines are available. A number of putative blood biochemical indicators of mineral status have been proposed. However, there is consensus that the use of multiple indicators is advised. Reliance on a single indicator may limit the sensitivity of the assessment of mineral depletion. Failure to standardize conditions for sample collection (e.g., fasting and before exercise) contributes to confusion about interpretation of mineral nutritional status.

Some emerging areas of research appear to be fruitful for additional investigation. These include confirmation that iron deficiency without anemia promotes anaerobic glycolysis and energy inefficiency during training and the interdependent roles of zinc, copper, manganese and selenium intakes on antioxidant stress and muscle damage during exercise.

References

1. Lukaski, H.C., Vitamin and mineral metabolism and exercise performance, in: *Perspectives in Exercise and Sports Medicine, vol. 12, The Metabolic Basis of Performance in Exercise and Sport*, Lamb, D.R. and Murray, R., Eds., Cooper Publishing Group, Carmel, IN, 1999, pp. 261-314.

2. Sauberlich, H.E., *Laboratory Tests for the Assessment of Nutritional Status*, 2nd ed., CRC, Boca Raton, FL, 1999.
3. Standing Committee on the Scientific Evaluation of Dietary Reference Intakes, Food and Nutrition Board, Institute of Medicine, *Dietary Reference Intakes for Calcium, Phosphorus, Magnesium, Vitamin D and Fluoride*, National Academy Press, Washington, D.C., 1997.
4. Standing Committee on the Scientific Evaluation of Dietary Reference Intakes, Food and Nutrition Board, Institute of Medicine, *Dietary Reference Intakes for Vitamin A, Vitamin K, Arsenic, Boron, Chromium, Copper, Iodine, Iron, Manganese, Molybdenum, Nickel, Silicon, Vanadium and Zinc*, National Academy Press, Washington, D.C., 2001.
5. Martin, L.J., Su, W., Jones, P.J., Lockwood, G.A., Trichler, D.L and Boyd, N.F., Comparison of energy intakes determined by food records and doubly labeled water in women participating in a dietary intervention trial, *Am. J. Clin. Nutr.*, 63, 483, 1996.
6. Briefel, R.R., Sempos, C.T., McDowell, M.A., Chien, S and Alaimo, K., Dietary methods research in the third National Health and Nutrition Examination Survey: underreporting of energy intake, *Am. J. Clin. Nutr.*, 65, 1203S, 1997.
7. van Beaumont, W., Greenleaf, J.E. and Juhos, J., Disproportional changes in hematocrit, plasma volume and proteins during exercise and bed rest, *J. Appl. Physiol.*, 33, 55, 1972.
8. Dill, D.B. and Costill, D.L., Calculations of percentage changes in volumes of blood, plasma and red cells in dehydration, *J. Appl. Physiol.*, 37, 521, 1974.
9. Cornelis, R., Heinzow, B., Herber, R.F.M., Christensen, J.M., Poulsen, O.M., Sabbioni, E., Templeton, D.M., Thomassen, Y., Vahter, M and Vesterberg, O., Sample collection guidelines for trace elements in blood and urine, *J. Trace Elem. Med. Biol.*, 10, 103, 1996.
10. Sunderman, F.W., Electrothermal atomic absorption spectrometry of trace metals in biological fluids, *Ann. Clin. Lab. Sci.*, 5, 421, 1973.
11. National Committee for Clinical Laboratory Standards, *Status of Certified Reference Materials Definitive Methods and Reference Values for Analysis*, National Reference for the Clinical Laboratory 7-CR, Villanova, PA, 1985.
12. Bowers, G.N. and Rains, T.C., Measurement of total calcium in biological fluids: flame atomic absorption spectrometry, *Methods Enzymol.*, 158, 302,1988.
13. Endres, D.B. and Rude, R.K., Mineral and bone metabolism, in: *Tietz Textbook of Clinical Chemistry*, 3rd edition, Burtis, C.A. and Ashwood, E.R., Eds., W.B. Saunders, Philadelphia, pp. 1395-1457.
14. Reid, I.R., Ames, R.W., Evans, M.C., Gamble, G.D and Sharpe, S.J., Long-term effects of calcium supplementation on bone mass and fractures in postmenopausal women: a randomized controlled study, *Am. J. Med.*, 98, 331, 1995.
15. Smith, E.L., Reddan, W. and Smith, P.E., Physical activity and calcium modalities for bone mineral increases in aged women, *Med. Sci, Sports Exerc.*, 13, 60, 1981.
16. Schwellnus, M.P. and Jordaan, G., Does calcium supplementation prevent bone stress injuries?, *Int. J. Sports Nutr.*, 2, 165, 1992.
17. Lukaski, H.C., Chromium as a supplement, *Ann. Rev. Nutr.*, 19, 279, 1999.
18. Vincent, J., Biochemistry of chromium, *J. Nutr.*, 130, 715, 2000.
19. Veillon, C. and Patterson, K.Y., Analytical issues in nutritional chromium research, *J. Trace Elem. Exp. Med.*, 12, 99, 1999.

20. Anderson, R.A., Polansky, M.M. and Bryden, N.A., Strenuous running: acute effects on chromium, copper, zinc and selected clinical variables in urine and serum of male runners, *Biol. Trace Elem. Res.*, 6, 327, 1984.
21. Lukaski, H.C., Bolonchuk, W.W., Siders, W.A and Milne, D.B., Chromium supplementation and resistance training: effects on body composition, strength and trace element status of men, *Am. J. Clin. Nutr.*, 63, 954, 1996.
22. Linder, M.C. and Hazegh-Azam, M., Copper biochemistry and molecular biology, *Am. J. Clin. Nutr.*, 63, 797S, 1996.
23. Lukaski, H.C. and Smith, S.M., Effects of altered vitamin and mineral nutritional status on temperature regulation and thermogenesis in the cold, in: *Handbook of Physiology, Section 4, Environmental Physiology*, Fregly, M.J. and Blatteis, C.M., Eds., Oxford University Press, New York, 1996, pp. 1437-1456.
24. Milne, D.B., Copper intake and assessment of copper status, *Am. J. Clin. Nutr.*, 67, 1041S, 1998.
25. Milne, D.B., Johnson, P.E., Klevay, L.M and Sandstead, H.H., Effect of copper intake on balance, absorption and status indices of copper, *Nutr. Res.* 10, 975, 1990.
26. Solomons, N.W., On the assessment of zinc and copper nutriture in man, *Am. J. Clin. Nutr.*, 32, 856, 1979.
27. Lukaski, H.C., Klevay, L.M. and Milne, D.B., Effects of copper on human autonomic cardiovascular function, *Eur. J. Appl. Physiol.*, 58, 74, 1988.
28. Chang, L.-Y., Slot, J.W., Geuze, H.J and Crapo, J.D., Molecular immunochemistry of the Cu, Zn superoxide dismutase in rat hepatocytes, *J. Cell. Biol.*, 107, 2169, 1988.
29. Marklund, S.L., Extracellular superoxide dismutase and other superoxide dismutase isoenzymes in tissues from nine mammalian species, *Biochem. J.*, 222, 649, 1984.
30. Milne, D.B. and Johnson, P.E., Assessment of copper status: effect of age and gender on reference ranges in healthy adults, *Clin. Chem.*, 39, 883, 1993.
31. DiSilvestro, R.A., Influence of copper intake and inflammation on rat serum superoxidase activity levels, *J. Nutr.*, 118, 474, 1988.
32. Olin, K.L., Golub, M.S., Gershwin, M.E., Hendricks, A.G., Extracellular superoxide dismutase activity is affected by dietary zinc intake in nonhuman primate and rodent models, *Am. J. Clin. Nutr.*, 61, 1263, 1995.
33. Kim, S.H. and Keen, C.L., Influence of dietary carbohydrate on zinc-deficiency-induced changes in oxidative defense mechanisms and tissue oxidative damage in rats, *Biol. Trace Elem. Res.*, 70, 81, 1999.
34. Davis, C., Effect of dietary zinc and copper on β-amyloid precursor protein expression in the rat brain, *J. Trace Elem. Exp. Med.*, 10, 249, 1997.
35. Davis, C.D., Milne, D.B. and Nielsen, F.H., Changes in dietary zinc and copper affect zinc-status indicators of postmenopausal women, notably extracellular superoxide dismutase and amyloid precursor proteins, *Am. J. Clin. Nutr.*, 71, 781, 2000.
36. Flohè, L. and Ötting, F., Superoxide dismutase assays, *Methods in Enzymology*, 105, 93,1984.
37. Marklund, S. and Marklund G., Involvement of the superoxide anion in the autoxidation of pyrogallol and a convenient assay for superoxide dismutase, *Eur. J. Biochem.*, 47, 469, 1974.

38. Crapo, J.D., McCord, J.M. and Fridovich, I., Preparation and assay of superoxide dismutases, *Methods Enzymol.*, 53, 382, 1978.
39. DiMauro, S., Bonilla, E., Zevani, M., Nakagawa, M and De Vivo, D.C., Mitochondrial myopathies, *Ann. Neurol.*, 17, 521, 1985.
40. Milne, D.B. and Nielsen, F.H., Effects of a diet low in copper on copper status indicators in postmenopausal women, *Am. J. Clin. Nutr.*, 63, 358, 1996.
41. Johnson, W.T., Dufault, S.N. and Thomas, A.C., Platelet cytochrome c oxidase is an indicator of copper status in rats, *Nutr. Res.*, 13, 1153, 1993.
42. Chrzanowska-Lightowlers, Z.M.A., Turnbull, D.M. and Lightowlers, R.N., A microtiter plate assay for cytochrome c oxidase in permablized whole cells, *Anal. Biochem.*, 214, 45, 1993.
43. Lukaski, H.C., Bolonchuk, W.W., Klevay, L.M and Milne, D.B., Maximal oxygen uptake as related to magnesium, copper and zinc nutriture, *Am. J. Clin. Nutr.*, 37, 407, 1983.
44. Lukaski, H.C., Hoverson, B.S., Gallagher, S.K and Bolonchuk, W.W., Copper, zinc and iron status of female swimmers, *Nutr. Res.*, 9, 493, 1989.
45. Lukaski, H.C., Hoverson, B.S., Gallagher, S.K and Bolonchuk, W.W., Physical training and copper, iron and zinc status of swimmers, *Am. J. Clin. Nutr.*, 51, 1093, 1990.
46. Singh, A., Deuster, P.A. and Moser, P.B., Zinc and copper status of women by physical activity and menstrual status, *J. Sports Med. Phys. Fitness*, 30, 29, 1990.
47. DeMaeyer E.M., Dallman, P., Gurney, J.M., Hallberg, L., Sood, S.K and Srikantia, S.G., Preventing and controlling iron deficiency anemia through primary health care: a guide for health administrators and programme managers, World Health Organization, Geneva, Switzerland, 1989, pp. 5-58.
48. Gillespie, S. and Johnston, J.L., *Expert Consultation on Anemia Determinants and Interventions*, Micronutrient Initiative, Ottawa, Canada, 1998, pp. 1-37.
49. Harrison, P.M. and Arosio, P., The ferritins: molecular properties, iron storage and cellular regulation, *Biochim. Biophys. Acta*, 1275, 161, 1996.
50. Milne, D.B., Gallagher, S.K. and Nielsen, F.H., Response of various indices of iron status to acute iron depletion produced in menstruating women by low iron intake and phlebotomy, *Clin. Chem.*, 36, 487, 1990.
51. Kondo, Y., Niitsu, Y., Kondo, H., Kato, J., Sasaki, K, Hirayama, M., Numata, T., Nishisato, T and Urushizaki, I., Serum transferrin receptor as a new index of erythropoiesis, *Blood*, 70, 1955, 1987.
52. Skikne, B.S., Flowers, C.H. and Cook, J.D., Serum transferrin receptor: a quantitative measure of tissue iron deficiency, *Blood*, 75, 1870, 1990.
53. Skikne, B.S., Circulating transferrin receptor assay — coming of age, *Clin. Chem.*, 44, 7, 1998.
54. Langer, E.E., Haining R.G., Labbé, R.F., Jacobs, P., Crosby, E.F and Finch, C.A., Erythrocyte protoporphyrin, *Blood*, 40, 112, 1972.
55. Haas, J.D. and Brownlie, T., Iron deficiency and reduced work capacity: a critical review of the research to determine a causal relationship, *J. Nutr.*, 131, 676S, 2001.
56. Viteri, F.E. and Torun, B., Anemia and physical work capacity, *Clin. Haematol.*, 3, 609, 1974.
57. Magnusson, B., Hallberg, L., Rossander L., Swolin, B., Iron metabolism and sports anemia. I. A study of several iron parameters in elite runners with different iron status, *Acta Med. Scand.*, 216, 149, 1984.

58. Celsing, F., Nyström, J., Pihlstedt, P., Werner, B and Ekblom, B., Effect of long-term anemia and retransfusion of central circulation during exercise, *J. Appl. Physiol.*, 61, 1358, 1986.

59. Magazanik, A., Weinstein, Y., Dlin, R.A., Derin, M., Schwartzman, S and Allalouf, D., Iron deficiency caused by 7 weeks of intensive physical exercise, *Eur, J. Appl. Physiol.*, 57, 198, 1988.

60. Newhouse, I.J., Clement, D.B., Taunton, J.E and McKenzie, D.C., The effects of prelatent/latent iron deficiency on physical work capacity, *Med. Sci. Sports Exerc.*, 21, 263, 1989.

61. Schoene, R.B., Escourrou, P., Robertson, H.T., Nilson, K.L., Parsons, J.R and Smith, N.J., Iron repletion decreases maximal exercise lactate concentrations in female athletes with minimal iron-deficiency anemia, *J. Lab. Clin. Med.*, 102, 306, 1983.

62. Rowland, T.W., Deisroth, M.B., Green, G.M and Kelleher, J.F., The effect of iron therapy on the exercise capacity of nonanemic, iron-deficient runners, *Am. J. Dis. Child.*, 142, 165, 1988.

63. Rowland, T.W. and Kelleher, J.F., Iron deficiency in athletes: insights from high school swimmers, *Am. J. Dis. Child.*, 143, 197, 1989.

64. Lukaski, H.C., Hall, C.B. and Siders, W.A., Altered metabolic response of iron-deficient women during graded, maximal exercise, *Eur. J. Appl. Physiol.*, 63, 140, 1991.

65. Zhu, Y.I. and Haas, J.D., Altered metabolic response of iron-depleted nonanemic women during a 15-km time trial, *J. Appl. Physiol.*, 84, 1768, 1998.

66. Hinton, P.S., Giordano, C., Brownlie, T and Haas, J.D., Iron supplementation improves endurance after training in iron-depleted, nonanemic women, *J. Appl. Physiol.*, 88, 1103, 2000.

67. Shils, M.E., Magnesium, in: *Handbook of Nutritionally Essential Mineral Elements*, O'Dell, B.L. and Sunde, R.A., Eds., Marcel Dekker, New York, 1998, pp. 117-152.

68. Elin, R.J., Assessment of magnesium status, *Clin. Chem.*, 33, 1965, 1987.

69. Altura, B.T. and Altura B.M., A method for distinguishing ionized, complexed and protein-bound magnesium in normal and diseased subjects, *Scand. J. Clin. Lab. Invest.*, 54 (Suppl 217), 83, 1994.

70. Elin, R.J., Magnesium: the fifth but forgotten mineral, *Am. J. Clin. Pathol.*, 102: 616, 1994.

71. Ryschon, T.W., Rosenstein, D.L., Rubinow, D.R., Niemela, J.E., Elin, R.J and Balaban, R.S., Relationship between skeletal muscle intracellular ionized magnesium and measurements of blood magnesium, *J. Lab. Clin. Med.*, 127, 207, 1996.

72. Elin, R.J., Status of the mononuclear blood cell assay, *J. Am. Coll. Nutr.*, 6, 105, 1987.

73. Liu, L., Borowski, G. and Rose, L.I., Hypomagnesemia in a tennis player, *Phys. Sportsmed.*, 11, 79, 1983.

74. Stendig-Lindberg, G., Shapiro, Y., Epstein, Y., Galun, E., Schonberger, E., Graff, E and Wacker, E.C., Changes in serum magnesium concentration after strenuous exercise, *J. Am. Coll. Nutr.*, 6, 35, 1987.

75. Fogelholm, M., Laakso, J., Lehto, J and Ruokonen, I., Dietary intake and indicators of magnesium and zinc status in male athletes, *Nutr. Res.*, 11, 1111, 1991.

76. Fogelholm, G.M., Himberg, J.-J., Alopaeus, K., Gref, C.-G., Laakso, J.T., Lehto, J.J and Mussalo-Rauhamaa, H., Dietary and biochemical indices of nutritional status in male athletes and controls, *J. Am. Coll. Nutr.*, 11, 181, 1992.

77. Cordova, A., Navas, F.J., Gomez-Carramiñana, M and Rodriguez, H., Evaluation of magnesium intake in elite sportsmen, *Magnesium Bull.*, 16, 59, 1994.

78. Lukaski, H.C., Interactions among indices of mineral element nutriture and physical performance of swimmers, in *Sports Nutrition: Minerals and Electrolytes*, Kies, C.V. and Driskell, J.A., Eds., CRC Press, Boca Raton, FL, 1995, pp. 267-279.

79. Lukaski, H.C., Siders, W.A., Hoverson, B.S and Gallagher, S.K., Iron, copper, magnesium and zinc status as predictors of swimming performance, *Int. J. Sports Med.*, 17, 535, 1996.

80. Conn, C.A., Schemmel, R.A., Smith, B.W., Ryder, E., Heusner, W.W and Ku, P.-K., Plasma and erythrocyte magnesium concentrations and correlations with maximal oxygen consumption in nine-to-twelve-year-old competitive swimmers, *Magnesium* 7, 27, 1988.

81. Deuster, P.A., Dolev, E., Kyle, S.B., Anderson, R.A and Schoomaker, E.B., Magnesium homeostasis during high intensity anaerobic exercise in men, *J. Appl. Physiol.*, 62, 545, 1987.

82. Manore, M.M., Merkel, J., Hellekesen, J.M., Skinner, J.S and Carroll, S.S., Longitudinal changes in magnesium status in untrained males: effect of two different 12-week exercise training programs and magnesium supplementation, in: *Sports Nutrition: Minerals and Electrolytes*, Kies, C.V. and Driskell, J.A., Eds., CRC, Boca Raton, FL, 1995, pp. 180-189.

83. Garber, C.C. and Miller, R.C., Revision of the 1963 semidine HCl standard method for phosphorous, *Clin. Chem.*, 29, 184, 1983.

84. Lukaski, H.C., Magnesium, phosphate and calcium supplementation and human physical performance, in: *Macroelements, Water and Electrolytes in Sports Nutrition*, Driskell, J.A. and Wolinsky, I., Eds, CRC, Boca Raton, FL, 1999, pp. 197-210.

85. Kreider, R.B., Miller, G.W., Schenck, D., Cortes, C.W., Miriel, V., Somma, C.T., Rowland, P., Turner, C and Hill, D., Effects of phosphate loading on metabolic and myocardial responses to maximal and endurance exercise, *Int. J. Sports Nutr.*, 2, 20, 1992.

86. Cousins, R.J., Zinc, in *Present Knowledge in Nutrition*, 7th edition, Filer, L.J. and Ziegler, E.E., Eds., International Life Science Institute-Nutrition Foundation, Washington, DC, 1996, pp. 293-306.

87. Smith, J.C., Butrimovitz, G.P., Purdy, W.C., Direct measurement of zinc in plasma by atomic absorption spectroscopy, *Clin. Chem.*, 25, 1487, 1979.

88. Dressendorfer, R.H. and Sockolov, R., Hypozincemia in runners, *Phys. Sports Med.*, 8, 97, 1979.

89. Haralambie, G., Serum zinc in athletes in training, *Int. J. Sports Med.*, 2, 136, 1981.

90. Dressendorfer, R.H., Wade, C.E., Keen, C.L., Schaff, J.H., Plasma mineral levels in marathon runners during a 20-day road race, *Phys. Sports Med.*, 10, 113, 1982.

91. Deuster, P.A., Day, B.A., Singh, A., Douglass, L and Moser-Veillon, P.B., Zinc status of highly trained women runners and untrained women, *Am. J. Clin. Nutr.*, 49, 1295, 1989.

92. Fogelholm, M., Rehunen, S., Gref, C.-G., Laakso, J.T., Lehto, J.J., Ruokonen, I and Himberg, J.-J., Dietary intake and thiamin, iron and zinc status of elite Nordic skiers during different training periods, *Int. J. Sports Nutr.*, 2, pp. 351-365, 1992.

93. Couzy, F., Lafargue, P., Guezennec, C.Y., Zinc metabolism in the athlete: influence of training, nutrition and other factors, *Int. J. Sports Med*, 11, 263, 1990.

94. Cordova, A. and Navas, F.J., Effect of training on zinc metabolism: changes in serum and sweat zinc concentrations in sportsmen, *Ann. Nutr. Metab.*, 42, 274, 1998.

95. Brun, J.-F., Dieu-Cambrezy, C., Charpiat, A., Fons, C., Fedou, C., Micallef, J.-P., Fussellier, M., Bardet, L and Orsetti, A., Serum zinc in highly trained adolescent gymnasts, *Biol. Trace Elem. Res.*, 47, 273, 1995.

96. Khaled, S., Brun, J.F., Micallef, C., Bardet, L., Cassanas, G., Monnier, J.F and Orsetti, A., Serum zinc and blood rheology in sportsmen (football players), *Clin. Hemorheol. Microcirc.*, 17, 47, 1997.

97. Keen, C.L. and Zindenberg-Cherr, S., Manganese, in *Present Knowledge in Nutrition*, 7th ed., Filer, L.J. and Ziegler, E.E., Eds., International Life Science Institute-Nutrition Foundation, Washington, D.C., 1996, pp. 334-343.

98. Freeland-Graves, J., Derivation of manganese estimated safe and adequate daily dietary intakes, in: *Risk Assessment of Essential Elements*, Mertz, W., Abernathy, C.O. and Olin, S.S., Eds., ILSI Press, Washington, D.C., 1994, pp. 237-252.

99. Friedman, B.J., Freeland-Graves, J.H., Bales, C.W., Behmardi, F., Shorey-Kutschke, R.I., Willis, R.A., Crosby, J.B., Trickett, P.C and Houston, S.D., Manganese balance and clinical observations in young men fed a manganese-deficient diet, *J. Nutr.*, 117, 113, 1987.

100. Davis, C.D. and Gregor, J.L., Longitudinal changes of manganese-dependent superoxide dismutase and other indices of manganese and iron status in women, *Am. J. Clin. Nutr.*, 55, 747, 1992.

101. Dreosti, I.E., Manuel, S.J. and Buckley, R.A., Superoxide dismutase (E.C.1.15.1.1), manganese and the effect of ethanol in adult and fetal rats, *Br. J. Nutr.*, 48, 205, 1982.

102. Davis, C.D., Ney, D.M. and Gregor, J.L., Manganese, iron and lipid interactions, *J. Nutr.*, 120, 507, 1992.

103. Néve, J. and Leclercq, N., Factors affecting the determinations of manganese in serum by atomic absorption spectrometry, *Clin. Chem.*, 37, 723, 1991.

104. Burk, R.F. and Levander, O.A., Selenium, in: *Modern Nutrition in Health and Disease*, 9th ed., Shils, M.E. et al., Eds., Williams & Wilkins, Baltimore, MD, 1999, pp. 265-276.

105. Boylan, M. and Spallholz, J.A., Selenium, in: *Sports Nutrition: Vitamins and Minerals*, Wolinsky, I. and Driskell, J.A., Eds., CRC, Boca Raton, FL, 1997, pp. 195-204.

Section Six

Clinical Assessment
of Athletes

15

Clinical Assessment of Athletes

Khursheed N. Jeejeebhoy

CONTENTS

I. Introduction

Athletic activities, both recreational and professional, are becoming increasingly popular as spectator and participatory sports. Young men and women train to excel and compete at sports. As well, older sedentary individuals are engaging in sports for the purposes of losing weight, reducing the risk of diseases and for correcting progressive muscle wasting referred to as sarcopenia. In the latter category an increasing number of individuals have risk factors for coronary artery disease such as obesity, diabetes and hypertension. In addition, many elderly subjects are taking up athletics for the first time at an advanced age. In both situations, it is necessary to initially assess people to determine whether they are in good nutritional and physical status to engage in athletic activities. The potential competitive athlete often is underweight and on a restricted diet high in supplements with a view to having a very low body fat content and improving performance. The potential elderly or sedentary recreational athlete may be, in contrast, overweight and on a cycle of dieting followed by binge eating. In both groups, conditions likely to increase the risk of cardiac events and injuries need to be identified prior to initiating training.

After starting training, ongoing assessment is desirable in both types of athletes. In the competitive athlete, there is considerable risk of malnutrition, especially in women. In the older athletes, the objective is to promote weight reduction and to document improvement in cardiovascular function and a gain in muscle or lean body mass and muscle function. The assessment has two main sections: (1) an assessment of the nutritional status and (2) assessment of the medical and physical status.

II. Nutritional Status

The clinical assessment of nutritional status attempts to identify the initial nutritional state and the interplay of the factors influencing the progression or regression of nutritional abnormalities. Therefore, a clinical nutritional assessment is a dynamic process that is not limited to a single "snapshot" at the moment of measurement, but provides a picture of current nutritional status and insight into the patient's future status. The clinical assessment of nutritional status involves a focused history and physical examination in conjunction with selected laboratory tests aimed at detecting specific nutrient deficiencies and persons who are at high risk for future nutritional abnormalities.

A. History

The nutritional history should evaluate the following questions:

1. Has there been a recent change in body weight and was the change intentional or unintentional?
2. Is dietary intake adequate? Persons should be questioned about their habitual diet and any change in diet pattern. Have the number, size and contents of meals changed? Are nutrient supplements being taken? A diary documenting food intake may be

useful when the history is inconclusive. In this context, the diet of competitive athletes may be inadequate despite normal biochemical parameters.[1]

3. What is(are) the reason(s) for the change in dietary intake? Has appetite changed? Is there a disturbance in taste, smell, or the ability to chew or swallow food? Has there been a change in mental status or increased depression? Has there been a change in the ability to prepare meals? Are there gastrointestinal symptoms, such as early satiety, postprandial pain, nausea, or vomiting? Is the patient taking medications that affect food intake?

4. Is there evidence of malabsorption? Is there any gastrointestinal disease? Has there been a change in bowel habits?

5. Are there symptoms of specific nutrient deficiencies including macrominerals, micronutrients and water?

B. Physical Examination

The physical examination corroborates and adds to the findings obtained by the history:

6. *Anthropometric assessment.* Current body weight should be compared with previously recorded weights, if available. Weight for height should be compared with standard normal values. A search for evidence demonstrating depletion of body fat and muscle masses should be made. A general loss of adipose tissue can be judged by clearly defined bony, muscular and venous outlines and loose skin folds. A fold of skin, pinched between the forefinger and thumb, can detect the adequacy of subcutaneous fat. The presence of hollow cheeks, buttocks and perianal area suggests body fat loss. An examination of the temporalis, deltoid and quadriceps muscles should be made to search for muscle wasting.

7. *Assessment of muscle function.* Strength testing of individual muscle groups should be made to evaluate for generalized and localized muscle weakness. In addition, a general evaluation of respiratory and cardiac muscle function should be made.

8. *Fluid status.* An evaluation for dehydration (hypotension, tachycardia, postural changes, mucosal xerosis, dry skin and swollen tongue) and excess body fluid (edema, ascites) should be made.

9. *Evaluation for specific nutrient deficiencies.* Rapidly proliferating tissues, such as oral mucosa, hair, skin and bone marrow are often more sensitive to nutrient deficiencies than are tissues that turn over more slowly.

III.   Medical Status

A. Medical History

Clinical assessment should start with a careful history that should inquire about factors that are likely to influence the risks and benefits of exercise. In younger competitive athletes it is necessary to look for factors that are likely to endanger health or even risk death with strenuous exercise.

1.   Competitive Athletes

Sudden cardiac deaths of young athletes associated with physical exertion are very uncommon, occurring in about 1/200000 high school athletes per academic year.[2] Preparticipation screening for cardiovascular disease, consisting of standard history and physical examination, is customary practice for most high school and college athletes in the United States.

Cardiovascular system. A history of palpitations suggestive of previous arrhythmias and a family history of cardiomyopathy should lead to further investigations, as sudden arrhythmias and hypertrophic cardiomyopathy are risk factors for the rare instances where exercise is followed by sudden death.

Respiratory system. A history of cigarette smoking and of asthma, particularly intensified by exercise, should be obtained.

Nervous system. A history of dizziness, especially induced by exercise or by lifting heavy objects, should be ascertained prior to starting a program of aerobic or strength training exercise.

Musculoskeletal system. A history of previous injuries or operations on joints as well as the residual functional limitations should be evaluated. A history of juvenile arthritis should be determined.

Metabolic conditions. Juvenile diabetes and, if present, the dose of insulin, control of blood glucose and episodes of hypoglycemia should be obtained.

2.   Sedentary and Elderly Athletes

In addition to the history suggested above, those who are proposing to start recreational exercise and athletics should be questioned about symptoms suggestive of:

10. Angina, dyspnea on exertion, strokes and hypertension.

11. Diabetes and renal disease.

12. Body weight changes of either weight gain or unexpected weight loss. The former increases the risk of exercise and the latter occurs with the onset of serious disease.

13. The existence of arthritis and limitations in mobility.

The previous exercise status and a drug history should be obtained. Drugs likely to influence exercise ability are:

- Beta-blockers, which cause fatigue and prevent exercise-induced tachycardia.
- Insulin action will increase with exercise and may cause hypoglycemia.
- Anti-hypertensive drugs may cause a fall in blood pressure.

B. Physical Examination

Weight and height are taken and the Body Mass Index (BMI) calculated.

Head and neck are examined for enlarged nodes or thyroid enlargement. Eyes are checked for central and peripheral vision and the cornea and conjunctiva examined for signs of vitamin A and riboflavin deficiency. Tongue and mouth are examined for glossitis and stomatitis, which can suggest iron, folate or vitamin B_{12} deficiency.

Respiratory system is examined for any abnormalities such as evidence of asthma, chronic bronchitis and emphysema.

Cardiovascular system is examined for obvious cardiac failure, cardiac enlargement, arrhythmias, evidence of valvular heart disease and hypertension. In cardiomyopathy, a soft murmur may be heard, but a valsalva maneuver will markedly intensify it and suggest the diagnosis.

Abdomen should be examined for enlarged organs and for any masses or tender areas.

Central nervous system is checked for cranial nerve function, general motor function, general sensory function and coordination.

Musculoskeletal system is examined for wasting, joint swelling, joint tenderness and mobility — both passive and active.

C. Hematology

Knowing the hemoglobin level is essential to determine whether the person has sufficient oxygen-carrying capacity to undertake exercise. Particularly in women, marginal iron deficiency is extremely common because of menstrual blood losses. The hemoglobin tends to be at the lower limits of normal but the mean corpuscular volume (MCV) is reduced and the serum ferritin levels are markedly low. Because iron is an important part of a number of mitochondrial constituents such as cytochrome, deficiency results in reduced muscle performance and fatigue even when the hemoglobin is only slightly reduced. On the other hand, with vitamin B_{12} and folate deficiency, the MCV is increased. An increase in the MCV should lead to measurements of blood B_{12} and folate acid levels. An increase in white blood count and platelet levels are indicative of any inflammation.

D. Blood Biochemistry

Blood glucose levels should be measured to exclude diabetes. Creatinine levels should be measured to exclude renal disease. Blood electrolyte levels, magnesium, calcium and phosphorus should be checked. Abnormalities in any of these levels can alter muscle performance. Protein status can be assessed by the levels of prealbumin and blood urea nitrogen (BUN). In protein deficiency both these parameters are reduced. The serum albumin level is not indicative of nutritional status and in adults hypoalbuminemia is an index of occult disease.[3] The levels of ferritin, vitamin B12 and folate should be measured. Finally, total cholesterol, LDL cholesterol and HDL cholesterol should be measured.

E. Micronutrient Levels

During athletic training, dietary intake may become imbalanced due to inadequate intake of foods providing micronutrients. Diets high in refined carbohydrates are often deficient in zinc, selenium, vitamins and perhaps in other minerals and vitamins such as magnesium. A recent study showed that there was significant vitamin B_6 deficiency in high performance athletes.[4] Therefore, if the diet of an athlete is unbalanced, micronutrient levels should be measured.

F. Urine Analysis

Urine analysis should be done to look for renal disease. The presence of protein, casts and red blood cells suggests kidney disease and should lead to further examination. Temporary abnormalities in the urine such as proteinuria, microscopic hematuria and casts may be seen after prolonged vigorous exercise due to reduced renal blood flow and dehydration.

G. Stool Examination

Stool examination for parasites such as hookworm may have to be performed in countries where this problem is endemic. Parasites cause iron deficiency, which, in turn, reduces exercise tolerance.

H. Electrocardiographic and Echocardiographic Examination

1. Competitive Athletes

There is much debate about the prescreening of individuals about to embark on a program of strenuous training. Although rare (as mentioned above) sudden death has received much public attention. Various unsuspected congenital cardiovascular diseases are usually responsible; the most common lesions are hypertrophic cardiomyopathy and several congenital coronary artery anomalies. Arrhythmogenic right ventricular dysplasia may be another common cause of these deaths. It may be difficult to distinguish between borderline increases in thickness of the left ventricular wall and mild morphologic expression of hypertrophic cardiomyopathy in some trained athletes. However, cardiomyopathy can often be distinguished from the physiologic consequences of athlete's heart by noninvasive clinical assessment and testing.

2. Sedentary and Elderly Athletes

The American Heart Association recommends exercise testing with an electrocardiogram before the start of a vigorous exercise program for all individuals older than 40 years, even if they are asymptomatic and free of cardiac risk factors.[2] However, a study of more than 3000 asymptomatic men aged 35 to 59 years with increased risk of coronary artery disease casts doubt on the value of this recommendation. Each subject had an exercise test on entry and annually for 7.4 years. Exercise proved safe in this group, with approximately 2% experiencing exercise-related cardiac events. Only 11 of the 62 men who experienced such events had abnormal exercise tests on entry, a sensitivity of only 18%. The cumulative sensitivity of annual tests was also low, at 24%.[5] However, exercise testing can be useful for detecting exercise-induced arrhythmias and for determining the maximal heart rate for the exercise prescription.

Echocardiography can be used to study the thickness of the ventricular wall, ventricular diameter and valve function. In addition, any injury to the myocardium can be assessed by changes in the motion of the ventricular wall. Patients who have any history suggestive of coronary artery disease, those with significant risk factors such as hypertension, hypercholesterolemia, family history of myocardial infarction below the age of 50, diabetes and obesity would be wise to have an echocardiographic assessment by a cardiologist prior to embarking on an exercise program for the first time after the age of 40.

I. Bone Mass

1. Competitive Athletes

In the competitive athlete, especially in women who undertake intense aerobic physical training, bone loss and even osteoporosis has been recognized.[6] In such women, the so-called triad of amenorrhoea, eating disorder and bone loss occurs. The reason is a combination of reduced estrogen levels, reduced body weight and fat and an imbalanced diet.[7] In these cases, it is important to document the initial BMI and changes with training. Marked reduction in BMI and the development of amenorrhea or disordered menstruation should lead to checking the bone mineral density (BMD) by the use of dual energy x-ray absorptiometry (DEXA). If the BMD in an individual is more than 2.5 standard deviations (SD) below the mean for a young matched (for age and sex) population, the diagnosis is osteoporosis. If the BMD is below 1–2.5 SD of the mean for a young matched population, the diagnosis is osteopenia.

2. Sedentary and Elderly Athletes

In these persons there may be existing osteopenia or osteoporosis on entry into the training program. In these subjects exercise has a beneficial effect and increases BMD.[8] During exercise training, in persons with osteopenia or osteoporosis, a yearly record of changes in BMD is essential. Recording reduced BMD in the hip is important, as it is especially resistant to treatment. In this situation, a combination of jumping, stepping, marching and side stepping exercise is one of the few techniques capable of increasing BMD of the hip.[9]

J. Muscle Function

1. Strength

Strength in nutritional studies have been clinically assessed in the upper limb with a handheld dynamometer and shown to be improved by nutritional supplementation.[10] Hand grip strength is simple and easy to do and is well correlated with skeletal muscle strength. Maximum grip strength and mean value of a 10-second sustained grip will be completed with the dominant hand according to the method outlined in Sunnerhagen et al.[11] Briefly, the patient would be seated in a chair without armrests and with the lowest rib level with the edge of the table. The shoulder is adducted and the elbow flexed to 90° to 100°. The other arm would rest on a table. The palm and fingers would be clasped around the handle and the force exerted against the transducer in the handle would be recorded.

Another way of measuring the effect of nutrition on the strength of different muscle groups is the maximal weight that could be lifted fully one time only (1RM).[12] This measurement can be done for different muscle groups of the upper and lower limbs. Other methods to measure strength are the vertical jump and isokinetic extension at different rates that correlate with performance.[13]

2. Endurance

In a nutritional study of anorexic patients,[14] the effect of feeding on endurance was tested by an ergometric bicycle protocol (3-min steps of 30 W) before and after 8, 30 and 45 d of refeeding. Before refeeding, the workload reached during the exercise was 49% lower in AN patients than in control subjects (P < 0.01) and was correlated with body weight, fat-free mass, and leg muscle circumference (P < 0.002). The performance improved dramatically during refeeding (P < 0.03), reaching normal values after 45 d of refeeding, despite fat-free mass and leg muscle circumference values that were still 20% lower in AN patients than in control subjects (P < 0.01).

3. Peak Performance and Duration

Peak performance can be tested by a modified Wingate protocol. In a study of nutritional supplements,[15] volunteers were subjected to a protocol in which they were tested for the duration of maximal performance at 110% of VO_{2max}. The subjects were tested for their VO_{2max} and then placed on a bicycle ergometer. The protocol consisted of a 3-min warm-up, 1 min of 40% VO_{2max} followed by 1 min of 110% of VO_{2max} for four trial times. Then the subject bicycled till exhaustion at 110% VO_{2max}. In this study, the supplement improved peak performance above that seen with placebo.

IV. Clinical Conditions Associated with Athletic Activities

1. Dehydration and Electrolyte Deficiencies

Prolonged exercise is associated with the loss of sweat and dehydration. Dehydration can be avoided by ingestion of fluids during endurance exercise. Hyponatremia, (serum sodium < 135 mmol/L) may occur due to excessive fluid intake rather than sodium loss. In a recent prospective study, dehydration accounted for 26% and hyponatremia for 9% of individuals who sought medical care during endurance exercise. Hyponatremia was the most common reason for hospital admission. There was an inverse relationship between post-race sodium concentrations and percentage change in body weight, supporting the suggestion that fluid overload is the cause of hyponatremia.[16]

Plasma potassium rises in healthy subjects by only 0.5 mmol/L when exercising at 40–50% of VO_{2max}. Hyperkalemia occurs during strenuous exercise and is especially likely to occur in patients with angina or hypertension on beta-blockers such as propranolol.[17] Acidosis can occur with exercise,[18] but feeding alkalinizing agents does not improve performance.[19]

2. Asthma

Exercise-induced asthma is a well recognized clinical condition. It has been shown to occur to a greater degree in athletes who pursue strength (3.5 times more common than the general population) and endurance exercise (2.2 times more common). It occurs more frequently in women and in those who train more than 20 h per week.[20]

3. Arrhythmia

Cardiac events during exercise occurs in about 2% of individuals over 40 years of age.[2] Even in those who are 75 years of age, exercise-induced arrhythmia occurred in ~ 24% of males and only ~ 7% of females, but had no lasting effects.[21] However, asymptomatic persons who develop ventricular premature depolarizations had 2.6 times the risk of coronary events on follow-up.[22] On the other hand, exercise training of patients who had had myocardial infarction was shown to be of significant clinical benefit.[23]

4. Renal Failure

Frank renal failure may occur with severe dehydration during endurance exercise. It may rarely occur due to muscle breakdown called rhabdomyolysis.[24] On the other hand, exercise improved physical functioning in patients on dialysis.[25]

5. Gastrointestinal Disturbances

Gastrointestinal disturbance is common among athletes during competition. These include nausea, vomiting, belching, heartburn, chest pain, bloating, abdominal cramps, urge to defecate, frequent defecation and diarrhea.[26] The incidence of bloating, abdominal cramps and diarrhea was higher with running. In contrast, all the above symptoms were equally likely to occur during bicycling.[20] Measurement of occult blood in the stools showed that, during endurance exercise, there was increased loss of blood in the stool.[27] The magnitude of the blood loss was small and did not alter ferritin levels. The cause of blood loss is uncertain, but a possible explanation is that, during intense exercise, blood is diverted away from the bowel to the muscles, resulting in ischemia of the intestine. Athletes often take nonsteroidal analgesic drugs (NSAIDS) and the intake of these drugs has been shown to increase intestinal permeability and have more adverse gastrointestinal symptoms.[28] Therefore, gastrointestinal symptoms are partly due to exercise and partly due to drugs taken to alleviate pain.

6. Anemia

Plasma volume expansion occurs in athletes and contributes to the commonly occurring normocytic and normochromic anemia.[29] This "anemia" did not reduce performance. In football players, a study showed that individuals with a lower hematocrit paradoxically had better aerobic capacity.[30] Iron deficiency does not occur simply due to exercise per se.[31] Anemia in athletes should not be dismissed as being due to exercise, without proper investigation. Anemic athletes, especially older persons, could have an underlying serious condition such as colon cancer. The ingestion of NSAIDS can be associated with peptic ulceration and blood loss. Anemia could also be due to menstrual losses in women[32] when combined with a diet low in iron.

7. Immune Deficiency

A heavy schedule of training has been shown to be associated with a depression of immunity.[33] The causes for immune depression are multifactorial. Imbalanced diet can influence immunity. During intense exercise the demand for carbohydrate by muscle is high and competes with the needs of macrophages and for purine and pyrimidine synthesis. A high carbohydrate intake may lead to reduced intake of proteins and lipids, which are important in the maintenance of immune function.[33] Intense training is also associated with reduced immunity due to excessive weight loss and reduced plasma glutamine levels.[34] Because glutamine is an essential nutrient for lymphocytes, the reduction of glutamine can interfere with lymphocyte function.

V. Summary

Clinical assessment of the athlete is a comprehensive process that involves an evaluation of the current nutritional status and the possible change in nutritional status with athletic activity. In addition, it is desirable to assess the medical condition of the person embarking on athletic activities. While doing do, it is necessary to differentiate the medical status required for the competitive athlete from those who are going to undertake recreational activities. Athletic activities can cause complications that the clinician should recognize and prevent or treat.

References

1. Ziegler, P.J.,Khoo, C.S., Sherr, B., Nelson, J.A., Larson, W.M. and Drewnowski. A., Body image and dieting behaviors among elite figure skaters. *Int J Eat Disord.* 24:421, 1998.
2. Maron, B.J., Cardiovascular risks to young persons on the athletic field. *Ann Intern Med.* 129:379, 1998
3. Klein, S., Kinney, J., Jeejeebhoy, K.N., Alpers, D., Hellerstein, M., Murray, M. and Twomey, P., Nutritional support in clinical practice: review of published data and recommendations for future research directions. National Institutes of Health, American Society for Parenteral and Enteral Nutrition, and American Society for Clinical Nutrition. *Am J Clin Nutr.* 66:683, 1997.
4. Rokitzki, L., Sagredos, A.N., Reuss, F., Cufi, D. and Keul, J.J., Assessment of vitamin B_6 status of strength and speed-power athletes. *Am Coll Nutr.* 13:87, 1994.
5. Siscovick, D.S., Ekelund, L.G., Johnson, J.L., Truong ,Y. and Adler, A., Sensitivity of exercise electrocardiography for acute cardiac events during moderate and strenuous physical activity. *Arch Intern Med.* 151:325, 1991.

6. Sanborn, C.F. ,Horea, M., Siemers, B.J. and Dieringer, K.I., Disordered eating and the female athlete triad. *Clin Sports Med.* 19:199, 2000.

7. Burrows, M. and Bird, S., The physiology of the highly trained female endurance runner. *Sports Med.* 30:281,2000.

8. Rutherford, O.M., Is there a role for exercise in the prevention of osteoporotic fractures? *Br J Sports Med.* 33:378, 1999.

9. Welsh, L., and Rutherford, O.M., Hip-bone mineral density is improved by high-impact exercise in postmenopausal women and men over 50 years. *Eur J Appl Physiol.* 74:511,1996.

10. Klidjian, A.M., Archer, T.J., Foster, K.J. and Karran, S.J., Detection of dangerous malnutrition. *J Parenter Enteral Nutr* 6:119, 1982

11. Sunnerhagen, K.S., et al., Muscular performance in heart failure. *J Cardiac Failure.* 4:97, 1998.

12. Fiatarone, M.A., O'Neill, E.F., Ryan, N.D., Clements, K.M., Solares, G.R., Nelson, M., Roberts, S., Kehayias, J.J., Lipsitz, L.A. and Evans, W.J., Exercise training and nutritional supplmentation for physically frailty in very elderly people. *N Engl J Med.* 330:1769, 1994.

13. Young, W., Wilson, G. and Byrne, C., Relationship between strength qualities and performance in standing and run-up vertical jumps. *J Sports Med Phys Fitness.* 39:285,1999.

14. Rigaud, D., Moukaddem, M., Cohen, B., Malon, D., Reveillard, V. and Mignon M. Refeeding improves muscle performance without normalization of muscle mass and oxygen consumption in anorexia nervosa patients. *Am J Clin Nutr.* 65:1845-51, 1997.

15. Hofman Z., Smeets R. and Kuipers H., Muscular efficacy and metabolic tolerance of MyoVive (ML-1), a nutritional supplement to optimize mitochondrial function and reduce oxidative stress. *FASEB J,* 14: A491, 2000.

16. Speedy, D.B., Faris, J.G., Hamlin, M., Gallagher, P.G., and Campbell, R.G., Hyponatremia and weight changes in an ultradistance triathlon. *Clin J Sport Med.* 7:180, 1997.

17. Smith, D.J., Bia, M.J., and DeFronzo, R.A., Clinical disorders of potassium metabolism. in *Fluid Electrolyte and Acid-base Disorders,* Arieff, A.L. and DeFronzo, R.A., Eds., Churchill Livingstone, New York, Volume 1, 1985, p.449.

18. Swenson, E.R., Metabolic acidosis. *Respir Care.* 46:342, 2001.

19. Schabort, E.J., Wilson, G. and Noakes, T.D., Dose-related elevations in venous pH with citrate ingestion do not alter 40 km cycling time-trial performance. *Eur J Appl Physiol.* 83:320, 2000.

20. Nystad, W., Harris, J. and Borgen, J.S., Asthma and wheezing among Norwegian elite athletes. *Med Sci Sports Exerc.* 32:266, 2000.

21. Kallinen, M., Era, P. and Heikkinen, E. Cardiac adverse effects and acute exercise in elderly subjects. *Aging* (Milano). 12:287, 2000.

22. Jouven, X., Zureik, M., Desnos, M., Courbon, D. and Ducimetiere, P., Long-term outcome in asymptomatic men with exercise-induced premature ventricular depolarizations. *N Engl J Med.* 343:826, 2000.

23. Hambrecht, R., Gielen, S. and Schuler G. Physical training as an adjunct therapy in patients with congestive heart failure: patient selection, training protocols, results, and future directions. *Curr Cardiol Rep.* 1:38, 1999.

24. Sharma, N., Winpenny, H. and Heymann, T., Exercise-induced rhabdomyolysis: even the fit may suffer. *Int J Clin Pract.* 53:476, 1999.

25. Painter, P., Carlson, L., Carey, S., Paul, S.M. and Myll, J., Low-functioning hemodialysis patients improve with exercise training. *Am J Kidney Dis*. 36:600, 2000.
26. Peters, H.P., Bos, M., Seebregts, L., Akkermans, L.M., van Berge Henegouwen, G.P., Bol, E., Mosterd, W.L. and de Vries, W.R., Gastrointestinal symptoms in long-distance runners, cyclists, and triathletes: prevalence, medication, and etiology. *Am J Gastroenterol*. 94:1570, 1999.
27. Rudzki, S.J., Hazard, H. and Collinson, D., Gastrointestinal blood loss in tri-athletes: its etiology and relationship to sports anemia. *Aust J Sci Med Sport*. 27:3, 1995.
28. Smetanka, R.D., Lambert, G.P., Murray, R., Eddy, D., Horn, M. and Gisolfi, C.V., Intestinal permeability in runners in the 1996 Chicago marathon. *Int J Sport Nutr*. 9:426, 1999.
29. Shaskey, D.J. and Green, G.A., Sports hematology. *Sports Med*. 29:27-38, 2000.
30. Brun, J.F., Bouchahda, C., Chaze, D., Benhaddad, A.A., Micallef, J.P. and Mercier, J., The paradox of hematocrit in exercise physiology: Which is the "normal" range from an hemorheologist's viewpoint? *Clin Hemorheol Microcirc*. 22:287, 2000.
31. Weight, L.M., Klein, M., Noakes, T.D. and Jacobs, P., Sports anemia — a real or apparent phenomenon in endurance-trained athletes? *Int J Sports Med*. 13:344, 1992.
32. Malczewska, J., Raczynski, G. and Stupnicki, R., Iron status in female endurance athletes and in non-athletes. *Int J Sport Nutr Exerc Metab*. 10:260, 2000.
33. Bishop, N.C., Blannin, A.K., Walsh, N.P., Robson, P.J. and Gleeson, M., Nutritional aspects of immunosuppression in athletes. *Sports Med*. 28:151, 1999.
34. Shephard, R.J. and Shek, P.N., Immunological hazards from nutritional imbalance in athletes. *Exerc Immunol Rev*. 4:22, 19.

16

Summary — Nutritional Assessment of Athletes

Judy A. Driskell and Ira Wolinsky

CONTENTS

I. Introduction

Practitioners and researchers in the nutrition, exercise and sports areas currently perform many types of nutritional assessments on athletes. These assessments are dietary, anthropometric, physical activity needs, biochemical and clinical in nature. Nutritional assessment is a key to determining the health and performance efficiency of athletes.

The healthcare, training, feeding and education of athletes are best accomplished by an interdisciplinary team of sports medicine practitioners, including physicians, athletic trainers, exercise and nutrition scientists, dietitians, psychologists and other health professionals. Sports nutrition is an emerging field of study. A credible sports nutritionist is, generally, a registered dietitian (R.D.) who has advanced preparation in exercise sciences, including exercise physiology. In the year 2000, only 21 universities in the United States offered graduate programs in sports nutrition.[1] Athletes will benefit when sports nutritionist professionals successfully integrate the knowledge and skill of a multidisciplinary athlete healthcare team. The nutritional assessment of athletes is a challenge that is best accomplished by having medical-, nutritional-, exercise- and sports-oriented professionals working together.

II.   Dietary Assessment of Athletes

Evaluating the food and nutrient intakes of individuals, including athletes, is difficult and time consuming. The most accurate technique is generally having the athlete keep a food record as food is consumed, measuring portions as accurately as possible, for several days. Dietary intakes of athletes are usually influenced by their training and competition seasons. Athletes frequently take a variety of dietary supplements. Estimates of nutrient intakes obtained through the use of computer software are only as good as the dietary information supplied by the athlete, as well as only as good as the coding techniques used in entering the dietary data into the software.

Many athletes realize that nutrition is related to physical performance and many are becoming more interested in improving their nutrient intakes. National standards and guidelines are frequently utilized in evaluating the nutrient adequacy of athletes' diets. For example, the United States and Canada have established Dietary Reference Intakes for healthy populations.[2-5] Athletes should try to achieve these standards and may need to further increase their intakes based on the demands of their sport and activity levels. Research indicates that performance and health of athletes can be compromised at low intake levels. Dietary intake patterns should also be evaluated to identify possible causes of inadequate intakes. These measurements should be validated against biochemical, clinical and anthropometric measurements to assess the nutritional status of the athlete.

Dieting and exercising to extremes can provoke injury or death. Disordered eating means eating — or not eating — more often in response to external rather than internal cues. Disordered eating does impair athletic performance as well as cause malnutrition and exacerbation of mental problems. These eating disorders include anorexia nervosa, bulimia nervosa and binge eating disorder, as well as the not yet formally recognized muscle dysmorphia, anorexia athletica and exercise dependence. Eating disorders have been frequently observed in the athletic population, especially in the aesthetic sports. Sports nutritionists can be effective in the prevention of eating disorders. Treatment for eating disorders involves a team of health professionals including psychiatrists, psychologists, neuroendocrinologists and nutritionists.

III. Anthropometric Assessment of Athletes

Anthropometry is the science dealing with the measurement of size, weight and proportion of the body. Various anthropometric methods are utilized in evaluating the growth and body composition of children, adolescents and adults. United States federal guidelines have been released for evaluating body weights utilizing the body mass index (BMI).[6] However, the application of these federal guidelines to the athletic population has been questioned. Anthropometric measurements should always be conducted by trained personnel using appropriate equipment that has been maintained and calibrated.

The nutrient requirements for children are associated with growth. The growth of child athletes should be evaluated regularly to assure maintenance of an appropriate growth pattern and to identify those at risk for disordered eating. Height, weight and BMI percentile measurements should be performed at least once a year on child athletes, with the BMI being utilized primarily as an indicator of the consumption of excessive calories. Body composition measurements can be utilized in evaluating the effects of training. Children should enjoy sports or physical activity while maintaining a healthy lifestyle.

Great variability exists among adolescents, including those who are athletes, with regard to values for anthropometric measurements. The variability in the timing of puberty influences these anthropometric values. Generally, growth spurts occur earlier in girls than boys, and these changes influence body mass and composition. This differential maturation at any given chronological age presents a challenge in assessing the body composition of adolescents. Bioelectrical impedance analysis, skinfolds and height:weight measurements are the most appropriate growth assessment techniques. These assessment methods need to be further developed for use with adolescent athletes.

Currently, anthropometric methods are utilized in estimating physique. Many studies have been published documenting the body dimensions of athletes in a variety of sports. Most of the earlier studies utilized males; however, studies have also been conducted in the last couple of decades using females. Changes in body composition are frequently evaluated during training and during seasons utilizing anthropometric methodologies as indicators. These methods are potentially useful in monitoring athletes who might be at risk for eating disorders.

Only male athletes were included in the first Olympic Games in 1896. A century later, women represented slightly over a third of athletes competing in the Games of the XXVI Olympiad. As a group, men retain a performance edge over women in all sports largely because of differences in body composition and developmental physiology. Men are usually stronger than women, and women usually have less of their body mass as contractile tissue and more as adipose tissue than men. Men generally possess a larger aerobic capacity than women, but the responses of women to aerobic training seem to be similar to those of men if the intensity, frequency and duration of the training, as well as initial fitness, are similar. Today, women's sports seem to be on a par with those of men.

IV. Physical Activity Needs Assessment of Athletes

Dietary intakes should provide sufficient energy to sustain life. This energy is measured in kilocalories (kcal) or kilojoules (kJ), with kilojoules being the preferred unit. The body can use carbohydrates, lipids (fats) and proteins for energy formation. The energy production from carbohydrates and proteins is about 17 kJ/g (4 kcal/g) and that from lipids about 37 kJ/g (9 kcal/g). Direct calorimetric methods, involving an individual's being in a closed chamber and the heat produced by the body being measured, were first used for estimating energy expenditure. Direct calorimetry is expensive, cumbersome and does not permit the individual to live a usual life. Today, indirect calorimetric methods are utilized in estimating energy expenditure. Indirect calorimetry involves a measurement of oxygen uptake or carbon dioxide expenditure. Indirect calorimetric techniques permit an individual to exercise unimpeded during the measurements. Indirect calorimetry is used in measuring the energy expended during a specific physical activity. Doubly labeled water methods are most applicable when estimating energy expenditure over several days. The estimated total energy expenditure of a person is calculated by summing the resting energy expenditure (24 hour), the expenditure based on lifestyle or occupation (daily activity factor) and the expenditure due to exercise.

In most cases, an adult athlete's energy intake and energy expenditure should be similar. Thus, energy expenditure needs to be estimated and generally, field methods rather than laboratory methods are used. These field methods are not as precise as laboratory methods but are more practical. Portable indirect calorimetry is probably the most accurate indirect field method for estimating energy expenditure. Utilizing multiple indirect measures of activity-related energy expenditure may improve the accuracy and feasibility of using field methods to estimate energy expenditure. Self-reported physical activity records or questionnaires are frequently utilized in estimating energy expenditure, as these methods are inexpensive and least burdensome, but problems may exist with regard to how well the instrument represents population-specific activity behaviors as well as recall and reporting biases. The accuracy and reproducibility of these field methods can be improved if standardized methods for assigning energy costs and objective measures, such as an accelerometer, are utilized.

V. Biochemical Assessment of Athletes

Biochemical assessment of athletes provides information about how well their bodies are utilizing nutrients. Aerobic physical activity is known to decrease circulating levels of high-density lipoproteins. Evidence exists that athletes need more protein than nonathletes. Both men and women, athletes and nonathletes, frequently do not consume recommended amounts of calcium, folic acid and vitamin E. Women, both athletes and nonathletes, frequently do not consume sufficient iron. Some supplementation trials have been published in the refereed scientific literature in which athletes were given one or more of the vitamins as a dietary supplement. Many times in these research studies, control or placebo groups, equally trained, were not included. Sometimes the athletes in the studies had inadequate status of the nutrient prior to supplementation and sometimes not; this might be responsible for some of the conflicting findings reported in the scientific literature. Evidence exists — though not conclusive — that athletes may benefit from increased intakes of some of the vitamins and minerals.[7,8] Athletes frequently take vitamin or mineral supplements.[9]

An excellent book by Sauberlich[10] details the various methodologies utilized in biochemical assessment of nutrient status. The Institute of Medicine, National Academy of Sciences, in setting the Dietary Reference Intakes for healthy populations in the United States and Canada, evaluated existing data on the influence of physical activity on nutrient status with regard to the various vitamins and minerals.[2-5] Dietary Reference Intakes for the energy-yielding nutrients is forthcoming. This group indicated that it is possible that the requirements of some of these vitamins and minerals is increased for individuals who are ordinarily very physically active, but the data are not available to justify adjusting requirements. The functioning of energy-yielding macronutrients and energy metabolism in sports nutrition has recently been described in detail.[11]

Favorable changes in serum lipids usually occur in individuals as a result of moderate to vigorous exercise. An increase in high-density lipoprotein cholesterol concentration and decreases in total cholesterol, low-density lipoprotein cholesterol and triglyceride levels are generally observed in exercising adults as compared with values when they were more sedentary. Possible lipid oxidation may also result from ultra-endurance activities. Exercise also likely exerts some influence on serum lipid concentrations that may last for a day. Changes in cholesterol ester transfer protein and lecithin-cholesterol acyltransferase appear to be consistent with increased high-density lipoprotein cholesterol levels. More research is needed on the possible changes in serum lipid concentrations in individuals who initially are sedentary and then become more and more physically active.

The use of protein by the bodies of athletes for energy formation is relatively small. Controversy exists as to whether aerobic or resistance exercises increase the need for dietary protein, and some evidence exists that aerobic exercise does. Reports also exist that habitual exercise lowers the need for dietary protein. Some evidence exists that strength-trained athletes may require more dietary protein than sedentary individuals. Published studies also indicate that strength training results in reduced protein requirements. In his chapter in this volume, Phillips recommends that endurance- and strength-trained athletes consume at least 10% but no more than 20% of their dietary energy as protein.[12] More research is needed on the protein requirements of athletes.

The vitamin status of athletes is often assumed based on dietary intake estimations rather than biochemical measurements. Assumptions made from dietary data do not take into account vitamin bioavailability or activity or interactions. Few studies have examined the influence of exercise, acute or chronic, on tissue (usually blood, blood components, or urine) vitamin levels. Hence, the vitamin status and requirements of athletes are not fully known. Acceptable vitamin extraction and quantification methods must be utilized. Appropriate precautions must be made to minimize the destruction of the vitamin while it is being measured. Sophisticated analytical instrumentation and skilled technicians are required for measuring tissue levels of most, if not all, the vitamins. In Table 13.2 of this volume, Löest and Haub list the biochemical parameters frequently utilized for assessing an individual's status of the various vitamins.[13] Exercise may influence the distributions of many of the vitamins in the various tissues. Research is needed to determine the influence that the vitamins, individually and in combinations, have on circulating and stored levels of vitamins in athletes of different training status and how the supplemental vitamins affect athletic performance.

As more information is becoming available on the roles that minerals play in the development and maintenance of physical fitness and performance, the need for assessment tools to evaluate the adequacy of the various essential minerals is realized. Many times, individuals conducting these biochemical measurements are unaware of the need to use appropriate procedures for collecting blood and performing analytical techniques. Appropriate guidelines are available. One should utilize multiple indicators of status for each of the minerals. In Chapter 14, Lukaski gives reference intervals for the various minerals and discusses the data available on athletes.[14] Carefully performed research is needed on the mineral requirements of athletes.

VI. Clinical Assessment of Athletes

Many people of all ages participate in various athletic activities. Some of these individuals either may be at risk for a chronic disease, or may have already been diagnosed as having one. Obese and sedentary elderly individuals should have a medical and physical examination prior to initiation of an exercise program. According to the American Heart Association, all individuals over 40 years of age should undergo exercise testing before starting a vigorous exercise program.[15] Ongoing clinical assessment is desirable for competitive athletes. Considerable risk of malnutrition exists among competitive athletes, particularly women. Eating disorders are frequently observed in competitive athletes, especially women.

Clinical assessment involves nutritional and medical histories as well as a physical examination along with selected biochemical tests aimed at detecting specific nutrient deficiencies and identifying individuals at risk of future nutritional abnormalities. Electrocardiographic and echocardiographic examinations are frequently advised for the prescreening of individuals prior to their initiating strenuous training programs. Bone mass and muscle function measurements have also been suggested for competitive athletes and physically active elderly adults. Clinical conditions that are often associated with athletic activities include dehydration and electrolyte deficiencies, exercise-induced asthma, arrhythmia, renal failure, gastrointestinal disturbances, anemia and immune deficiency. As stated by Jeejeebhoy in Chapter 15, "Athletic activities can cause complications that the clinician should recognize and prevent or treat."[16]

VII. Summary

As more and more individuals of all ages and sizes are participating in exercise and sports activities, the importance of nutritional assessment of these individuals is becoming better recognized. The nutritional assessment has five major components: dietary, anthropometric, physical activity needs, biochemical and clinical measurements. Nutritional assessment, which is a key to determining and monitoring the health and physical performance of professional, collegiate and recreational athletes, is best accomplished by a team of health professionals.

References

1. Moffatt, R.J. and Cheuvront, S.N., Introduction to nutritional assessment of athletes, in *Nutritional Assessment of Athletes*, Driskell, J.A. and Wolinsky, I., Eds., CRC, Boca Raton, FL, 2002, pp. 3-13.
2. Institute of Medicine, National Academy of Sciences, *Dietary Reference Intakes for Calcium, Phosphorus, Magnesium, Vitamin D and Fluoride*, National Academy Press, Washington, D.C., 1997, 432 p.
3. Institute of Medicine, National Academy of Sciences, *Dietary Reference Intakes for Thiamin, Riboflavin, Niacin, Vitamin B$_6$, Folate, Vitamin B$_{12}$, Pantothenic Acid, Biotin and Choline*, National Academy Press, Washington, D.C., 1998, 564 p.

4. Institute of Medicine, National Academy of Sciences, *Dietary Reference Intakes for Vitamin A, Vitamin K, Arsenic, Boron, Chromium, Copper, Iodine, Iron, Manganese, Molybdenum, Nickel, Silicon, Vanadium and Zinc* (prepublication copy), National Academy Press, Washington, D.C., 2001.

5. Institute of Medicine, National Academy of Sciences, *Dietary Reference Intakes for Vitamin C, Vitamin E, Selenium and Carotenoids*, National Academy Press, Washington, D.C., 2000, 506 p.

6. National Heart, Lung and Blood Institute, National Institutes of Health, Clinical Guidelines on the Identification, Evaluation and Treatment of Overweight and Obesity in Adults: The Evidence Report, http://www.nhlbinih.gov/nhlbi/news, June 26, 1998 (accessed July 2, 1998).

7. Wolinsky, I. and Driskell, J.A., *Sports Nutrition: Vitamins and Trace Elements*, CRC, Boca Raton, FL, 1997, 235 p.

8. Driskell, J.A. and Wolinsky, I., *Macroelements, Water and Electrolytes*, CRC, Boca Raton, FL, 1999, 256 p.

9. Krumbach, C.J., Ellis, D.R. and Driskell, J.A., A report of vitamin and mineral supplement use among university athletes in a division I institution, *Int. J. Sport Nutr.*, 9, 416, 1999.

10. Sauberlich, H.E., *Laboratory Tests for the Assessment of Nutritional Status*, 2nd ed., CRC, Boca Raton, FL, 1999, 486 p.

11. Driskell, J.A. and Wolinsky, I., *Energy-Yielding Macronutrients and Energy Metabolism in Sports Nutrition*, CRC, Boca Raton, FL, 2000, 337 p.

12. Phillips, S.M., Assessment of protein status in athletes, in *Nutritional Assessment of Athletes*, Driskell, J.A. and Wolinsky, I., Eds., CRC, Boca Raton, FL, 2002, pp. 283–315.

13. Löest, H.B. and Haub, M.A. Assessment of vitamin status in athletes, in *Nutritional Assessment of Athletes*, Driskell, J.A. and Wolinsky, I., Eds., CRC, Boca Raton, FL, 2002, pp. 317–338.

14. Lukaski, H.C., Assessment of mineral status in athletes, in *Nutritional Assessment of Athletes*, Driskell, J.A. and Wolinsky, I., Eds., CRC, Boca Raton, FL, 2002, pp. 339–369.

15. Fletcher, G.F. , Balady, G., Froelicher, V.F., Hartley, L.H., Haskell, W.L. and Pollock, M.L., Exercise standards: a statement for healthcare professionals from the American Heart Association, *Circulation*, 91, 580, 1995.

16. Jeejeebhoy, K.N., Clinical Assessment of Athletes, in *Nutritional Assessment of Athletes*, Driskell, J.A. and Wolinsky, I., Eds., CRC, Boca Raton, FL, 2002, Chap. 15.

Index